Julianne S. Oktay, LCSW, PhD

Breast Cancer
Daughters Tell Their Stories

Pre-publication
REVIEWS,
COMMENTARIES,
EVALUATIONS . . .

"This is a powerful account of the experiences of daughters who lived through the diagnosis and long treatment of their mothers' cancer, or of losing their mothers to cancer. The research results reported in this book give voice to a neglected group of women who not only lived through and experienced the uncertainty, suffering, fears, and hopes of their mothers, but also lived with fears of their own futures. These daughters describe in their own words how their mothers' diagnosis, treatments, and experiences living with cancer affected the very fabric of their own existence and hopes for the future. It profoundly changed, altered, or enhanced their connections with others in their lives, their assessment of their own risks, and their actions in leading a healthy or risky lifestyle, as well as whether they performed self–breast exams or agreed to undergo genetic testing. For some, they became fatalistic; for others, their mothers' experience ignited their spirituality.

This is an exceptional study with credible interpretations of findings, thoughtful analyses, and presentations of themes in the lives of daughters who lived through and/or lost a mother with breast cancer. It is a book about a slice of women's lives with an illness that transforms the lives of patients, as well as their daughters.

This is a book that should be on the must-read list of any student in the health or social science field (e.g., nurses, physicians, sociologists, psychologists, and social workers), as well as any professional who cares for women with cancer and/or their families. It is also a fine example of qualitative research methodology and its power in humanizing research findings."

Afaf I. Meleis, PhD, DrPS(hon), FAAN
Professor of Nursing and Sociology
and Margaret Bond Simon
Dean of Nursing,
University of Pennsylvania

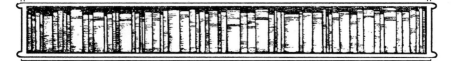

More pre-publication
REVIEWS, COMMENTARIES, EVALUATIONS . . .

"**A**s a daughter of a breast cancer mother, and myself a thyroid cancer survivor, I found the book to be a fascinating account of how a breast cancer diagnosis affects the entire family, especially the daughters.

Since my mother's first diagnosis when I was 15, to her second diagnosis when I was 30, I have always worried about getting breast cancer and possibly dying from it. Now a mother of four, I occasionally find myself daydreaming about myself, dying of cancer, saying good-bye to my children. I try to put these thoughts out of my mind, knowing that it is not healthy.

This book allowed me to reach deep inside to my inner child and heal some of my old wounds. Some of the stories brought tears to my eyes, but mostly they brought me a sense of comfort, knowing that I was not alone in my feelings. I offer my deepest thanks and praise to those women who have poured their hearts and souls into these pages."

Andrea Leonard-Bruno, CPT, CSCS
President and Founder,
The Breast Cancer Survivors' Foundation;
President, Leading Edge Fitness;
Adjunct Faculty Member,
American Council on Exercise

The Haworth Press®
New York • London • Oxford

Breast Cancer
Daughters Tell Their Stories

THE HAWORTH PRESS®
Gerontology and Women
J. Dianne Garner, Editor

Whistling Women: A Study of the Lives of Older Lesbians by Cheryl Claassen

Breast Cancer: Daughters Tell Their Stories by Julianne S. Oktay

Still Going Strong: Memoirs, Stories, and Poems About Great Older Women edited by Janet Amalia Weinberg

Other titles of related interest:

Relationships Between Women in Later Life by Karen A. Roberto

Women and Aging: Celebrating Ourselves by Ruth Raymond Thone

Women As They Age, Second Edition by J. Dianne Garner and Susan O. Mercer

Women and Healthy Aging: Living Productively in Spite of It All edited by J. Dianne Garner and Alice A. Young

Feminist Perspectives in Medical Family Therapy edited by Anne M. Prouty Lyness

Prevention Issues for Women's Health in the New Millennium edited by Wendee M. Wechsberg

Cancer Resources on the Internet edited by M. Sandra Wood and Eric P. Delozier

Handbook of Cancer-Related Fatigue by Roberto Patarca-Montero

Minding the Body: Psychotherapy in Cases of Chroinic and Life-Threatening Illness edited by Ellyn Kaschak

Women and Cancer edited by Steven D. Stellman

Understanding and Assisting Low-Income Women with Cancer by Emma Jean Tedder

The Application of Problem-Solving Therapy to Psychosocial Oncology Care edited by Julia A. Bucher

Breast Cancer
Daughters Tell Their Stories

Julianne S. Oktay, LCSW, PhD

The Haworth Press®
New York • London • Oxford

For more information on this book or to order, visit
http://www.haworthpress.com/store/product.asp?sku=5286

or call 1-800-HAWORTH (800-429-6784) in the United States
and Canada or (607) 722-5857 outside the United States and Canada

or contact orders@HaworthPress.com

The Haworth Press, Inc., 10 Alice Street, Binghamton, NY 13904-1580.

PUBLISHER'S NOTE
Identities and circumstances of individuals discussed in this book have been changed to protect confidentiality.

The research described in this book was supported by a grant from the National Cancer Institute #RO3 CA 70605-02.

Cover design by Marylouise E. Doyle.

Library of Congress Cataloging-in-Publication Data

Oktay, Julianne S.
    Breast cancer : daughters tell their stories / Julianne S. Oktay.
        p. cm.
    Includes bibliographical references and index.
    ISBN-13: 978-0-7890-1451-1 (hc. : alk. paper)
    ISBN-10: 0-7890-1451-3 (hc. : alk. paper)
    ISBN-13: 978-0-7890-1452-8 (pbk. : alk. paper)
    ISBN-10: 0-7890-1452-1 (pbk. : alk. paper)
    1. Breast—Cancer—Patients—Family relationships. 2. Breast—Cancer—Psychological aspects. 3. Breast—Cancer—Social aspects. 4. Children of cancer patients. 5. Mothers and daughters. I. Title.

RC280.B8O369 2005
362.196'99449'00922—dc22

                                        2004014891

To my parents
Nadine Lewis Shaberman
and
Harry Louis Shaberman

and to all of the breast cancer survivors, mothers and daughters

ABOUT THE AUTHOR

Dr. Julianne S. Oktay is Professor and Director of the doctoral program at the School of Social Work at the University of Maryland. Since earning a PhD in Sociology and Social Work at the University of Michigan, Dr. Oktay has conducted numerous research studies in the field of psychosocial health care. In 1991, she co-authored *Breast Cancer in the Life Course: Women's Experiences* with Carolyn A. Walter. She has published widely in such journals as *Health and Social Work* and the *American Journal of Public Health*. She participates actively in the American Cancer Society and the Komen Foundation, as well as professional societies such as the Association of Oncology Social Work, the American Psychosocial Oncology Society, the Society for Social Work Research, the Council on Social Work Education, and the National Association of Social Workers.

CONTENTS

Foreword

In a nation where breast cancer receives widespread attention, its devastating impact on family members, especially daughters, remains a surprisingly unexplored terrain. Although any life-threatening illness brings tremendous stress to loved ones, breast cancer carries an additional source of concern due to its tendency to be passed down through a family's female members. Thus, a daughter has more to fear than the suffering and possible death of her mother. In an era of genetic testing and counseling, these women carry a burden that poses continuing questions and decisions about the likelihood of cancer in their own lifetimes.

In this book, Julianne Oktay explores this frontier using qualitative methods to chronicle the stories of forty-one adult daughters whose mothers had breast cancer. Approximately one-third of the mothers survived the illness; the others did not. These daughters, an ethnically diverse group, range in age from nineteen to fifty-two and have experienced maternal breast cancer at a variety of ages and stages of development. Not surprisingly, their experiences include intense grief, loss, and anger but also resilience and a will to live life to the fullest. Amid this, they must appraise their personal sense of risk and make decisions about genetic testing, more frequent mammograms, and other strategies to protect their health.

Oktay's study stands as an exemplary demonstration of the grounded theory methods pioneered by Glaser and Strauss (1967). Each step of the study, beginning with training interviewers and continuing through data analysis and write-up, is presented clearly and succinctly. In this way, the flexible, iterative nature of qualitative inquiry unfolds before the reader's eyes. Attention to methods is balanced (but not overshadowed) by attention to ethical concerns, since these interviews invariably dealt with emotionally laden content and raised questions concerning each woman's decisions about her future. Working inductively from multiple interviews carried out with each woman, Oktay and her colleagues are meticulous in coding the interview transcripts early on, developing a provisional model, then testing it further using iterative sampling just as the originators of grounded theory envisioned. The emergent themes rest upon a firm empirical foundation carefully built and tested for its strength.

As a fellow social work researcher, I was especially gratified to see Oktay conclude the study with concrete, feasible recommendations for counseling and other interventions designed to serve the needs of future generations of women at risk. Medical, nursing, social work, and other providers are given guidelines tailored to the various situations these women must confront, including communicating with other family members, supporting caregivers, and making difficult decisions regarding genetic testing.

The National Cancer Institute made a wise decision to fund this study. It is still rare to see rigorous qualitative research; this book represents an important addition to our expanding archive of knowledge about the psychosocial effects of breast cancer. Whether this devastating disease is experienced firsthand or through the life of a loved one, breast cancer remains a mystery in many ways, particularly in its subjective impact. Oktay and her team of researchers have opened the door to greater understanding.

Deborah K. Padgett, PhD
Professor, New York University School of Social Work
President, Society for Social Work Research (2004-2006)

REFERENCE

Glaser, B. and Strauss, A. (1967). *The discovery of grounded theory.* Chicago: Aldine.

Acknowledgments

This book (and the research project that led to it) has been a central focus of my life for the past eight years. During that time, many people have contributed, although, naturally, I bear final responsibility. The project itself was generated by a call for proposals based on the National Action Plan on Breast Cancer, which came about due to the advocacy of the National Breast Cancer Coalition—a hardworking group of breast cancer advocates. The funding was provided by the National Institutes of Health, under the supervision of the National Cancer Institute. I am most grateful for this support, and thankful to the advocates who worked so hard to "humanize" the breast cancer research agenda. I hope that this book will ultimately lead to improved services for women and daughters, and justify their efforts.

The daughters who so generously shared their stories are the real heroines of this book. My goal is to make their voices heard. The forty-one women interviewed for the book were enthusiastic, giving of their time and energy, and eager to share their experiences in the hope of helping others. I have so much admiration for these women, who so honestly shared their experiences and their ideas. I apologize to them that I had to cut out many of their stories, and hope that the final representation accurately reflects the core of their experiences. If the book ultimately helps other daughters, I know they will forgive my lapses and will feel that the time and effort they gave to this project was worthwhile.

The "Daughters Project," as it came to be known, was a team effort from the start. Central to its success was the work of Susan McFeaters. Susan was a student in the doctorate program at the University of Maryland at the time. Because of her background in health care social work, she was assigned to me for a graduate research assistantship. She was just beginning the assistantship when I learned that the grant application would be funded. This was a stroke of luck for me, because Susan provided excellent organizational skills that were needed to get the project off the ground and to keep it well organized. She did a wonderful job of recruiting informants, organizing meetings, office management, and undertaking the computerized aspects of the analysis. Susan's people skills were also invaluable to the project, and her clinical skills made her an outstanding interviewer. We all learned so much about interviewing by reading her interviews and by the gentle teaching techniques she used in the team meetings. Her astute analytical abilities were also central to the development of the themes. The rest of the team—Julia Rauch, Michelle Jones, and Carolyn Walter—all made major contributions, both as interviewers (Julia and Michelle) and through sharing their ideas and contributing to the process of identifying the themes. I am so grateful to them for contributing so generously to the project.

I also am most grateful for the help and support of the advisory board, made up of providers and advocates. These busy professionals gave generously of their time, attending board meetings, reading and responding to early drafts, and helping to recruit good informants. Thanks especially to Jessica Heriot, Maimon Cohen, Miles Harrington, and Marsha Oakley, Lillian Brooks, Rebecca Latham, Shawishi Yvonne Martin, Michele Better, Sandra Fink, and Joan Weiss. Special recognition and appreciation goes to Annette Drummond, who was such a strong believer in the power of research to provide the answers to breast cancer. As a member of the advisory board, she was dedicated to this project and so many other advocacy activities. Her passing is a loss to her family and friends, and to the entire breast cancer community.

Another team played an important role with the second part of the project—the actual writing of this book. First, Hannah Cosdon worked on the literature search that frames the discussion of those daughters whose mothers died. Hannah is also an experienced social worker, and she brought to the project a clinician's understanding of children and adolescents that I lacked. Hannah identified the relevant literature, tracked down obscure articles, and, most valuable, wrote thoughtful, intelligent comments long after her official role was completed. I appreciated her insights. Hannah provided an understanding of a population with which I had little experience and of the theories that underlie clinical practice with traumatized children and adolescents.

Kathryn Adams, a recent PhD graduate on the "mommy track," read this manuscript carefully and patiently, and helped me with critical decisions. Katy writes beautifully, with a musical ear. Her reading of the final manuscript greatly improved the flow of the writing. Liz Fisher, another doctoral student, handled correspondence with the daughters, worked on the references, created the diagrams, and read the final manuscript. I am most grateful for her patience, accuracy, and constant cheerful attitude. Gwen Young contributed in so many ways. She transcribed most of the interviews with accuracy and sensitivity, and handled many of the secretarial tasks of the project. She typed the completed manuscript, remaining always cheerful and patient as I worked and reworked the chapters to get them to reflect what I wanted to say. I am most grateful for her constant good humor, speedy and accurate work, and gentle support.

The University of Maryland School of Social Work has provided me so much support: stimulating and supportive colleagues, access to critical resources, a sabbatical to write, and the most wonderful dean any faculty member could hope for (Jesse Harris). I am also grateful to my students, who have shared their own experiences with illness in classes, and who have contributed in many ways to the development of my ideas. Special thanks also are due to the Albin O. Kuhn Library at the University of Maryland Baltimore County, for providing me with the study carol where this manuscript was written. I know I could have never completed a project of this magnitude without a space free of the distractions of home and office. Finally, I must acknowledge the support of my two Sony VAIO laptop computers: Viola and Violetta. Viola gave her life to this book, and it was a sad day when she could no longer "boot up" and welcome me to work with her happy sound. Fortunately, Violetta has proved an able replacement.

It is difficult to acknowledge the support of my family, because it is so constant, so indirect, and so important to me. In the years since I started this project, my family has gone through several important transitions. Both of my daughters have gotten married, and I am a grandmother! I thank them for their love, and for helping me to understand the power and the complexity of mothering. My parents were healthy, independent elders when I began work on this project, but sadly, my father had a stroke two years later, and my mother's memory began to decline. In March 2003, my father passed away. I know I will never be as special to anyone as I was to him, and I thank him belatedly for all his love. My mother provided me with a model of a strong, intelligent, and capable woman who used all of her abilities to nurture and support her family. I only hope that I will be able to do the same. To my husband, Erol, I cannot find words to express my appreciation. I know that he is happy to see this project concluded (too many cheese-and-crackers dinners), and, even so, is proud of my accomplishment.

Chapter 1

Background and Introduction

Breast cancer is a major killer of American women, with approximately 212,000 diagnosed and 40,000 dying every year (Jemal et al., 2003). Although currently no cure or prevention has been found for the disease, improved survival rates have resulted in increasing numbers of breast cancer survivors. The National Cancer Institute (NCI) estimated recently that there were 8.9 million cancer survivors in the United States. About one-third of the female cancer survivors are breast cancer survivors (NCI, 2002). Many services are now available for breast cancer survivors, including individual counseling, support groups, educational programs, and mentor programs. However, the needs of another group of survivors have been largely ignored—the family members of women with breast cancer. Although the term *breast cancer survivor* is generally used to refer to living women who have been diagnosed with breast cancer, family members are also survivors, whether they have a mother, wife, sister, or daughter who has been diagnosed with the disease. Little research has been done on the impact of breast cancer on these "survivors," and few services are available to them.

The impact of breast cancer is most profound in one group of these other breast cancer survivors: daughters. The daughters are a particularly important group to study for several reasons. Daughters not only have a parent of the same sex with a serious illness, but also may lose that parent to a female-related illness. Those who lose a parent when they are young are generally thought to be at risk for long-term psychological consequences. However, little research has been done focusing specifically on daughters who lose their mothers; consequently, little is known about their experiences.

It has long been known that there is a genetic aspect to breast cancer, but the discovery (in 1994) of mutations in two genes (BRCA1 and BRCA2) offered new hope for identification of at-risk women, and eventual prevention or successful treatment. This new knowledge focuses attention on daughters who are at risk of inheriting the disease from their mothers. Although the genetic form of breast cancer applies to only a small proportion of breast cancer diagnoses (5 to 10 percent), daughters in families that carry these mutations have a higher than normal probability of getting breast cancer in their lifetimes than do other women. Because of their increased risk, daughters are prime candidates for the genetic counseling and testing increasingly available for this disease. An awareness of their experience with their mothers' illness is key to understanding their future needs in the genetic counseling and testing situation.

Another important reason to study daughters is that the mother-daughter relationship is both highly complex and extremely important to women. A better understanding of the mother-daughter relationship and how it is affected by breast cancer is important for providing better services to women who are diagnosed with the disease, to their daughters, and to other family members.

PREVIOUS RESEARCH

Research on daughters of women with breast cancer is quite limited, but research on the impact of cancer on the family is more readily available. The literature increasingly recognizes that serious illnesses affect the entire family and not just the member who is ill (Rolland, 1994). Studies of families during the illness show that "a significant number of families are seen to function more poorly than other families in the same community" (Lederberg, 1998, p. 981). These studies also find that psychological problems, such as anxiety and depression, are common in family members of cancer patients (Ell et al., 1988; Kissane et al., 1994; Northouse, 1984). Many studies point to the importance of open communication in the family in preventing psychological problems and family destabilization (Cohen, Dizenhuz, and Winget, 1977). Studies on bereavement also point to the long-term impact of cancer on family members (Kissane et al., 1994; Kissane, Bloch, Onghena, et al., 1996).

Studies of cancer's impact on specific family members have concentrated on two groups: spouses and young children of cancer patients. Studies of young children show that "they show vegetative disturbances, psychological symptoms, acting-out behaviors, and school problems, as well as long-term changes in cognitive performance and personality attributes, such as self-esteem" (Lederberg, 1998, p. 984). These studies also emphasize the importance of open communication (Rosenheim and Reicher, 1985). In addition, children of different ages have varying abilities to understand and cope with information about a parent's cancer (Christ, 2000; Patenaude, 2000).

Lewis and her colleagues have done extensive research on the impact of breast cancer on the family unit (Lewis, 1996). In studies of families of newly diagnosed breast cancer patients, and those in which family members already have adapted to the cancer diagnosis, they found that the illness results in depressed mood in both parents; this affects marital adjustment, coping, and, ultimately, household functioning (Lewis and Hammond, 1992). Later research focused on the impact of a mother's breast cancer on her young and adolescent children. Analysis showed higher levels of behavior problems, lower coping efficacy, and low self-esteem scores in these children (Armsden and Lewis, 1994), although these factors were not essentially different from those of children of women with other serious diseases. This is attributed to the impact of illness on the parents' depressed mood and the resultant marital strain, which leads to self-absorption and inaccessibility. Lewis, who studied children of both sexes, suggests that attachment theory be used to differentiate the impacts on girls and boys.

Unfortunately, research that focuses specifically on women whose mothers had breast cancer is very limited. In a review of the literature, Wellisch, Hoffman, and Gritz wrote (1996),

> A curious reality emerges if one surveys the psychological literature about the breast cancer patient and her family members. A very substantial literature now exists on the problems of the patient. A smaller but growing literature exists on the impact of breast cancer on the patient's spouse or significant other. Where the breast cancer patient's daughter is specifically concerned, the psychological literature becomes minuscule. This is grossly out of proportion to the potential size of this population. (p. 28)

The earliest study on daughters (Lichtman et al., 1984) found that although many mother-daughter relationships improved, breast cancer created special problems in some mother-daughter relationships.

Wellisch has focused much of his research on the impact of breast cancer on daughters (Wellisch et al., 1991, 1992, 1996). While much of this research examines issues of risk and risk behavior, Wellisch has also studied psychological impact of the disease on daughters. On many mental health dimensions, Wellisch and his colleagues found little or no difference between women whose mothers had breast cancer and women not affected by breast cancer. However, they found that the following factors correlated with "psychologically high-risk" daughters: daughter's age and mother's survival status. This research also identified the special problems experienced by some adolescent girls when mothers have breast cancer, and established women whose mothers die when they are adolescents as most likely to experience psychological stresses later in life (Wellisch, Hoffman, and Gritz, 1996).

OVERVIEW OF STUDY

A qualitative study was conducted to gain a better understanding of the experiences of women whose mothers had early breast cancer (under age fifty). This study focused on the younger breast cancer daughters, those whose mothers were under age fifty at their diagnosis. Several reasons for this exist. Because breast cancer strikes young women and it is a significant cause of death in young adulthood, it is sometimes forgotten that breast cancer is more common in older women. With increasing age, the prevalence of breast cancer increases. For this reason, the largest group of breast cancer daughters are women whose mothers are elderly. I chose to focus on the subset of daughters of younger mothers because the genetic forms of breast cancer are more likely in women who are diagnosed at younger ages. Daughters whose mothers were diagnosed at younger ages also are more likely to be interested in genetic testing, because they themselves will be young enough for the results to impact their reproductive decision making. (A woman who is diagnosed in her seventies is more likely to have daughters who are past childbearing age.) Another reason this study focuses on daughters of younger mothers is that loss of a mother in middle age is normative, and the experience of caring for and losing elderly parents has been extensively studied. Many services for caregivers and the bereaved are now available for women in midlife. However, having a seriously ill mother, and losing a mother, when a daughter is still a child, or a young adult, is not common. I wanted to focus my study on the youngest daughters, since they are the ones who could be expected to be most adversely affected, and for whom few services are available. Approximately 33,000 women under the age of fifty are diagnosed with breast cancer each year. About 10,000 women in this age group die (U.S. Cancer Statistics Working Group, 2003). These cases tell the stories of the women's daughters.

This book describes the study, presents the elements of a theoretical model developed from the study, and summarizes the findings. Chapter 2 offers a description of the methodology that was used in the study. A "grounded theory" approach was used to create a theoretical model that describes the experiences of breast cancer daughters (Strauss and Corbin, 1998). The most important factors that distinguish the experience were found to be daughter's age and mother's outcome (death or survival). The concept of "illness phase" was also used to organize the findings. Illness phases were "family background" (period prior to the mother's illness), "period during illness and treatment," "period following mother's death" (if mother died), and "long-term impact." This framework, which is described in detail in Chapter 3, is used to organize the material in Chapters 4 through 8. Chapters 4 through 7 describe the cases of women whose mothers died, each chapter being devoted to daughters in a common age category. Chapter 8 describes the experiences of women whose mothers survived. Chapter 9 discusses the concept of risk. It identifies themes related to how breast cancer daughters think about their own risk and what they do to deal with this. In Chapter 10, the results are examined by phase of the experience, and common themes for each phase are identified. The results of the study are summarized, and recommendations are made for practice, in Chapter 11.

BACKGROUND

This research is part of a fairly new perspective for medical studies, focusing on the experience of the patients and families. Traditionally, medical research has emphasized the biomedical characteristics of a disease, and not how it feels to those who have the disease. To the patient, of course, both are important. However, an overemphasis on the biomedical has led to services that are often insensitive and sometimes even ineffective. If a health practitioner is not aware of what the patient is thinking and feeling, how can he or she provide information, answer questions, facilitate decision making, and help a patient or family member cope with the disease? As chronic illnesses have become predominant in the developed world, patient behavior has become increasingly important in both the prevention and successful treatment of disease. In the case of breast cancer, women are encouraged to conduct monthly self-exams, have regular mammograms, follow up on suspicious findings, eat properly, exercise regularly, and handle stress well. These behaviors are ideally based on a view of disease that is compatible with the biomedical view. Recently, we have learned that even when the biomedical cause of disease is known and the behaviors to prevent it are well understood, as is the case for heart disease (not so for breast cancer, unfortunately), most people do not do what is recommended to prevent the disease. Teenagers (and adults) still start smoking (because it is "cool"), fail to use condoms to prevent human immunodeficiency virus (HIV) infection, and drive while intoxicated. Adults who smoke do not quit, even when they are fully aware of the dangers (e.g., lung cancer, heart disease). (Some people with advanced stages of emphysema and lung cancer continue to smoke.) It is increasingly recognized that to successfully prevent and manage disease, the patient experience must be taken into consideration. The research described in this book is compatible with a biopsychosocial model of illness (Rolland, 1994). This view suggests that an increased understanding of the experience of breast cancer daughters will ultimately lead to better medical care for all women.

This study is a direct descendent of a previous study that I conducted (with Carolyn A. Walter) on the experience of women who have breast cancer (Oktay and Walter, 1991). Carolyn and I set out to examine how women's life-course development impacted on the breast cancer experience. We interviewed about forty women who ranged in age from their twenties to their late eighties at the time of their breast cancer diagnosis. We found strong support for issues of life-course development as an important (and often overlooked) factor in how women experienced breast cancer and in how it impacted their lives, and also found some unexpected consistencies across the age span. It was clear from this study that the mother-daughter aspects of the illness were important for all age groups in our study:

> We found evidence of conflict between mothers and daughters throughout the life course, with breast cancer serving to complicate this already highly complex relationship further. . . . In many cases, a kind of power struggle seemed to be going on, with both parties wanting both nurturance and independence, or control. . . . Guilt concerning the possible genetic nature of the disease often made direct communication between mothers and daughters even more difficult. (Oktay and Walter, p. 196)

Those women with breast cancer who were mothers were especially concerned about the possible impact of the disease on their children. If they had young children, they were terrified about what might happen to the children if they died. If they had daughters, they worried about passing on a genetic link to the disease. If their mothers were living, they focused on how their disease might affect them, or on what they expected from them regarding care and nurturing. The women handled these issues in different ways. Some tried to hide the diagnosis from their children and/or mothers and to carry on as normally as possible. Some made plans for children, in case of their death. Regardless of age, issues such as maternal guilt, poor communication, and mutual protection bore directly on the quality of life of both the cancer survivors and their daughters.

My interest in studying these issues further was sparked by the National Breast Cancer Coalition (NBCC). In the early 1990s, this group of breast cancer activists identified a set of priorities, called "The National Action Plan on Breast Cancer." They were successful in getting the National Institutes of Health to supplement the traditional breast cancer research agenda and to provide some funding for research on these issues. One of the priorities dealt with the psychosocial aspects of the new genetic discoveries in breast cancer. In response to the call for proposals of the National Breast Cancer Coalition and the National Cancer Institute (NCI), I developed a proposal to do a qualitative study on daughters, focusing broadly on their experiences and not only on risk. The value of this type of study is precisely that it does *not* define the question narrowly in advance. This leaves the researcher open to explore the issues raised by the women themselves. In contrast, most research, especially funded research, sets up a very specific set of research hypotheses based on previously developed research and theory. These hypotheses are then tested, usually based on data from very specific questions on a structured questionnaire. This type of research (quantitative research) is valuable when there are well-substantiated theories, strong prior research, and good instruments that measure what is being studied. The women of the NBCC convinced the federal research establishment to listen to survivors and advocates; the NCI funding makes it possible to study the experiences of the daughters, whose voices had not yet been heard.

This research also has roots in the feminist concept that an important goal of research is to give voice to women (Reinharz, 1992). Gilligan (1982a,b) and Miller (1986) have emphasized the importance of research that is based on women telling their life stories. Other feminist researchers have argued that women's voices have often been silenced, leading to the further oppression of women (Belenky et al., 1986). By listening to these stories, and allowing daughters to use their own voices, it is hoped that this research empowers them, and at the same time, informs others (professionals, policymakers, etc.) who can use this knowledge to provide better services. Another aspect of both feminist and qualitative research is the recognition that I am a real embodied person, not an objective, national, uninvolved scientist. This book necessarily reflects my own voice (not just the voices of the daughters) and my own experiences. Therefore, I use my own voice to bring in my own experience as I reflect on the experiences of daughters. I hope that this will allow the reader to assess the validity of my conclusions, and to separate my voice from the voices of the women I studied.

It is important to note that this study does not judge the daughters, nor does it attest to the accuracy of the material. No indication was evident that these women were trying to deceive us, nor did they have any reason to do so. Also, no attempt was made to identify psychological processes, such as denial or projection, or inaccuracies in knowledge. The goal was to present the perspectives of the daughters and to allow them to speak in their own voices. When Hope Edelman (1994) published her influential book, *Motherless Daughters: The Legacy of Loss,* some reviewers said that the women sounded "whiny" and suggested that they "get over it!" However, such comments are judgmental and suggest that there is a correct way to react to a life tragedy such as the early loss of a mother. There isn't. What is important is the way women react, and not whether they "measure up" to some cultural ideal. In addition, this book does not make any attempt to diagnose the women. The goal here is to break away from the pathological perspective that is used in medical professions and to allow the women to speak about their experiences.

PERSONAL BACKGROUND

Qualitative research of this type requires the researcher to identify themes that emerge from the data (interviews). In so doing, I make use of my own personal experience, in addition to my professional background and theoretical frameworks, in the process. I have not had breast cancer myself. However, I was diagnosed with rheumatoid arthritis when I was thirty-two. At the time, I had two young daughters, ages eight and four. As I slowly learned how to live with a chronic illness, I tried to keep the illness from interfering in my children's lives. I worried that I would be less of a mother, because I often had less energy and was sometimes self-absorbed. I also worried that I would be unable to give them an optimistic, hopeful, and confident worldview. I realize now that the mother-daughter aspects of my earlier study were so compelling to me because of their connection to this experience in my own life.

My experience as a daughter also played an important role. My mother was an extremely strong and competent woman, and conflict was always a component of our relationship. For years, I took her for granted and did not recognize how special she was or how lucky I was to have her in my life. I rolled my eyes and complained to my friends about her, secretly proud of her accomplishments. She was extremely healthy until her early eighties. Around the time this study got underway, she began to show signs of memory impairment. I watched helplessly as she declined gradually, fighting for control, covering up her failings, pretending, denying. She was, for the first time in my life, vulnerable, and I became her protector. I learned to pretend (deny) along with her, trying to preserve her dignity. During the time I was writing this book, she went from a fiercely independent woman to one who sits quietly, frustrated that she is so "useless," made helpless and fearful by even the most basic of life's daily activities. I have been changed by this experience in many ways and have gained more understanding of the feelings of the daughters in my study.

SUMMARY

Daughters, regardless of whether their mothers survived breast cancer, constitute an overlooked group of breast cancer survivors. This remains true, in spite of the fact that many studies show that breast cancer impacts the family as a whole and children in particular. Previous research has found that daughters are at high risk for psychological complications later in life, particularly if they were adolescents at the time of diagnosis and if their mothers did not survive. Recently, the discovery of two breast cancer genes (BRCA1 and BRCA2) has focused increased attention on daughters, because they are at higher-than-average risk. Because their mothers' illness was a life-altering experience for these women, they are different than other populations that are at high risk for this disease. To provide appropriate health education and genetic counseling for this very special group of high-risk women, their experiences with their mothers' illnesses need to be better understood. They enter the health system with a history of serious illness and, in many cases, with the loss of a key attachment and identification figure—a mother.

To provide effective services to these women, this previous life experience must be taken into consideration. An increased understanding of daughters' experiences also can help mothers who have been diagnosed with breast cancer as they deal with their own daughters' reactions. It also can help daughters whose mothers have been diagnosed better understand the dynamics of their relationship under the stress of a life-threatening disease. Finally, it has the potential to help health professionals and planners design services that may prevent future problems in breast cancer families.

Chapter 2

How the Study Was Done

The following chapters present the results of a qualitative research project on the experiences of women whose mothers had breast cancer before the age of fifty. Qualitative research is a methodology that developed out of the fields of anthropology and urban sociology. It was the prevalent form of social science research in the days before quantitative methods became the "gold standard" in most social science fields. Although quantitative methods (e.g., surveys, questionnaires, statistical analysis) dominated social science research for many years, recently the pendulum has begun to swing back.

Quantitative research involves a search for knowledge of a "reality" using methods based on quantification, or measurement. Scales and indexes are used to measure such social science constructs as self-esteem, satisfaction, depression, and quality of life. These indexes often are used to evaluate interventions in practice fields such as social work and psychology. They also are used extensively in the social sciences to test theories about the correlates, causes, and consequences of these concepts. Qualitative researchers in the social sciences began to challenge this paradigm in the 1960s and 1970s. They critiqued the idea of a single, knowable reality, recognizing that there are multiple realities depending on the viewpoint of the observer, and pointing out how seemingly objective scientists often let their social and political notions influence their research. In addition, they recognized that in social science, the units that are studied (i.e., personalities, families, relationships, communities, societies) are highly complex, and cannot be fully understood using simplistic measures and statistical models. Qualitative researchers have developed a number of methodologies and techniques that aim to describe complex realities, and to build theories that can incorporate relationships and interactions that are multifaceted, constantly changing, and viewed differently by different parties.

The research that was used in this study adheres to this view and utilizes some of these methods. It is based on the assumption that reality is "constructed" by the people who experience it. Instead of trying to sort out a single "truth," it tries to describe the viewpoint of the individual, recognizing that the same situation will be viewed differently among participants. The qualitative researcher's goal is to describe the view of "reality" of the "insider." The position taken in this type of research is that the viewpoints of those who live through what is being studied (in this case, the daughters) are important and valid, regardless of whether they are substantiated by others. For example, in this study, the viewpoints of the daughters are presented. It is understood that the views of the mothers, fathers, physicians, grandparents, and brothers could be quite different. But this does not make the daughters' views any less valid or important.

Many characteristics of qualitative design flow from this worldview or epistemology. For example, although research questions are developed at the start of the study, they are treated as tentative and are refined as the study progresses. This is necessary because the researcher does not understand the "insider's" view at the start of the study, and as he or she comes to understand this construction of reality, the research questions may change. Similarly, decisions about the sample, the study settings, and the data analysis also may change as the study progresses because as the researcher gets closer to the viewpoint of the participants, his or her ideas will change and early views will seem naive or unrealistic (Maxwell, 1996). This chapter describes some details of how this particular study progressed.

As discussed in Chapter 1, this research evolved from a previous project that presented the views of women with breast cancer (Oktay and Walter, 1991). In their voices existed a strong concern about the impact of their illness on their families, especially their children, and, because they were female and at risk of the disease themselves, most particularly their daughters. I decided to study daughters whose mothers had had breast cancer to see if the mothers' concerns were well founded and to help both mothers and daughters manage the challenges of this dreaded disease.

PROJECT STRUCTURE

The study that forms the basis for this book was funded by the National Cancer Institute, under an initiative that was put into place in response to pressure by breast cancer advocates (National Action Plan on Breast Cancer). One requirement of this funding resource was that the researchers collaborate with "consumers" in the community. In response, I created an advisory board of health professionals and breast cancer survivors and advocates and met with this board periodically throughout the project.

I started the project by recruiting a respected colleague and friend, Julia Rauch, to serve on the project team. I also included two doctoral students, one of whom also served as project manager. I wanted to have an African-American interviewer on the project to be able to match interviewer and respondent, and Michelle Jones, the second doctoral student, was hired to meet this need. Michelle became a strong member of the team who not only related well to the African-American women she interviewed but also contributed in very significant ways to the development of the study hypotheses and themes. The final member of the team was Carolyn Walter, co-author of my previous study of women with breast cancer, who served as a "peer debriefer" for this project. She met with the team periodically and led discussions of problems or potential problems throughout the study. She also met with me and served as a sounding board as I developed the basic ideas and themes of the study. Carolyn and I tend to shift easily back and forth from discussion of professional issues to personal ones, and this proved invaluable in a project of this nature; using our own experiences as mothers and daughters, while not allowing them to overwhelm the voices of the respondents was very helpful.

To prepare for our first interviews, the research team of four interviewers had a daylong session with our peer debriefer. Carolyn asked each of us to talk about our own relationships with our mothers and our previous experiences with illness in the family. We worked as a team to identify areas in which each of us could have difficulty interviewing. We shared ways we could ask difficult questions and reviewed how to approach problems if they arose.

RECRUITMENT

My aim was to recruit informants who were split fairly evenly across a wide age distribution, and to have approximately half be women whose mothers survived and half whose mothers had not. This "sampling" strategy was based on the notion that these two factors would be important in understanding daughters' experiences. Because I was interested in studying women who might be interested in genetic counseling at some point, I set the cutoff for their mothers' diagnoses at "premenopausal." However, most daughters did not know their mothers' menopausal status, so this language was changed to "mother's age at diagnosis was under fifty." For the same reason, I limited the study to those daughters who did not have breast cancer themselves. I accepted only those over age eighteen and those whose mothers had been deceased for at least two years. Most of the women met this criteria; exceptions were made when very good informants whose mothers had died more recently volunteered.

This study is retrospective because it is based on the remembered experiences of women who are reporting on past events. Although the analysis includes chapters on children and adolescents, no actual children or adolescents were interviewed. All respondents were adult women recalling experiences they had when they were youths.

Although the basic assumptions of the study (that the daughter's age and whether or not the mother survived would be important variables) did not change as the study progressed, I found that breast cancer had a much lower impact on women whose mothers survived than on those whose mothers died. Therefore, over the course of the study, I focused increasingly on women whose mothers had died and stopped recruiting women whose mothers had survived. (In technical terms, saturation was reached with those whose mothers survived much sooner than for those whose mothers died.) Also, locating women whose mothers died when they were children or young adolescents proved difficult. This is partly because the incidence of breast cancer increases with age, and partly for reasons that will become clear in Chapter 4. As the study progressed, I stopped accepting women into the sample who were in late adolescence or early adulthood, and continued to search for more women who were young adolescents or children at the time of mother's death.

Forty-one women participated in the study, recruited through a combination of referrals from advisory board members (42 percent), other health professionals and advocacy group members (7 percent), newspaper advertisements (26 percent), and a recruiting brochure (16 percent). Approximately 9 percent of participants were self-referred.

SAMPLE DESCRIPTION

The analysis suggested that the important age for those whose mothers died was the daughter's age at mother's death, while for those whose mothers survived, it was their age at time of mother's diagnosis and treatment. Sixty-three percent of the women interviewed lost their mothers to breast cancer. Regarding age at mother's diagnosis, I initially grouped the women into four categories: the youngest group (one to ten years old) made up 27 percent of the sample, 27 percent were between eleven and seventeen, 31 percent were between eighteen and twenty-five, and the remainder (15 percent) were over twenty-five. The age categories were adjusted during the course of the analysis as themes were developed. In the final analysis, the age groupings were changed to one to nine, "children" (17 percent); ten to fifteen, "young adolescents" (20 percent); sixteen to twenty-two, "late adolescents" (28 percent); and over twenty-three "young adults" (35 percent). Most were white (73 percent), but outreach to the African-American community resulted in 27 percent who were African American. The ages of the participants at the time of the study ranged from nineteen to fifty-two, with an average of thirty-three years.

INTERVIEWING

After screening for eligibility, women were matched to one of four interviewers by race (white, African American), age (under forty, forty and older) and religion (Jewish, non-Jewish) to increase the rapport between informant and interviewer. Interviews took place in the women's homes, generally lasting from one to two hours; the longest interview was four hours. Interviews with women whose mothers died were almost always longer than those with women whose mothers survived.

The study was designed so that each woman would be interviewed three times. The first interview was primarily an opportunity for each woman to "tell her story." The purpose of the second interview was to fill in areas that had not been explored fully in the first interview, to explore in more depth special areas relevant to the case, to present our beginning ideas to the respondents, and obtain their feedback. During the third interview, discussion focused on a questionnaire (based on the theoretical model) that the informant completed prior to the third interview. This third interview was primarily confirmatory.

Each interview was shared with the team shortly after it was completed and then reviewed briefly before the second interview. The interviewers wrote up summaries of each interview (see Appendix I for an example), and shared them with the informants at the following interview. The researchers conducted a total of 103 interviews; all were audiotaped and transcribed.

A basic interview outline was used to guide the interviews (see Appendix I), but the interviewers always started with very general questions, designed to elicit a woman's story in her own words. (For example, "I understand that your mother had breast cancer. Could you tell me something about how that was for you?") Respondents tended to be eager to share their experiences. Some women spoke for an hour or more in response to a general question followed by further probes (e.g., "How did you feel about that?" or "Tell me more about . . . " or "Then what happened?"). Probes were simple "pumps" that encouraged a respondent to say more, questioned feelings, or requested information on other family members ("How did this affect your father?") (Weiss, 1994). Appendix II provides a detailed description of a typical interview conducted by the author.

The interviewers copied the tapes, and the project manager sent these to one of the several study transcribers. The original tapes were stored in the locked project file. Transcriptions were returned within a week, and the interviewers reviewed them while listening to the tapes, so that corrections could be made while the interview was still fresh. Once corrected, the transcription was entered into a computer database.

The interviewers contacted each woman by phone within a few days of the interview, to ask how she was feeling, see if she had anything to add, and follow up on any referrals made. In most cases, these calls were fairly insubstantial. However, in several cases, women raised important areas that had been "forgotten" during the interview. Sometimes an additional interview was done; more often, the interviewer made a note to bring up these areas at the next scheduled interview. During these phone contacts, most women indicated that they had enjoyed the interviews and were happy to be involved in the study.

TEAM MEETINGS

The biweekly team meetings continued throughout the active phase of the study. In these meetings, the team (myself and three interviewers, one of whom was project manager) discussed each case, identifying areas that hadn't been fully explored, as well as "themes" that seemed to characterize each case. As the study progressed, the team identified more prominent themes as cases were compared and contrasted.

These discussions also provided an opportunity to improve interview techniques, and to address problems that came up as the project progressed. The meetings provided a venue in which the team could support the interviewers, and helped each of us learn from our mistakes. After the third set of interviews, team meetings offered an opportunity to identify which parts of the model had been validated and to explore any needed changes to the model.

ADVISORY BOARD MEETINGS

The advisory board, which met twice a year, gave generously of their time and played a major role in recruitment of daughters and in helping interpret the findings. I shared with them case studies, emerging problems, and early interpretations of findings. They responded honestly and with humor, demonstrating their professional and personal experience. The advisory board was a major asset to the project, and I am forever grateful to these individuals.

CODING AND ANALYSIS

This study used grounded theory methodology and techniques (Glaser and Strauss, 1967; Strauss and Corbin, 1998) to produce a theory that is derived inductively—that is, developed out of the data. A grounded theory study contains several important components. One of these is the notion of "constant comparison," which means that the ideas constituting the theory are developed and refined throughout the project. As concepts are formed, they are compared to new data and refined until a point of saturation is reached.

"Theoretical sampling" is another concept used in grounded theory research: the sample's characteristics are determined as the study progresses, and new cases are sought on the basis of theoretical development. For example, in this study, one of the important variables that emerged from the data was the birth-order position of the daughter. Many of the women in the study were older daughters, and so, as the study progressed, we sought women who were younger sisters to determine how their experiences differed. Women were sought in each of the four age categories until we believed that we were no longer getting new material (had reached saturation).

Each interview was read and coded line by line. Codes and comments were noted in the margins. Each transcript was then coded on the computer, creating an analytical "tree," using the Non-Numerical Unstructured Data Indexing, Searching, and Theorizing (NUD*IST) software (see Appendix I). The conceptual framework was revised based on constant comparisons between the coding scheme and the data as new data were coded. I met weekly with the research project manager to review the coding process and revise the conceptual framework. As the project progressed, the coding categories became more stable and few new categories were added.

Analysis moved to identification of broader concepts and categories and to identification of prominent themes over time. Because the major variable in our analysis was daughter's age at time of mother's illness and death, a matrix which crossed these concepts and categories with the age categories was eventually created. The same was done for the two main categories: mother survived and mother died. This matrix forms the basis for the chapters that follow.

Another important technique of the grounded theory method is "negative case analysis." This means that as the theory develops, the researcher searches for cases that do not fit the theory. When such cases cannot be found, the researcher can conclude that the theory building is adequate. Finding "negative cases," on the other hand, suggests that additional theory building is necessary. For example, in this study, one finding was that the impact of breast cancer on women whose mothers survived often was fairly minimal. To test this, we searched for cases of women whose mothers survived who felt that their mothers' breast cancer had had a major impact on them. When we found these negative cases, we used them to more fully develop the model (see Chapter 8).

TRUSTWORTHINESS

Qualitative studies are subject to three types of bias: researcher bias, respondent bias, and reactivity (Padgett, 1998). This study employed several devices to reduce bias. We interviewed our respondents three times, over a period of eighteen to twenty-four months, providing what is called "prolonged engagement." Over this time period, the interviewers became respondents fairly well acquainted with the respondents and gave them opportunities to bring up information and ideas that they may not have raised had we done only one interview. It was not uncommon for women to remember information between the first and second interview. (They often said that the interview got them thinking, and talking to relatives, to clarify their impressions of events that occurred long ago.)

Triangulation (using multiple sources of data) was also used to increase validity. Our study had four interviewers, and all four read transcripts and interview summaries and identified possible themes and areas for further exploration. This made it difficult for any researcher to allow preexisting ideas to define the direction of the study. Peer debriefing throughout the project provided external validation for developing ideas. Other forms of external validation occurred when we shared our emerging model with the advisory board and when we gave presentations on the project to varied audiences. These presentations also provided validation for emerging ideas and alerted us to important issues that we had not examined.

Member checking was probably the most important device we used to ensure trustworthiness. We routinely asked our respondents for their feedback during the interviews and in the questionnaires and focus groups that took place at the end of the project. Six separate questionnaires were developed, one for each category in the matrix model. The questionnaires were sent to the informants in advance of the third (final) interview. In the final interview session, interviewers and respondents discussed the questionnaires; interviews noted respondents' reactions to the model, placing particular emphasis on identifying topics the women disagreed with or areas that were missing from the model. (This is also triangulation of method.)

Throughout the project, I kept a journal, recording ideas, problems, and progress of the study. (A sample journal entry is shown in Appendix I.) The journal and the record of the "nodes" developed in the N4 (NUD*IST) program made it possible to trace the emergence and development of ideas, creating what is called an "audit trail."

WRITING

All writing for the project was done by the author, with the help of several editors, at the conclusion of the grant. At that time, we had created a report that presented the basic findings for the National Cancer Institute. After The Haworth Press offered me a book contract, I worked on the manuscript over the next four years, as time from administrative responsibilities and parent caregiving allowed.

I began by developing case studies for each of the women in the study. Here, the term *case study* is used to refer to the women's stories. This allowed me to read and become familiar with all of the cases, including the ones in which I was not the interviewer. Case studies were written in order of the daughter's age at the mother's diagnosis, and included all cases, whether the mother did or did not survive. Although I knew that I wanted to organize the book by age of daughter, I had difficulty deciding where to draw the lines between age categories, as some cases seemed to belong in more than one category (e.g., child and adolescent). Eventually, I divided the adolescents into two categories: young adolescent and late adolescent. However, situations were not always neat, and in writing the chapters, I often had to refer to cases from other chapters to provide support for the themes. I wanted to include all of the case studies in the chapters themselves, but to conserve space some cases were moved to Appendix III, in an abbreviated form.

Another dilemma was how to present the women whose mothers survived. I considered the idea of including them in the chapters with the women whose mothers died, because they contributed to the themes in the section on "experience of mother's illness." However, I decided to create a separate chapter for them. I initially placed it before the chapters on women whose mothers died, thinking that it would be better to start with the lower emotional intensity of these cases. However, this created problems because in discussing the themes for those whose mothers survived, I wanted to make comparisons to cases whose mothers died, and these cases appeared later in the book. Therefore, I have placed the chapter on women whose mothers survived after the chapters on those whose mothers died. Conclusions about the common themes for each are developed in Chapter 10.

The placement of the material on risk also created some difficulty. Ideally, this material would have been part of the section on long-term impact for each age category. However, I did not identify differences in how daughters perceive their risk by age at diagnosis or by mother's survival status. Therefore, the material on risk is presented in the case studies in Chapters 4 through 8, and it is discussed in a single chapter later in the book (Chapter 9).

Once case studies were developed, I identified major themes in each of the three phases of the daughters' experiences. I also did some literature review at this point, to connect the findings to other researchers' writings. This is different than the process of quantitative research, in which the literature review is done at the beginning of the project and used to identify the problem. In contrast, qualitative research is inductive, starting with the data (daughters' experiences) and going on to the literature only after the themes have been identified inductively. A wonderful research assistant, Hannah Cosdon, helped extensively with locating relevant literature and commenting on the case studies from her clinical background. This helped me to connect the findings to the research literature and to identify implications for clinicians. Another research assistant, Dr. Kathryn Adams, helped me edit the case studies, and to connect them to the discussion of themes, creating draft chapters.

After deciding which cases would be used in the text, I sent copies of the case studies to the women to read. I am sensitive to the fact that seeing one's own (often) very painful memories in print can be a difficult experience. I wanted the women to approve their case studies before publication. I also wanted them to be able to choose pseudonyms if they so wished. I made most changes in the case studies that the women requested, even when it meant that material had to be omitted. However, when respondents wanted me to omit material that was key to the analysis, I attempted a compromise, omitting something they thought might hurt the feelings of a family member, but leaving in the substance.

CONCLUSION

This chapter described the methodology of the qualitative research study that forms the basis of this book. Qualitative research uses an inductive model that focuses on the view of the insider—in this case, the daughter of a woman with breast cancer. Intensive interviews were conducted with adult daughters who were of various ages at the time of mother's diagnosis or death. From these interviews, broad themes that described the experiences of each category of women were identified. These themes were checked with the research participants, as well as with an advisory board of health professionals and breast cancer advocates. Trustworthiness of the study was ensured by a number of methods. Appendix I includes some examples of the methodology used in this study. Appendix II offers a typical interview description. Appendix III includes additional case study material in an abbreviated form. Appendix IV offers additional resources for those interested in delving into these topic areas.

Chapter 3

A Daughter's Experience of Her Mother's Breast Cancer: Theoretical Model

A primary goal of this study is to build a theoretical model (see Chapter 2). This chapter presents the basic structure of the model that was developed from analysis of the interviews with women whose mothers had breast cancer. This study identified three factors that are absolutely critical to understanding a daughter's experience. Table 3.1 illustrates the three factors and their major categories.

MOTHER'S SURVIVAL

The first factor was whether the mother survived the breast cancer. This factor is almost so obvious that it hardly needs mentioning; however, it forms a basic pillar of the theoretical model that was developed. In addition, although this factor is so basic, many studies on daughters do not take this into account and simply group all daughters of women with breast cancer together (Wellisch et al., 1992).

Although this factor seems easily defined, it was not always so in the study. Obviously, it was known whether a woman's mother died. However, when a mother had had breast cancer and was a survivor, there was no guarantee that she would remain cancer free. In fact, several equivocal cases occurred. For example, Ramona's mother was diagnosed when she was eight. At the time of the first interview, Ramona was in her early forties, and her mother had recently died after a recurrence of her breast cancer. Even though her mother had died, she was considered to be in the "mother survived" category for the purposes of the study, because her experience throughout her young adulthood (the end cutoff of the study) was that of a woman

TABLE 3.1. Major factors and their categories in the theoretical model.

Factor	Categories
Outcome of mother's illness	1. Mother survived
	2. Mother died
Daughter's age	1. Child
	2. Young adolescent
	3. Late adolescent
	4. Young adult
Phases of experience	1. Period before mother's illness
	2. Period during mother's illness and treatment
	3. Period following mother's death (if mother died)
	4. Long-term impact

whose mother survived. Two other women had mothers who were without health problems at the time of the first interviews but had recurrences by the time of the later interviews. These cases too were classified as "mother survived," because the data from our interviews were of a woman whose mother had survived up to that time. The reasoning was that any one of the other women whose mothers survived could have a recurrence of the cancer in the future. This is the meaning of the "mother survived" category, which could more accurately be titled, "mother survived to the point of the interviews."

DAUGHTER'S AGE

The second critical factor was the age of the daughter. The daughter's age was central in determining her experience when her mother got breast cancer. Because our study focused on women whose mothers were under age fifty at time of diagnosis, daughters ranged in age (at mother's diagnosis) from one year to the early thirties.

The experience of illness and, possibly, death of a mother is very different for a child than it is for a young adult. Age had a special importance in the period after death for women whose mothers died. The cognitive and emotional capability of a young child is limited and precludes a complex understanding of the meaning of death. In addition, a younger child is much more dependent on the mother; her loss can be much more threatening. An older child may have the capacity to understand the illness and death cognitively, but may not be able to handle the emotional impact. A family may seek to rely on an older adolescent or young adult daughter to help the mother, or other family members, thus replacing some of the mother's functions. This is less likely to occur with a younger daughter. As with the outcome of the mother's illness, this factor also is quite obvious and hardly needs extensive explication. Even so, the division of the sample into age groups was not always clear-cut. A daughter of eleven, for example, might be similar to younger children, but in other ways her experiences could more closely resemble those of young adolescents. Initially, I had expected to divide the sample into four groups: children, adolescents, young adults, and adults. However, the experience of the adolescent group could not be described clearly, because those who were young adolescents had quite different experiences from those who were close to adulthood. I tried many ways to divide the population, and ended up separating the adolescents into two groups: young adolescents and late adolescents. This worked well with my sample and helped clarify themes in each of the groups. However, any division is to some extent arbitrary, because age is not a set of clearly differentiated stages; instead, everyone experiences a unique progression. Developmental age is not the same as chronological age, and movement from one stage to another is gradual, not sudden. The subjects of the study are real people and not theoretical "ideals"; cases in each category often reflect themes of other age categories. For example, the case of a daughter who is placed in the "early adolescent" group may demonstrate themes from children and late adolescents.

Another important consideration regarding age is that the daughters who were children when the mother was diagnosed or when she died were adolescents and young adults before we interviewed them. All respondents were over eighteen at the time of the interview, although the age range was wide (up to the early fifties). Thus a woman who was a child during her mother's illness may describe experiences from her adolescence and early adulthood that reflect themes of women whose mothers were ill at a later point in the daughters' lives. Although a woman who was a child at the time of her mother's illness may relate to some themes discussed in the sections on early adolescence, late adolescence, and young adulthood, the reverse is not true. (A woman whose mother was diagnosed when she was a young adult is less likely to find the themes of those who were children and young adolescents relevant to her situation.)

Another reason it was difficult to divide the sample into clear age categories is that the duration of the breast cancer varied widely. If the cancer was discovered late and the mother's period of illness was short, the mother's cancer likely took place while the daughter was within a single age category. However, if the mother survived for many years, the daughter may have gone through several age categories. I tended to classify these daughters by their age at mother's death because the death was such a significant event in the daughter's life. These cases may be used to illustrate themes in earlier chapters (e.g., Janice, Chapter 6; Nancy, Appendix III).

Daughter's age at the time of diagnosis is helpful to understanding the experience of illness and treatment for cases in which the mother survived. However, experience after the illness is more complex. Mother and daughter continue to age and to interact with each other at different stages in their lives. The mother-daughter relationship evolves as they go through various developmental stages. The woman who was a child at her mother's diagnosis continues to interact with her mother throughout her adolescence and adulthood. The daughter matures and the mother feels less vulnerable as years of survivorship increase; the mother often is more likely to share with her daughter. Because the ages of both mothers and daughters are constantly changing, the patterns in their relationships do not get fixed at the point of diagnosis (or death) as they do for those whose mothers died. For this reason, Chapter 8 is not subdivided into age categories. The themes in these mother-daughter relationships are very similar, regardless of the daughter's age at her mother's diagnosis.

Age was identified as a central organizing concept for the entire theoretical model. Daughters confirmed the importance of this factor. Ninety-two percent rated daughter's age as "very important" or "somewhat important" on the administered questionnaire.

PHASES OF THE BREAST CANCER EXPERIENCE FOR DAUGHTERS

The third factor central to understanding the experience of the daughters was the identification of critical phases. The phases that demark the experience of women whose mothers have breast cancer are

1. period prior to mother's illness (family background),
2. period during mother's illness and treatment,
3. period following mother's death (if mother dies), and
4. long-term impact.

These four phases apply to all age groups, although the issues that were most salient in each of these phases differs for each age group. The first three phases generally are clearly demarcated for women whose mothers die, while the shift from "period after mother's death" to "long-term impact" is more of a gradual process, and may be more psychological than temporal.

For women whose mothers survive, no clear demarcation exists between the period of mother's illness and treatment and long-term impact. At the end of treatment, women are monitored for signs of recurrence. Although most recurrences happen within three to five years of the original diagnosis, they (or a new breast cancer) can occur at any time. Therefore, although the probability of a recurrence or a new diagnosis declines over time, it never completely disappears. For this reason, phases 3 and 4 blend together into a single phase, "experience following mother's illness," for cases in which the mother survies.

Phase 1: Experience Before Mother's Diagnosis (Family Background)

The first phase (period before mother's illness) differs from the others in that it is not a defined period; it is a description of the context in which the illness occurred. The impact of this period, referred to as a "passive" period, is not discussed extensively in the following chapters. However, it identifies an important set of background factors that can help practitioners prevent problems before they become obstacles.

This study identified three characteristics of the family that were especially important in shaping the daughters' experience. These were family configuration, family communication style, and prior family problems.

Family Configuration

The family configuration was an important component of family background. Daughter's birth-order position was identified as an important predictor of her experience. If the daughter was an only child, an only daughter, or an oldest daughter, regardless of her age, she tended to carry more responsibility and often assumed a mothering role with younger siblings. Younger daughters often learned from their older siblings on how to behave, and what to feel and think.

Gender of siblings also was an important factor. Women with sisters found great comfort in sharing with them and, if the mother died, in mourning their loss. Women who had brothers generally did not find the same comfort in these relationships. Youngest daughters whose siblings had already left home at the time of mother's illness may have experienced a sudden role shift, and for the first time carried heavy family responsibilities.

Another important component of the family configuration was the presence of a marital partner. In two-parent families, fathers may have been able to care for their wives, so these tasks may not have fallen on daughters. However, in single-parent families, daughters took much more responsibility for mother's care. This also occured in two-parent families in which the father had never played a role in child rearing. Breast cancer is always a major threat to a family's stability, but in these families, the threat was even greater. In addition, in some cases, the father had died before the mother became ill. Daughters knew that they could lose their mother too. Not surprisingly, daughters in these families tended to be especially fearful.

Communication Style

Communication style also emerged as an important famly characteristic. Many of the women in our study identified "lack of open communication" as a problem in their families even before the mother's illness. A history of secrecy created an atmosphere that made it difficult to share information and feelings. In these families, daughters experienced feelings of foreboding and even extreme fear. They never felt certain that they had been given all the information about the illness and often suspected that things were happening without their knowledge.

Prior Family Problems

Closely related to family communication style was whether the family had experienced problems in the past. The presence of past family problems often made it more difficult for daughters whose mothers died to successfully resolve their loss, resulting in complicated mourning. If the family had a chaotic lifestyle and little stability for the children, breast cancer may have been seen as just another in a series of crises. For example, if the family had a history of alcoholism or drug abuse, this would have an effect on the daughter's experience when mother was diagnosed. For example, in one family with a heavily drinking father, the mother tried to protect the children from him and to cover for his lapses. When the mother died, she could no longer do this and the children lost a buffer between themselves and their addicted father. In another case, a history of child sexual abuse and a lot of secrecy surrounding it existed in the family. When the mother died, the daughter felt she lost her only opportunity to learn about her family history and gain an understanding of the forces that had shaped her childhood. Another case involved depression and alcohol abuse in the mother. In this case, the daughter had a very conflictual relationship with the mother, and when the mother got breast cancer, the cancer became part of the ongoing conflict. When the mother died, the daughter was left with much unresolved guilt and anger. Finally, one mother used her cancer diagnosis to induce guilt on her daughter. The daughter did what her mother wanted but felt furious about it. This type of situation can make for complicated grief, and the effects of these family problems can reverberate in the families for many years.

When the final questionnaire was sent to the informants, 100 percent of those whose mothers survived said that "daughter's birth order and gender of siblings" was important, as did 96 percent of those whose mothers died. For the factor "family communication patterns," the figures were 100 percent (mothers survived) and 92 percent (mothers died). For "prior family problems," the figures were lower: 70 percent and 86 percent respectively. This is not because they believed that prior family problems were less important, but because some families did not have prior family problems.

Phase 2: Experience of Illness and Treatment

The second phase of daughter's experience when the mother was diagnosed was the period during the mother's illness and treatment. This phase comprises several components, which vary by age of the daughter and are discussed in detail in Chapters 4 through 7.

Illness and Treatments

The characteristics of the breast cancer itself and how early it is diagnosed are important factors in understanding daughter's experience. Breast cancer can spread (metastasize) beyond the breast, where it is much harder to treat. When women are initially diagnosed, their breast cancer is "staged," and this determines which treatments are recommended. Women with early stage disease have less aggressive treatment (lumpectomy and radiation), while women with later-stage disease are more likely to have a mastectomy followed by chemotherapy. Breast cancer is not like a flu; once it is gone, the illness is not over. The disease can recur at any time after treatment, but, as stated earlier, most recurrences occur within five years of the initial diagnosis.

The treatments the mother had held an importance in the daughter's experience. Many mothers discussed in our study had mastectomies. The main impact of this surgery on the daughters was the separation due to hospitalization. For younger daughters, this may have been the first time that the mother was away from home, and the separation was often frightening. Another item of interest for many daughters was the mother's mastectomy scar. Some mothers in our study had radical mastectomies and were left with major scarring and deformity of the chest wall. These women often covered themselves and did not allow their daughters to see the scars. Daughters who had previously had free access to the mother's body and private space found it painful to be closed out of her room or bathroom for the first time. Other daughters were upset when they caught glimpses of the mother's scar. In some cases, when mothers had prostheses, very young daughters played with them. In contrast, older daughters often helped mothers find the prostheses and attractive clothes.

Chemotherapy was especially traumatic for daughters. This treatment usually results in hair loss, and seeing the mother this way made the illness real to daughters. Young adolescents were particularly disturbed if the mother lost her hair, weight, or interest in taking care of herself. When the mother was too weak or ill from the chemotherapy to perform household tasks, daughters often took on chores such as cooking, doing laundry, and supervising siblings.

For women whose mothers do not survive, two additional phases are identified: phase 3 (experience after mother's death) and phase 4 (long-term impact). The components of these phases are presented in Chapters 4 through 7. Because the phases are experienced differently by daughters (whose mothers die) of different ages, separate chapters have been written for each age group.

INTERACTIONS OF OUTCOME, AGE, AND PHASES OF DAUGHTER'S EXPERIENCE

The central components of the theoretical model of daughters' experience when mother has breast cancer cannot be considered separately, as they are intricately interrelated (see Figure 3.1).

Relationship Between Outcome of Mother's Breast Cancer and Phases Experienced by the Daughter

The phases a daughter goes through are determined by the outcome of her mother's illness. Although the first two phases (experience prior to mother's illness and experience during illness and treat-

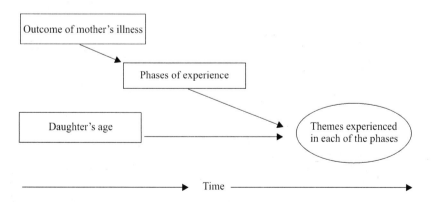

FIGURE 3.1. Relationship between the major factors identified in the study.

ment) are the same regardless of whether the mother survived, the next two stages are very different for the two groups of daughters.

For women whose mothers died, the phases are period before mother's illness (family background), experience of mother's illness and treatment, experience following mother's death, and long-term impact. For women whose mothers survived, only three of the phases are relevant: period before mother's illness (family background), experience of mother's illness and treatment, and long-term impact.

Young girls, adolescents, and young adult women whose mothers survived experienced the illness phase similarly to those whose mothers died. When a child's mother dies, the daughter's age at the time has a long-term impact. However, when a mother is diagnosed with breast cancer and survives, the mother's status as a survivor continues; this fact impacts the daughter throughout life's stages. In these cases, the mother-daughter relationship continues to evolve as mother and daughter go through various developmental stages and life experiences. The woman who was a child at her mother's diagnosis interacts with her mother through her young adolescence, late adolescence, and young adulthood. Her relationship with her mother evolves as she develops, and the breast cancer may remain an issue in their relationship. In cases of suvival, mothers and daughters have many opportunities to fix problems that may have developed when the mother was diagnosed; old issues can be renegotiated at any time. As a daughter matures, she may be more comfortable asking her mother about her past illness, and as a mother feels less vulnerable as cancer-free years increase, she may be more willing to open up to her daughter. Because the ages of the women and their mothers are constantly changing, the patterns do not get fixed at the point of diagnosis (or death). For this reason, the age of daughter at mother's diagnosis is less of a defining factor for women whose mothers survive than it is for those whose mothers die.

For women whose mothers survived, there is no clear period after the illness. Many daughters of women who survived did not appear to detect major changes in their mothers after the illness, and generally described a fairly quick "return to normal." This is probably because the mothers were successful in protecting their daughters from their worst fear. (This issue is discussed further in Chapter 8.)

Relationship Between Daughter's Age and Phases

The different phases of the experience of mother's cancer are also very different for daughters depending on their age. Although the basic components of the phases are somewhat similar, the way they occur for daughters of different ages is very different. The daughter's age influenced what happened to her in each of the phases of the experience. For example, it influenced what information was shared with her, what role she played in the illness, and how profoundly she was affected by family changes if her mother died. For example, one characteristic of the illness phase is "increased responsibilities." All daughters experience increased responsibilities, but the new role of a child is very different from the new role of the young adult.

STRUCTURE OF THE BOOK

The first three chapters of this book have provided the background of the study and the framework of the theoretical model that was developed. The structure of the rest of this book is based on the combination of these three factors: mother's outcome, daughter's age, and phases of the experience. The next section deals with the experience of women whose mothers died (Chapters 4 through 7). Each of the chapters deals with a single age group: children (Chapter 4), young adolescents (Chapter 5), late adolescents (Chapter 6), and young adults (Chapter 7). Each chapter is organized by the phases of the experience. Women whose mothers survived are discussed in Chapter 8. While the four chapters on women whose mothers died discuss the critical phases or time periods, the chapter on women whose mothers survived focuses on the experience following mother's illness (see Table 3.2). This is because the period during mother's illness is virtually the same as it is for women of the same age whose mothers died.

Chapter 9 addresses daughters' risk, because breast cancer has a genetic component. Daughters must not only experience their mothers' illness, but face the possibility that they are at risk for breast cancer. Chapter 10 reorganizes the early material to focus on each of the critical phases (see Table 3.3). This chapter identifies broad themes for each phase, and describes patterns based on comparisons of the four different age categories. Finally, Chapter 11 summarizes the results and considers the implications of the study for health professionals, advocates, and breast cancer patients and their families.

TABLE 3.2. Major factors and organization of Chapters 4 through 8.

Daughter's age	Outcome of mother's Ilness	
	Mother died	**Mother survived**
Child	Chapter 4—Phases of Experience • Period before mother's illness • Mother's illness and treatment • Period following mother's death • Long-term impact	
Young adolescent	Chapter 5—Phases of Experience • Period before mother's illness • Mother's illness and treatment • Period following mother's death • Long-term impact	Chapter 8—Phases of Experience • Period before mother's illness • Mother's illness and treatment • Experience following mother's illness
Late adolescent	Chapter 6—Phases of Experience • Period before mother's illness • Mother's illness and treatment • Period following mother's death • Long-term impact	
Young adult	Chapter 7—Phases of Experience • Period before mother's illness • Mother's illness and treatment • Period following mother's death • Long-term impact	

CONCLUSION

This research provides an illustration of the experiences of women whose mothers had breast cancer. The study identified three factors as central to understanding a woman's experience with her mother's

TABLE 3.3. Organization of Chapter 10.

Phases of experience	Mother's outcome	Age of daughter
Period before mother's illness	All daughters	All age groups
Period of mother's illness and treatment	All daughters	Child Young adolescent Late adolescent Young adult
Period following mother's death	Daughters whose mothers died	Child Young adolescent Late adolescent Young adult
Long-term impact	Daughters whose mothers died	Child Young adolescent Late adolescent Young adult

breast cancer: her age, whether her mother survived, and the phases of the daughter's experience. Four age groups were analyzed: women who were children (one to nine), young adolescents (ten to fifteen), late adolescents (sixteen to twenty-two), and young adults (twenty-three and up) at the time of mother's illness. Four phases of the experience were identified: the period before mother became sick (family background); mother's illness and treatment; experience following mother's death (if mother died); and long-term impact on daughter. Issues related to daughter's risk are also discussed.

Chapter 4

Experience of Young Daughters When Mothers Die from Breast Cancer

This chapter presents the stories of women who were children (under age ten) when their mothers died from breast cancer. It begins with three case studies: Rita and Carol, whose mothers died when they were eight, and Nora, whose mother died when she was nine. Each of the case studies has six sections. The first follow the phases described in Chapter 3, and the remaining two discuss risk and current situation. Major themes are identified and discussed following the case studies.

CASE STUDY #1: RITA

Age at Her Mother's Breast Cancer Diagnosis: 5;
Age at Time of Her Mother's Death: 8

Background

As a young child, Rita lived with her mother, father, and older brother. Rita's mother, a biology teacher, had left work after her children were born, but when Rita was about five, her mother took a part-time job at a hospital.

> My mother was very career-focused. She was very smart. My father was a scientist. He was a nice guy, and made a decent living and everything, but he was out of it, in a way. She was very child-centered and she made decisions based on what the family would need. He went along with her. He never argued or disagreed with her or anything like that.

Experience of Her Mother's Illness

When Rita was five and her brother was eight, her mother found a lump that was diagnosed as cancer. She had a mastectomy. Rita's only memory of this was going shopping to buy the "fake breasts." "I'd play with them, you know, like little kids would do." She also remembers trying to see her mother's mastectomy scar.

> Once I remember I was lying with her, and I tried to look and I did see some scar. I don't think I saw the whole thing—just the top part. But I was very aware of it. I was very curious, but I wasn't much of a talker. So I would, like, lift somebody's shirt up, but not ask them.

Rita knows little about her mother's treatment after the mastectomy, but she remembers that

> she was pretty sick sometimes. I remember when she had hair growing on her face from something she was taking. She used to put on this white lotion to take the hair off, and my brother and I would make fun and say she looked like Santa Claus. She liked that.

She also remembers that her mother had "something pretty gross right by her belly button. We couldn't really see it. She had bandages and tape."

From the beginning, Rita's mother was expected to die.

> I know the day she was diagnosed, she came home and told my father. My brother was there, and he started crying. And I said [to him], "What's cancer?" I ran after him. "What's cancer? What's cancer?" And he said, "Mom's gonna die." Then I remember asking her, "Are you going to die?" And she said she didn't know. I don't remember ever having a conversation about it again over the next three years. There was an immediate reaction that she was going to die. It was just one of those things—that cancer meant death. I think my father felt that way too. I think everybody just thought it was a matter of time. I don't recall being told, but I heard a lot. I didn't talk, but I was very attentive. If anybody was having a conversation, I heard it. But you can tell by the mood of a house, and my father was very expressive in his face. He was not verbal, but I could read his body language.

The doctor Rita's mother worked for encouraged her to stop working.

> He told her that she would live longer if she didn't work. But she was very insistent on continuing to work. I guess she thought she would die, and she wanted to make sure that there was money for her kids to go to college. She wanted to get the maximum number of hours for So-

cial Security insurance for dependents, which she did do. I think it was a very smart decision. It paid for me to go to college.

Rita and her brother were raised to be very independent.

My mother was like this even before she was sick, but I think it went to an extreme when she got sick. Once we had to walk to our elementary school in a hurricane. And she was saying, "You have to be able to do this on your own. Come on!" The wind was blowing, and my brother said, "This is crazy!" But we went. If he went, I went. I just pretty much followed him. I had to be like an adult. It was to an extreme. I think she was really freaked out. Like when she was gonna die, what was going to happen to her kids? Were they going to survive? Like it was survival of the fittest. She was doing the best she could do. And she thought, *Well, I've got to make these kids capable of taking care of themselves.* She couldn't count on my father being around. . . . When they found she had cancer, it had spread, but she did live three years. She had cancer in other areas too. It spread other places. She had it in, like, seven different parts of her body when she died.

Rita has a strong memory of the last time she saw her mother before she died.

I was supposed to go to Girl Scouts after school, and for some reason I just had to be home. I don't think I even knew why. Maybe I did. I must have known she was home and was sick. I said, "I have to go home." I must have known things were going on, but I can't really remember them. I went in to see my mother and she was really sick. She was lying on the bed. She couldn't really say anything. But I went in, and then I went back out and went to my Girl Scouts meeting. I'm so glad I did that.

Because Rita was prepared, she states, "I wasn't . . . shocked when my mother died."

Rita and her brother did not attend their mother's funeral.

My brother decided he didn't want to. And I just did whatever he did. I was shocked that my brother didn't want to go. I thought for sure he would, 'cause he was really close with my mother. Very close. But for some reason he didn't. I didn't want to go to the funeral 'cause I had been to a funeral when I was five. My cousin had to stand up there with her mom, and I just remembered that. I was shy. I didn't want all that attention. It was too much. [Now] I think we both should have [gone]. My father should have had the sense. You see, he left everything up to us. We were our own parents, in a way. We made the decisions. I stayed at the house with my friend and my Girl Scouts leader. Then people came over, of course. I was running around, playing games and stuff.

People don't know how the hell to act. [They were] trying to be nice; I felt it was somewhat insincere. I wasn't interested in it.

Experience Following Her Mother's Death

Rita does not remember the period after her mother died as a particularly sad time:

I feel like I should say, "Oh, it was terrible; it was terrible!" It really wasn't. Like, I don't remember crying or anything. My father did rearrange his work hours, so he went to work earlier and came home around four-thirty. He was nice. There were fun times. My father was fun. He made Hungry-Man dinners, and salads, which were very good.

Rita took pride in her independence:

It was different. I stepped on a bee once, and I just kept on walking. I became an instant tomboy! I was my own parent. I really was totally in control of my life. He [father] was nice, but he was emotionally unavailable to a great extent, especially with me. I got his credit card to go shopping. I decided what clothes I wore. I decided what I did, what time I went to bed at night. If I wanted to sleep at my friend's house, I would just tell him, "Dad, I'll be over at Jenny's." I took my own showers, washed my hair. And I loved hanging out with Jenny's family. I ate dinner at her house every night. I had my place at their dinner table. They took trips on Sundays, and I went with them. I had a great time!

Rita enjoyed the freedom from parental control:

One of the things I liked was—my mother [had been] putting me in these outfits. Once I wore a white shirt to a birthday party, and I got it dirty, so I got yelled at. So after she died, I was wearing whatever the hell I wanted, and I was a tomboy, so I was wearing jeans and tank tops and comfortable clothes that I could get dirty in and not be yelled at. I played football with my brother and his friends. I was really good. They could never get me down! No matter what they did, I'd hold on! I loved playing football! We had the freedom to have people come over, and we played in my backyard. My father was at work, or whatever. That was fun!

Rita was just starting third grade when her mother died, and her grades dropped from A's to C's: "I don't know if I developed learning disabilities or if it was because I wasn't paying attention in school. I don't even know how I got through school, 'cause I don't remember doing any homework." At school, Rita felt different from other kids:

We [Rita and her brother] didn't want to do anything that anybody was gonna say, "Oh, they're like that because their mother died" [about]. You feel like someone's always on the verge of saying, "Oh well, her mother died." It's like something is wrong with you, and that's the reason for it. I didn't want there to be anything wrong with me. I didn't want to mess up. It's that kind of thing.

Soon after her mother's death, Rita's father began dating. Rita remembers that before her death, her mother tried to fix her father up with a divorced friend, but it didn't work out. Rita was not upset by her father's dating, but she became very angry when he decided to remarry.

He dated all kinds of women, and they were okay. Some of them were better than others. He did get married two years later, and he ended up with the worst situation possible. The difficulties were that she was very strong willed, and so was I. She was domineering. She was very controlling. And I felt more intelligent than her. I'm pretty damned sure that at nine years old, I was smarter than she was. And I had a sense of myself. I had been raising myself, and I felt that I did a decent job and if somebody else was gonna try to tell me what to do, it would have had to have made intellectual sense to me. If you're gonna tell me, "Rita, you should go to bed early," you should have a good reason why. She was the opposite of my mother. My mother wanted me to be an adult when I was five years old. But [Rita's stepmother] wanted her kids to be children when they were forty. And I picked up on it immediately.

Rita and her stepmother-to-be fought especially about religion because her stepmother was more religious than Rita's mother had been, and she wanted Rita to be more involved in religion. They also fought about clothes.

She bought a jacket for me, but didn't ask me what kind of jacket I'd want. Now I'd been used to buying my own clothes. This jacket was ugly. I was not going to wear this jacket. She said, "You have to wear this jacket." And I'm like, "No, I don't." And I had a fit, let me tell you. My father never witnessed this before. I had been nice to every woman he brought in that house; I really was. So that's when it all started unraveling. When she got engaged to my father, she started, "You're doing this" and "You're doing that," without any consideration of what I wanted.

Rita tried to talk to her father about her objections to this marriage:

He was painting his bedroom. I said to him, "Dad, can I talk to you? There's something about this [stepmother's name]. I think something's wrong with her personality." He never got off his chair. I don't even think he looked at me. He just kept painting and said, "Well, if you don't like it, you can leave in eight years. You can leave when you are eighteen." And I walked out of there and I didn't cry or anything. I didn't scream. I just said, "Oh, shit! I'm really on my own." And I was.

After her father remarried, things got worse:

People would hear me screaming three houses down. It was a war zone. That's what it was. You might as well [have] put on camouflage suits when you walked through that door. Believe me, he [father] was on the firing line. He was not having a happy time. I told my father to drop dead when I was eleven. I threw a grapefruit at his head. I said, "It doesn't matter if you're dead or alive. You do nothing for me emotionally. You do nothing for me financially." I was cold. But that was the truth. I called it as I saw it. I took my father at his word. That's the way he felt. That was fine. I never wanted a goddamn thing from him. If he handed me five dollars, I told him to keep it.

Once, when she was in high school, Rita's father tried to get the family to go to a therapist; after one session her stepmother refused to go back.

In addition to losing her mother and her positive relationship with her father, Rita lost her maternal grandparents.

My grandparents moved away, which they would not have done [if mother was alive]. She [grandmother] went from seeing her grandchildren once a week or every other week to once a year. She didn't go to any of our graduations, or birthday parties, or anything like that. And you know, Passover, Hanukkah, any of those things. Even Christmas.

Rita spent most of her time with her friend's family. Conflict later developed between her friend's mother and Rita's parents:

My friend's parents were very nice. Because I didn't have any clothes, I was wearing jeans that were three sizes too big. I wore three pairs of long underwear underneath them, to hold them up. Everybody would laugh during gym. They [friend's parents] were trying to give me things, and [Rita's stepmother] would call and say, "Don't take Rita shopping." She [stepmother] would ground me from everything. She was trying to break me down. She was trying to take away my friends, because I made them into my family.

Rita's parents didn't allow her to go to Girl Scouts camp, which she loved. Her Girl Scouts leader called her father and tried to convince him to let her go:

[The leader said] "How do you not let a kid go on a Girl Scouts camping trip? This kid did nothing wrong." But it didn't work. I never missed school, 'cause I got out of the house. I almost won an award for missing the least amount of days of school. I was surviving. I was not one of those kids [who was] falling apart. I was gonna make it. I was gonna make it without a goddamn thing from them. Nothing. I knew what I was doing. I knew I had that Social Security money, when I turned eighteen. That was a big thing.

One especially sad time for Rita was her eighth-grade graduation:

I was hysterical crying, and I didn't know why. Probably because my mother wasn't there. Also, probably because of being treated like dog shit. You know, if my mother was alive, it wouldn't have been perfect, but I wouldn't have been treated like a fucking piece of shit!

Three weeks before her high school graduation, the day that Rita turned eighteen, she packed her things and moved into her friend's house. She is proud that at her high school graduation she did not cry at all:

I was vice president and I gave an awesome speech. I don't even know how the hell I pulled that whole thing off. I was wearing boxer shorts and a T-shirt under my robe because my father wasn't going to buy me an outfit. I got away with it.

Long-Term Impact

Rita said the major impact of her mother's death is her expectation that she also will die young:

Maybe the most identifiable thing to me is just my inability to believe that I will have a future. I felt that I was gonna die when I was in my early thirties. It made me very focused. Because of my mother's death, because of this whole childhood experience I had, I felt that it had to have been . . . that I had to make it worth something (my mother's life). [I'm] constantly fighting against the clock, never really enjoying anything. It's just crazy. I had to make something out of my life, because there's no way I suffered that much for nothing. And if I was going to die by the time I was thirty-five, I had to do it before then.

Rita feels her mother's death led her to seek a PhD, and later, to start a tutoring program for low-income children.

Risk

One reason Rita expects to die of cancer in her thirties is because she sees personality similarities between her and her mother. "I think that I have the personality of somebody that gets cancer. My personality is similar to my mother's. And we both had really bad childhoods. That's more likely to give me cancer than anything else."

Rita has had several medical problems. An ovarian cyst was discovered when she was twenty-four. "I was on the [examining] table, and they told me and I started hysterically crying. I thought, *Okay, I'm dead.* To me, anything like that means you're dead." She went to two or three doctors before one found a defect on her cervix.

> It turns out that I was born with a defect and I had an extra piece on my cervix that would have most likely turned into cancer in ten years if I had not removed it. I was born with a genetic defect. My mother was obviously born with one too.

Recently, Rita has had problems with bladder spasms. She is convinced these problems are also genetic. "I do not honestly believe that I have any control over this anymore. I think that whatever is going to happen is a done deal at this point."

Despite this belief, she has altered her diet. "I eat very little sugar, and I'm eating mostly vegetables. I feel better, and that's why I'm doing it." She states that cancer-preventing diets must "start when you're young. It's already set in stone. It takes ten years or something for cancer to actually come out. I think it's more psychological." Rita was thirty when we interviewed her, and her mother was diagnosed with cancer at thirty-one. "It should be a fun year next year," she said sarcastically.

Given Rita's views about genetic predisposition, it is not surprising that she sought out genetic counseling:

> You know, it was a very nerve-racking experience. I'm sure I made more out of it than a normal person would have. I've been thinking about this since [I was] eight years old. They made me feel a little better actually, because really it's only one person in my family—only my mother. They showed me my numbers. I thought about genetic testing, but I haven't done it. The problem is that even if you have it,

even if you get your breast removed, you can still get breast cancer. And knowing my luck, that's exactly what's gonna happen to me anyway. And since I have a predisposition to cancer, I gotta get all my body parts removed. I feel like any day now, they're gonna tell me I have cancer anyway. I'm gonna get cervical cancer. That's the way I feel. I'm not even worried about breast cancer anymore.

In addition to annual mammograms, Rita sees her gynecologist every three months. At one of her checkups, her doctor thought she had a cyst in her breast. "They sent me for a mammogram, and there wasn't [a cyst]. But then everybody said, 'Oh, my God, you shouldn't have gotten a mammogram with a predisposition to breast cancer. You'll get too much radiation!'"

Current Situation

Rita had recently completed her PhD in social work and was working on establishing an agency for tutoring low-income children. She was about to be married and had no plans for children.

I'm not going to have kids, thinking I'm gonna die. What would happen if I had small children? That is a major concern. There's no question about it. I want to adopt anyway. I can love children who aren't my own. I can help other kids—set up a college scholarship fund. Plus I don't see the point of why everybody has to have kids anyway.

Rita rarely mentions her mother's death to others. "I don't go into it too much. It's not my nature. I might have said a couple of comments over the years." She finds Mother's Day particularly hard; she spends it alone or "hanging out with my dog." At the time of our interview, she was planning her wedding. "I'll probably have a song, maybe, dedicated [to my mother]. I'm not going to cry or anything like that. It's just obvious that there's somebody not there."

After the study was completed, Rita was diagnosed with thyroid cancer at age thirty-four. This was the age at which her mother died. Rita had her thyroid removed. "As you can imagine, it was an emotional roller coaster."

CASE STUDY #2: CAROL

Age at Her Mother's Breast Cancer Diagnosis: 5;
Age at Time of Her Mother's Death: 8

Background

Carol was the youngest child in a large Christian family. When Carol was five, all of her older siblings were in school. She was able to spend special time alone with her mother. "I was kind of her buddy when the other kids were gone. I was very quiet and well behaved because there were so many of us. I remember being very close then." Carol has happy memories of her mother taking her shopping and to restaurants. Carol remembers dancing around the kitchen with her mother when her mother learned she was pregnant again: "Mother was a lot of fun."

Experience of Her Mother's Illness

Carol's mother had a mastectomy when Carol was five. She does not remember being told her mother had breast cancer, or the operation, but she does remember her embarrassment when her mother showed her a fake breast. She also remembers seeing her mother's scar once, when her mother was wearing a nightgown and leaned over:

> It was bruised and nasty-looking. That was kind of scary. I think that has terrified me since. The idea of being cut on. It's terrifying. . . . Sometimes I'll have pains in my left breast and that's what I visualize. I'll have some anxiety build up, and that's what I envision. That radical mastectomy that left her scarred and disfigured below her nightgown.

Carol thinks that her oldest brother and sister knew more about mother's illness than she did.

When Carol was eight, her father gathered all of the children and told them, "Your mother is very sick. We should pray for her." Carol was not alarmed, because the children often prayed for those who were sick. They all assumed that their mother would get well. Her mother went to another city for radiation treatments and chemotherapy. While she was in the hospital, relatives visited and cared for the children. Later, Carol felt guilty that she had had so much fun playing while her mother was so ill. After five weeks of chemotherapy, her mother decided to discontinue treatment. "She just said, 'Enough. I've had it. Let me go home.'" When Carol's mother returned home, she looked visibly ill for the first time, with dark circles under her eyes. Despite this, Carol's main memory from that time is a positive one: "I would come in after school every day and she'd always have a big smile for me."

One day, a neighbor picked up the children after school and took them to her home. This was unusual. Carol's father later came to the neighbor's home and told the children, "God has taken your mother." Carol did not know what he meant, but she realized that something horrible had happened when she heard her older brother let out a high-pitched cry. Carol looked over at her house and saw what looked like a casket being carried from their home. "That was the first realization that, 'This is death. This is death.'" Carol began to cry, kicking and screaming until the neighbor took her outside and told her to calm down.

Carol did not mention her mother's funeral in her interviews.

Experience Following Her Mother's Death

Shortly after her mother's death, Carol's father began dating a longtime family friend who was a widow. They were married several months after Carol's mother's death. Carol's stepmother had four children of her own, so Carol experienced many changes. She had to give up her bedroom, and the family got rid of her dog after her stepmother's dog attacked him. Carol recalls, "There were so many things going on that year, you have to survive the moment [chuckling]. We were moving on, and you'd better jump on the train, or you'll miss it." Carol's older siblings had a difficult time accepting their father's remarriage, so Carol tried not to make things worse, even if this meant hiding her own feelings. She felt that it was her job to "pitch in and make the new blended family work."

Carol did not do any grieving for her mother. She explains,

> Maslow's hierarchy of needs was there. You have to survive! So, forget your grief, because now you've got to try to get along with a boy you knew in school who is now suddenly your brother. I mean, there were so many things going on that year that it was kind of like . . . grieving was the last thing on the list.

Carol liked her stepmother. She tried not to show any negative feelings (e.g., sadness), because her stepmother was trying hard to make everyone happy. Carol's mother and stepmother had been friends, and it was not taboo to talk about her mother in Carol's family: "What she became was the ethereal being. She was an angel." Still, Carol sensed that her stepmother would be hurt by expressions of grief. For example, one time Carol's older brother created a memorial in honor of their mother. Carols sensed that this memorial made her stepmother uncomfortable: "Her vocation in life was to make things happy for children. That was her deal. 'I'm going to make you all happy.'" Whenever Carol had to discuss losing her mother with others, she always said, "Yeah, my mom died, but I have a wonderful stepmother," because she didn't want people to feel sorry for her. She explains: "I mean, I grew up in a beautiful home with everything a kid could dream of. And my stepmother was wonderful. So even losing my mother, I felt like, I should feel better than this."

Carol felt her father did not grieve fully for her mother for many years. "He eventually did grieve, in his way. He tended to intellectualize it." Carol remembers having many long, philosophical talks with her father when she was a teenager, on the meaning of God and why evil existed in the world. "He probably knew that I was just scared and grieving, and putting all that anxiety and fear into my head, just like he did."

Carol took many risks during her youth:

> I was in this death wish, risking kind of stuff. I was someone who had fear, but I always turned it into something I was going to do. I taught horseback riding. [I was] scared to death of horses after a bad experience when I was younger, but I forced myself to do it. It was my way of saying, "I'm not afraid of death." I did think about death a lot growing up. I wanted to know about death. Teenagers get a little morbid and do that kind of thing. But I probably did it more than the average teenager because I was really scared of death. I figure I'm gonna die in my thirties.

It was not until Carol left home that she began to deal with her long-ignored grief.

> When I moved away, I had the opportunity to put enough distance from my stepmother to actually grieve the loss of my mom. One night, I just had this horrible sense of missing my mother. I suddenly felt overwhelmed with the need to know more. I realized that I didn't even know the day that my mother died. I didn't know her birthday. I hadn't visited

her grave since the funeral. So all these things kind of came crashing
in on me, and all of a sudden it mattered.

Carol called her older sister and learned that the anniversary of their
mother's death was only three days away. The next time she was
home, she visited her mother's grave, and has since observed the anniversary of her mother's death.

Long-Term Impact

Carol occasionally has a sense of panic, especially at times of transition. Sometimes she is depressed ("I've had bouts of depression—
nothing that would be diagnosable—and anxiety, but nothing that I
didn't handle") and experiences insomnia: "When I'm going through
a transition, it's hell. I have terrible, terrible insomnia." She also has
had difficulty with intimate relationships. "I didn't think I was capable of making that bond, and I had an irrational fear that I would bring
bad things to someone." On the positive side, Carol feels that she lives
her life fully. Because she expects to die young (thirty-six, the age at
which her mother died), she feels her experience has made her a lot
more sensitive. "It's a cliché, but in some ways I'm a lot happier. Everything tastes better. I want to embrace all that, live it! Go ahead and
take that vacation!"

Carol feels that the biggest impact on her has been "very spiritual
and philosophical. It drew me into a field where I was going to have to
deal with things, and I love what I do."

Risk

When Carol was in college, one of her sisters was diagnosed with a
rare cancer. Carol lived near her at the time. They often discussed
their mother's cancer. "I tended to be the caregiver. Unlike Mama, she
talked about her pain. She was very uncomfortable." Then, several
years later, Carol's brother was diagnosed with another rare (but
treatable) cancer. Shortly before the study began, Carol's father had
been treated for cancer. "So cancer is definitely a theme in my family." Because of her family history, Carol expects to get cancer. "It
was just another block to add to the fear column. Something that is
going to happen to me someday. Cancer is something that we have
learned to live with. It's bad, but there's hope in what we've seen. All

but my mother are living and doing well." In spite of the intellectual knowledge that cancer can be survived,

> I still have a hard time imagining that I'll live. I mean, I believe I will intellectually, but there's that piece of me, that irrational side—and it's not totally irrational, because of course I know the genetics, and I know I could be a genetic time bomb.

Carol stays active in an effort to prevent cancer. "I believe that staying active is a good cancer-fighting agent. I try to limit dairy products and fat. But I have a real sweet tooth, which [her mother] had. I'm not as good about that, but I try to watch my diet. I try to practice stress management. I'm a big believer in that."

Current Situation

Carol was thirty-one at the time of interview, working as a counselor (she has also worked with homeless youth for a religious agency). She has since earned a social work degree.

To her surprise, Carol defied her own predictions and got married. She found a soul mate in her husband. "We've both kind of been through some stuff, and we worked on it alone. So each of us figured that the other one can handle it [adversity]." Carol feels that her husband is teaching her to "slow down and live life as if it's not about to end."

At the time of the interviews, Carol was thinking about having children.

> I've been very anxious about getting pregnant. I want to have a baby more than anything in the world, right now. My husband wanted to wait. Wait for what? Wait for me to have a child that's so young that [he or she] loses me? I don't have time to wait anymore.

Today, Carol has two children and is happy to report that many of her fears about death and difficulty with transitions have diminished greatly.

> I now have moved away from being primarily "the daughter" to "the mother," and my new role puts old fears in the past. For instance, I can picture myself growing old, instead of fearing I will not reach old age. My concerns now are giving my children a happy childhood so that they will want to live life fully and to want to make me a grandmother one day. I feel I have a lot to look forward to. I have an abundant life, with or without cancer.

CASE STUDY #3: NORA

Age at Her Mother's Breast Cancer Diagnosis: 1; Age at Time of Her Mother's Death: 9

Background

Nora lived in a small house with her mother, father, and an older sister. Nora's grandmother had emigrated from Ireland, and her mother was the first in the family to attend high school. Her father had a civilian job with the U.S. Navy. The two girls went to Catholic schools. Nora's sister was an excellent student who was very involved in extracurricular activities, such as Girl Scouts and sports. "She was so bright and pretty and clean and neat. She was certainly the good little girl in the house. I was not."

The family was part of the Catholic community in a small town where people knew one another well. Nora's mother was active in her church and the community. "She was very religious—incredibly religious. We went to church all the time. Within the community, she [her mother] gave of her time. She worked at the school. She worked in the church when she could. Everybody respected her." Nora's father was abusive toward her and her sister, but he was always devoted to their mother.

> He was very abusive to us as kids, physically, verbally, whatever. And also, he was an alcoholic. My father and I never got along very well. When we were little, he would just beat us with a belt. My sister would say, "Don't cry because it really makes him mad." Well, I'm stupid, so I didn't cry, and so he would just beat the shit out of me.

Nora's mother had a sister and a brother, but neither lived in the area. All her grandparents were deceased.

Experience of Her Mother's Illness

Because her mother was diagnosed when Nora was very young, she has only vague knowledge of the details of her mother's illness.

> I think my mother had a lump in her breast. From what I can figure out, it was pea-sized, because I once heard someone saying offhandedly, "It's amazing how something that small can kill you." I just put that together years later.

Nora does not have clear memories of her mother's treatment. "I imagine they did a mastectomy. I remember one of [her operations]. I must have been three or four years old, and I was sitting on the lawn of the hospital while she was undergoing some major surgery." Once, her sister heard a doctor saying, " 'While we were in there, we took her appendix out.' So I know they did a hysterectomy." Nora also remembers her mother having a reaction to one of her medications, and having to wear an eye patch and wash her eye out frequently. "I'm assuming that was all in response to the chemotherapy."

Nora once picked up one of her mother's prostheses, and said, "Boy, this is funny!" Her mother replied, "Well, it wouldn't be funny if I didn't have one." Nora explains, "I remembered that comment, and for years later, I was mortified [because] I realized what it was and what I had done." However, at the time, Nora accepted her mother's illness as normal.

> I don't think I noticed that she didn't have any breasts. I don't think that was striking to me in any way. That was just her. My mother was in bed all the time. I remember her being very frail. But it never dawned on me that she was any different from any other mother. My sister was four years older, so she was much more impacted by what life was like while she was sick. I was oblivious to it all. There was a chair next to my mother's bed and I would just sit there for hours and talk to her. I have some memory of that. I just sat there, waited on her, and did whatever [I] had to do. I was perfectly comfortable just sitting there. My sister couldn't stand that. I guess because she know more of what was going on.

Nora remembers that her mother often was away. "When she would get sick, she would have to go out to [the military hospital], and we rarely visited other than Sundays. We wouldn't see her for long periods of time." Sometimes Nora's aunt stayed with them when her mother was ill.

> She would come down, and once they realized just how sick she was going to be, she would stay a month, two months, three months at a time. But my father's edict was that she was there to take care of her sister, and we were not to ask anything of her. So we were pretty much on our own.

Her aunt did not provide supervision during these periods. "I remember going places in the winter dressed in shorts. I just looked in my drawer and I put on whatever I put on, you know."

Nora was nine when her mother died. The death was a complete surprise to Nora.

> I remember that I prayed every night that my mother would get better. I think one time it hit me that, what if she didn't? But then denial kicked in and I said, "Well, that's dumb. Of course she will!" And until she died, I had no idea she was going to die.

Nora was playing with her sister one day when her father came in and said, "Go upstairs and say good-bye to your mother."

> So I [said], "Okay," and I went upstairs. I had no idea. I just assumed she was going to the hospital again. She was very frail. She was, my aunt said, like, eighty-five pounds. But she was able to speak. She sat up. She said, "Good-bye!" My sister said she knew because my father was upset, and he never got upset. But I didn't notice it at the time.

The children were sent to a neighbor's house for a while and later were allowed to return home.

> When we walked in the door, my father took the homework my sister had with her, and said something like, "Oh, let me put this down for you." And I said [to myself], "Whoa, something is wrong!" I knew right away something was up, because Dad was nice to us. Of course, all the neighbors were there. The priest was there. When they told us, they said, "Your mother passed away." Well, I had no clue what that meant. None in the world. I had no idea. Nobody cried. We all just sat there. So I sat there, perfectly still, trying to figure out what was going on. The priest was picking at some sort of a candle while he was talking to us. I had no idea what he was talking about. I remember he said, "Your mother passed away on us," like it was her fault. I thought, *Did she move?* Everybody was sitting there quietly. They were so concerned about [not] showing us [their] grief. It was hard to pick up a clue as to what was happening. Then I saw my aunt was in the back [of the house]. I looked down the hall, and I saw her crying. Then I thought, *That's what happened. She died!* Because she was crying. That's how I figured it out.

Later that evening, Nora saw her mother being carried out. "They didn't even bring a stretcher. They just carried her [body] out."

Experience Following Her Mother's Death

The week following her mother's death was very difficult for Nora.

> It was just a horrendous week. We just sat around and did nothing. We never talked about her. They shielded us from any emotion. They didn't let us go to school. I just remember sitting for five days doing nothing. We did two nights of viewing. So we stood there. I had my little image of how, "Oh, she's not dead. I can see her eyes. She blinked." I kept it to myself, but I thought, *I'm the only person here who realizes she's not dead.*

Nora remembers little about the funeral, but, "I stood there and greeted everybody. They tell you what to do, and you kind of get through it all." Later, she remembers her aunt saying to her, "I watched you during the funeral. You were so brave." "And I thought, *Christ! I'm nine years old. I know what to do.*" Nora said that after her mother's funeral, she hated the smell of carnations and incense. After the burial, the family did not go to visit the graveside or perform other mourning rituals.

The silence in Nora's family continued after her mother's death.

> We never spoke her name. He [father] got rid of all of her things . . . her wedding rings—he lost those. I don't know what the hell he did with them. He just got rid of it all. None of that had any meaning to him whatsoever. That was just it. She was dead, and she was gone, and it was pretty much as though she had never been there. It's not that he denied that she was ever there. But he certainly wasn't going to talk about it. He was never going to bring it up. Every now and then, I would see something [of hers], and I would just take it.

Nora's mother died in early December, so she didn't return to school until after Christmas vacation:

> When I got back, no teacher said a word to me. I was in fourth grade. When I got to fifth grade, my teacher had no idea my mother was dead. This was very hard, because I had to tell people, and I just couldn't. I didn't know what to say or how to say it. Once I was hanging around after school, and the teacher said, "Oh, does your mother work?" And that was so hard for me. I thought, *Couldn't someone have told them?* When I was bad, which was frequently, the nuns [unaware that her mother was dead] would say to me, "I talked to your mother last night, and I told her what you did." Well, you know [chuckling], their credibility was shot.

When Nora's aunt visited, "We would take her to the grave." Sometimes, Nora went by herself. "I went on my own, 'cause we could walk there. It was maybe a mile and a half away. I would go every now and then."

Regarding discussing her mother's death with friends, Nora said,

> My sister and I were the only kids in that school who came from a one-parent home. Everybody else had intact families. Then, another child's mother died in the sixth grade. He was this incredibly smart, geeky guy. A kid said, "Well, maybe now he won't be so smart 'cause his mother's dead." I thought that was pretty awful, and I punched her. You know, my own internal rage just made me deck her. He and I have been friends ever since. I just know it was that bond.

After her mother died, Nora had almost no parental supervision.

> My father was oblivious to having children. He had no clue. I think having girls was hard for him. We went to a school that had uniforms. Thank God! Or we would have had nothing to wear. When I got bigger than my sister, I had no clothes that fit me. When I turned thirteen, I got a job and so did my sister, and we bought our own stuff, because he had no idea.

Nora's father drank more heavily after her mother's death. "The drinking was just prominent. He was drunk all the time, you know." According to Nora, his behavior deteriorated. "He was drinking more. He was much more abusive. But he was much more pathetic. I think that we started to see that this is not our fault, you know. This guy is really just out of control."

By this time, Nora was drinking too.

> I was drinking by the time I was eleven. It was good that he was drunk, because [that way] he didn't know I was drunk. My friends, you know, we bought it, or we got someone to buy it for us. We just hung out with older kids and they bought it. And we stole it. We stole a lot. We'd break into houses and steal. I wouldn't steal anything from my father, because he'd kill me. I didn't need to be killed more than I was.

Nora addressed whether her drinking interfered with her school or work:

> Not for a while. But then, I would drink at school in elementary school. Certainly by the ninth grade, it interfered a lot. I was getting high, and yeah, it interfered. I used pretty much whatever I got my hands on, and we started getting high five, six, seven times a day. And that lasted awhile. It got pretty ridiculous. I was an awful student. We [Nora and her friends] wouldn't do homework for months, and then we would take speed and stay up all weekend and get just enough done so we didn't fail. That was our mode of staying in school. My father never threat-

ened not to pay the tuition, because it was my mother's deepest desire that I go to a Catholic school. So I wasn't worried about that.

When Nora was eleven, she was sexually assaulted by a sixteen-year-old boy. She blamed herself, and did not tell anyone. Around this time, her father began to date.

He definitely went out right away. He remarried when I was twelve. When I was thirteen, I started working. So I pretty much had money all the time. I worked in a grocery store, bagging groceries every night after school and on Saturdays and during the summer. So I made a fair amount of money for the time.

Growing up, Nora did not have any information about her mother's illness. Once, several years after her mother's death, she and her father were fighting, and she yelled at him, "You never even told me why my mother died!" She recalls, "About two weeks later, we were driving in the car, and he looked at me and he said, 'Cancer.' And I said, 'What?' And he said, 'Your mother died of cancer.'"

Long-Term Impact

Nora believes she is a much more self-sufficient person because of her mother's death.

I think I'm much more independent, obviously. For many years, I expected people to die. My aunt [father's sister-in-law] died a year and a day later, which was pretty eerie. Then, my mother's best friend died of cancer within a year of my mother dying. She had breast cancer. And then, seven months later, my grandfather died.

Nora's father was in a serious automobile accident that same year. "I think my sister and I were just like, 'This is just what happens.'" Nora remembers her sister discussing how they might have to stay with one of their aunts if their father died. "She was like, 'Yeah, they're just gonna die. They're old anyway and they're just gonna die, so it doesn't really matter which aunt we go to, 'cause she's just gonna die anyway.'"

Nora has had three fairly serious depressions, one a postpartum depression, and one when she was working on a dissertation for her doctorate. While in therapy for the depressions she realized that she had not dealt with her mother's illness and death, and that this was affecting her as an adult. Nora recognizes that she was angry as a child, but her anger was directed at her father, not her mother or herself. "I wasn't angry at myself. I could blame him and he was easy to blame, so I did." Another effect of this experience is that even as an adult, Nora is uncomfortable if she perceives that someone is trying to "mother" her.

Risk

Nora did not discuss her risk in the interviews, but she affirmed many of the risk issues on the final questionnaire. Responding to a question which asked if she thinks she will get breast cancer at the same age which her mother did, Nora checked "Yes."

> I worry about it more than I think I will [get it]. You know, I am the age as we speak. And my awareness is just heightened. I don't think about getting it, but it's certainly a possibility. It's a real clear possibility. Am I fearful? Absolutely. And that's just being realistic. There's so much we know, but you're just gonna get it anyway. There's very little you can do about it. I wouldn't say it's inevitable, but certainly my risks are high. So I've kind of told myself, "Don't freak out. Do the right things. You'll catch it as early as you can and you'll live with it." She [Nora's mother] lived nine or ten years when treatments were pretty barbaric. So I figure, "Hey, if you get it, you get it. You'll deal with it."

Nora has taken actions to prevent breast cancer. For example, she has avoided birth control pills and decided to have her children early in life. "I certainly wanted to do that as early as I could. That was a reason. That wasn't the driving force, but certainly, when I thought about having them later, that was on my mind."

Nora does monthly breast exams most of the time. "There are some months [when] it's pretty scary. It's a weird feeling. It's no big deal most of the time, but every now and then I get this little panic thing. 'Do you understand what you're looking for?' That's very scary." Sometimes she decides not to do an exam if she misses the "window," telling herself that she wouldn't be able to be sure what she was feeling. "I can hear my other self talk and I realize that it's just a lot of fears." Nora has mammograms on her own initiative and at her own expense. "My sister working for the cancer society keeps me very aware. I'm lucky in that sense. My physician wouldn't push it. So I just go, and have them send her the records. I don't even ask anymore. I just go when I think I should go."

Current Situation

Nora was thirty-seven at the time of interview. She was married and had converted to her husband's religion, Judaism. She has two children, a son and a daughter. Because Nora had her children at a much younger age than her mother did, her children were now past the age that Nora was when her mother died.

> My daughter is four years past where I was, and my son's a little further along. I always knew they'd be okay if they could get as far as I had gotten. That was almost a relief. When my daughter hit nine, I thought, *You know what? If something happens to me, I know she's gonna be okay because I'm okay.* And after that point, it was a gift. Just being able to see them get older and older is just such a pleasure and such a gift. I could never be as bad a parent as my father was. Most people couldn't be. So it's like, "I'm doing all right." That's almost comforting. I might have a horrible day and say something horrible to them or do something really insensitive or whatever, and I know I shouldn't. But I can never be that bad.

Nora works as a counselor at a mental health center. Her father and stepmother moved to Florida, and she sees them infrequently. They do not discuss the past. Nora's sister works for a cancer advocacy organization. Nora has invited her sister to join a group for "motherless daughters," but her sister is not interested. Nora herself has participated in the group; as a result, she would like to find out more about her mother as a person.

DISCUSSION

This section discusses three phases of daughters' experience: Experience of mother's illness and treatment, experience following mother's death, and long-term impact. Box 4.1 presents the major themes identified in each of these phases. (Another important factor, risk, is discussed in Chapter 9.)

In addition to the cases of Rita, Carol, and Nora, the discussion includes references to an additional case (Marci, Appendix III). Also, because women whose mothers survive breast cancer experience the first phase of the illness in the same way as do women whose mothers ultimately die, the section on the experience of mother's illness and treatment makes reference to Ramona (Chapter 8) and Chloe (Ap-

---

BOX 4.1. Themes Found in Daughters Whose Mothers Died When They Were Children

Phase I: Mother's Illness and Treatments

1. Lack of communication
2. Am I still safe?
3. Independence

Phase II: Following Mother's Death

1. Loss of the family
2. Survival

Phase III: Long-Term Impact

1. Seeking information
2. Delayed grieving
3. Mental health impact
4. Strong, independent personality

---

pendix III), whose mothers survived. In addition, because the line between children and young adolescents was not always a clear one, when younger adolescent cases (presented in Chapter 5) had experiences that reflect themes discussed in this chapter, they are referred to here.

Daughter's Experience of Her Mother's Illness

Three themes were identified in this phase for children. These are lack of communication, am I still safe?, and independence.

Lack of Communication

Lack of communication about the illness is a theme that appears in the stories of women who were children when their mothers were diagnosed. Rita recalls only one conversation with her mother about breast cancer, but she listened attentively and was sensitive to body language and facial expressions. Carol was told that her mother was ill and was asked to "pray for her." She always assumed that her mother would get well again, and it was only when she saw her older brother's reaction to the news that God "had taken" their mother that she realized her mother had died. Nora does not remember her mother before the cancer diagnosis. She simply accepted the illness as normal for her mother, completely unaware that her mother was seriously ill. When told to say "good-bye," Nora did not realize her mother was on her deathbed. She didn't understand the meaning of "your mother passed away," and it wasn't until she saw her aunt crying that she realized that her mother had died.

Another respondent, Marci (see Appendix III), was only a baby at time of diagnosis, but she is bitter not only that she was not told about her mother's illness but that even her mother was not told. This was common practice at the time (circa 1960) when having cancer was perceived as a "death sentence." Marci has no memory of anyone telling her about her mother's illness, even after her mother's death. However, she suspects that someone told her that her mother "went to sleep," because she now suffers from insomnia.

In contrast to most children in our sample, communication was more open in Ramona's case (see Chapter 8). Ramona was eight at the time of diagnosis; her mother survived for about thirty-five years. Her mother (a biology teacher) took a scientific approach and explained how cancer cells function but did not share the more emotional aspects of her diagnosis. She tried to protect Ramona from negative comments about cancer by strangers, and presented a positive, optimistic picture. Ramona understood the seriousness of the illness, however, when she saw her father crying while talking on the phone. "That was the first time I really knew this was really, really, really serious."

These daughters, children at diagnosis, often were not told about their mothers' illnesses, or were given only limited, reassuring information. However, in spite of efforts to protect them, they were aware that something was wrong. As Nora says, "You can tell by the mood of a house." They were especially sensitive to nonverbal cues and to any changes in routine. They sensed that something was wrong, for example, when they were sent to a neighbor's house after school or when a relative came to stay. Even when given factual information (as Ramona was), the emotional aspects of the illness were rarely discussed. This lack of communication had some negative consequences. The daughters in this study were quick to percieve signals that something was amiss—they sensed a threat, and felt the emotions of their family members. They overheard information, or misinformation, and tried to piece together the story—which often occurred much later. At the same time, they realized that the illness and the emotions surrounding it had to be hidden. They learned not to ask questions and to hide their own emotions. Because of this "code of silence" they did not get help with their own emotions from adults or siblings. Instead of learning that strong emotions can be expressed and survived, they had no opportunity to express their fears or their love. Later, as adults, they lacked important information. If their mothers died, they had to seek out family members or try to locate medical records to learn what they died from. As adults, these women sometimes perpetuate a pattern of silence in their own families, not telling *their* children about their pasts, or about other traumatic events in the family.

Some research has shown that open communication is an important factor in the adaptation of the child when a parent is ill (Ell and Northern, 1990; Vollman et al., 1971). In addition, children's level of anxiety is related to the quality of family communication (Kroll et al., 1998). Evidence also suggests that children experience better adjustment when emotional expression is tolerated (Berlinsky and Biller, 1982).

Why is communication between adults and children often so poor? One reason is that it is very difficult for parents to effectively explain serious illness.

> Parents may fear that they cannot be as solid, articulate, and certain about the path and outcome of the disease to their children as they would like to be. They find it difficult to emphasize hope for the future while also being honest about the inherent uncertainty of the situation. (Patenaude, 2000, pp. 239-240)

When a woman learns she has breast cancer, she fears the negative impact on her child. She might attempt to protect her child from this impact by avoiding the issue altogether. This lack of communication may be well intentioned; parents often seek to shield children from potentially painful subjects. They do not want to overwhelm the child. Some may think that by not telling the child, they will minimize the harm. They also may think that by showing their own fear, they will create fear in the child. Parents fear being overcome by emotions and losing control. They also may feel guilty (Oktay and Walter, 1991) if they believe they have failed to protect their children from the impact of the illness. In addition, some may think that to admit the possibility of death might make death more likely. Parents also may be in denial or have a belief system that emphasizes using prayer instead of dwelling on facts.

In *Healing Children's Grief: Surviving a Parent's Death from Cancer,* Christ (2000) illustrates the dynamics of poor communication between adults and children.

> Because most of the children [six to eight years old] were reluctant to reveal their fears about the parent's possible death, especially to either parent, parents could not be guided by the children's questions when trying to decide when and what type of information they needed to provide. (p. 74)

Christ stresses how difficult this task is. "Just how difficult it was for young parents facing the death of a spouse to discuss the illness and its prognosis with their children cannot be overemphasized" (p. 76).

The failure to communicate with children may also be related to what is happening in the patients' marital relationships. Some evidence suggests that breast cancer is more difficult on husbands than wives (Baider, Rizel, and De-Nour, 1986). Partners of the patient often become isolated, fearing they will "say the wrong thing." This can inhibit communication (Wortman and Dunkel-Schetter, 1979) between husband and wife. (In our study, some mothers were not even told of their diagnosis—a sure way to block communication!) When communication between marital partners is blocked, children likely will be isolated. Parents who cannot talk to each other about their emotions will not be able to discuss how to tell the children. Also, in most families, the wife/mother is the emotional caregiver. When illness prevents her from performing this role, it is unlikely that the father or siblings will take over. As a result, communication of an emotional nature simply does not take place.

The children in breast cancer families may experience something similar to siblings of terminally ill children (Fanos, 1996). In these families, healthy siblings generally are not told about the illness; sometimes even the ill children are not told (Fanos and Wiener, 1994).

This lack of communication impacts not only the adaptation of individual family members but also affects the relationships between members. . . . This enforced silence negatively impacts both the parent-child and sibling relationships and may even threaten healthy development for healthy siblings. (Fanos, 1996, p. 8)

Although it is beyond the scope of this study to analyze why communication with children may be lacking in breast cancer families, it is important to emphasize that this causes problems for the children. They realize that something is happening, and that they are not being told. As adults, they experience long-term problems related to their lack of information about the mother's illness. For example, some experience guilt and regret that they did not express their love, as they were not aware of the situation. (This is discussed further in Chapter 11.)

Am I Still Safe?

The youngest daughters in our study were not especially bothered by the symptoms of the mother's illness, but were more disturbed by changes in routine. The most upsetting part of the illness for children was the separation from their mothers due to hospitalization. Although not always aware of their mothers' cancer, the children in our study were aware of (and upset by) changes in mothers' functioning. Nora remembers her mother being away for long periods and her aunt staying at her family's home. Marci (Appendix III) focused on how her mother came in and out of her life, and eventually never came back. Kara (Chapter 5) described how upset she was when she was not allowed to visit her mother in the hospital.

The literature on child development suggests that young children need to develop trust in their caregivers (Bowlby, 1980; Erikson, 1964). Trust is dependent on the child knowing that he or she can count on the caregiver (usually the mother) being available and responding to his or her needs. When a mother is hospitalized, it is very frightening for a child. Children are by nature self-centered; this situation makes them lose confidence that they will receive the care they need. This belief can affect their level of trust in the parents. If very young, they may never develop a sense of trust, and if they are older, their sense of trust may be threatened.

While hospitalization results in a physical separation, children also may feel abandoned by a mother who is physically present but not psychologically engaged with them. One of the effects of serious illness is a tendency toward self-absorption (Oktay and Walter, 1991). A woman diagnosed with breast cancer must absorb the very scary information she is given and make difficult treatment decisions. It may not be possible to fulfill the "mother role"—such as providing the type of unlimited attention that is needed by a young child—under these conditions. In a previous study (Oktay and Walter, 1991), mothers with young children often sent the children to alternate caregivers, such as grandmothers, until they got through the crisis stage. In the current study, it was this withdrawal of attention that children seemed most sensitive to. They are especially disturbed by the mother's absences due to hospitalizations or the children being sent to be cared for by family, friends, or neighbors. Many children were sent to neighbors' or relatives' homes during the terminal phase. (Some of these children, such as Carol and Kara, later felt guilty that they had been playing and having fun while their mothers were suffering.)

Some children did not notice the mother's symptoms; when they did notice, they usually were not disturbed. Instead, they accepted mother as she was. They seem to adapt to Mom being in bed, having scars and prostheses, or losing her hair. Nora never noticed that mother did not have breasts. She accepted mother being in bed much of the time as normal. Some even have happy memories of their mothers' illness. Nora and Rita enjoyed playing with their mothers' prostheses. Chloe (Appendix III) has happy memories of visiting her mother in the hospital, where she was allowed to sit for hours after school, drawing and doing homework. Nora enjoyed her mother's attention as she sat by her bedside and chatted happily. Ramona (Chapter 8) remembers her mother getting gifts, and her own reprieve from a painful treatment for fever.

When they did observe the physical effects of treatments, especially the mastectomy scar, most were not upset by it. Rita, who snuck a look at her mother's scar, remembers to a greater extent how funny her mother's facial hair remover was. An exception was Carol, who did report being disturbed by her mother's mastectomy scar; however, memories of her mother welcoming her home from school seemed stronger than her concern about her mother's physical appearance. As long as a mother is still able to "be a mom," the children do not look ahead with fear. They tend to live in the moment and accept the explanations they are given. The symptoms themselves are not imbued with ominous meaning. A couple of the women remember wondering if mothers could die, quickly concluding that they couldn't. Carol, for example, was sure the family's prayers would work. Nora also prayed for her mother every night and didn't let herself imagine that she might not get well. Kara (see Chapter 5) wondered, "Do mommies die?" She quickly answered her own question: "No. It doesn't happen."

Christ (2000) also found that the younger children in her study were more concerned with "changes in the caregiving parent, that parent's preoccupation, and the frequent separations, not the illness" (p. 48). These young children were accepting of changes involving medical equipment in the home, because they did not connect these with the terminal nature of the parent's illness.

More than anything else, the women in this study needed their mothers to be there for them. They were most disturbed when separated from the mother, even if they were well cared for by relatives or neighbors. It mattered little to the young daughters if mother had symptoms from the treatments. The daughters' main concern seemed to be their own safety. Separation from the mother threatened that safety.

Independence

Although the possibility of death may not have been openly discussed, some children sensed that their mothers were preparing them to survive without her. Rita's mother made her walk to school in inclement weather. Ramona (Chapter 8) felt rushed to grow up fast. She recalls that she was the first in her class to learn about menstruation, puberty, and sex. "She [Ramona's mother] worried that my father would not know how to raise a girl." Kara (Chapter 5) describes herself as "up underneath my mother"; she realized only later that her mother had been preparing her children for life without her. "She had us making our lunches for school. She was preparing us [for her to leave] and we didn't even know it." As with Ramona, Kara's mother taught her about menstruation, and showed her how to wear a sanitary napkin, to her great embarrassment.

Some mothers encouraged their young daughters to function more independently, without discussing this with the daughters. Daughters generally were unaware of the reasons for these actions at the time, but they were sensitive to being "pushed out of the nest." Mothers seemed particularly concerned about their girls' sexual maturation and wanted to be sure they were prepared. Mothers also tried to impact their daughters' futures in several ways. For example, Rita's mother worked for as long as she could to be sure that her children would get Social Security survivor's benefits. Rita was very grateful for the assistance she received with college expenses. Nora's mother insisted the children continue in Catholic schools after her death, and Nora's father honored this request.

Experience Following Her Mother's Death

Two themes were identified for the period after mother's death for the youngest age group in the study: loss of the family and survival.

Loss of the Family

After mother's death, most fathers of the young daughters remarried—sometimes only months later. The daughters soon found their fathers unavailable to them and unsympathetic to their problems with new stepmothers. Whether they liked or disliked their stepmothers, they often rejected their authority and their roles as "mother." Rita actively resisted her stepmother's attempts to parent her, and virtually went to war with both her father and stepmother, doing what she could to make their lives miserable. Nora, whose father did not remarry for three years, seemed to raise herself. When her father did remarry, his new wife did not even try to discipline Nora, who was by this time quite uncontrollable. Nora replaced her family with a group of kids who, like her, were lacking parental supervision. Marci (see Appendix III) describes her stepmother as cold and jealous. "She was also very jealous, particularly of me because I was the youngest and . . . the most like my mother." Marci's housekeeper was more of a mother figure than was her stepmother. Bettina's case (Chapter 5) is probably the most extreme, because her stepmother was abusive and alcoholic. "She beat me up. I had big welts and bruises on my back. This is as old as Cinderella." Bettina was sent halfway across the country to live with an aunt, where she was expected to do strenuous farmwork.

Exceptions to the "Cinderella" pattern also existed. Carol's father married a widow and good friend of the family, and Kara's (Chapter 5) father also married a woman who had known (and grieved for) Kara's mother. In these cases, the stepmother was able to mourn along with the family, encourage reminiscence, and even love the little girl because of (not in spite of) the fact that she was a living reminder of her mother. Even so, Kara turned to her aunt (mother's sister), not her stepmother, for mothering. Carol buried her emotions to promote harmony in her new stepfamily. Unfortunately, a family such as that of Cinderella, with a "wicked stepmother" (from the perspective of the bereaved daughter) was a common outcome. The introduction of the stepmother (and subsequent loss of family) enraged most daughters, and they focused their anger on the father and/or stepmother. However, the women in the sample did not direct their anger at their mothers for abandoning them (at least not consciously). Instead, most developed an idealized image of the mother and of how their lives would have been if she had lived.

Some dealt with conflict and rejection at home by seeking to escape. Escapes used by young girls included: finding a surrogate family, usually the family of a friend (Rita, Marci); using substances such as alcohol and drugs (Nora); and becoming very active in school and after-school activities (Rita). Their goal was the same: to stay out of the house as much as possible.

There is very little research on what happens to families after a mother's death. Although our understanding of stepfamilies in general has increased as more and more children are being raised in "custodial" families, bereaved families form only a small proportion of such families today (less than 5 percent). Even among bereaved stepfamilies, in most cases it is the father who is deceased, due to higher death rates among men. Only 2.5 percent of custodial families involve the death of the mother. Also, bereaved fathers are more likely to remarry, and they do so sooner than do bereaved mothers. Therefore, children who lose a father are less likely to live in stepfamilies than are children who lose a mother (Mills, 1988). While studies of the bereaved maternal stepfamily are rare, evidence that supports the experience of the daughters in our study exists. For example, children in maternally bereaved stepfamilies are reported to feel abandoned by their fathers, hostile, and resentful. Some researchers (Ihinger-Tallman and Pasley, 1987; Mills, 1988; Clingempeel, Brand, and Ievoli, 1984) speculate that the father's remarriage poses a major threat to the father-daughter relationship. This research found stepmother-stepdaughter relationships more problematic than stepmothers' relationships with stepsons. "From the child's perspective, stepmothers were detached and uninvolved in nearly every facet of the child's upbringing" (Santrock and Sitterle, 1995, p. 285). In addition, general literature on children in stepfamilies (not limited to those in bereaved families) suggests that daughters in stepfamilies have more problems than do sons, that higher marital satisfaction in the stepparents is associated with poorer stepdaughter adjustment, and that relationships between stepchildren and stepmothers are far more problematic than are those with stepfathers. Stinson (1991) speculates that this is because those in the mother role are the disciplinarians and usually enforce the rules.

In our sample, bereaved daughters often fought with their stepmothers; however, it is not clear that this was always an issue of a power struggle. Issues of identity seemed at least as important. That is, stepdaughters did not want stepmothers to be able to define who they were, for example, through clothing choices. The bereaved daughters identified strongly with their mothers—not with their stepmothers. Allowing the stepmother to set the rules or make decisions for them seemed to these young daughters a betrayal of their mothers.

Santrock and Sitterle (1995) suggest that the reason for the strong antagonism toward the stepmother found in *divorced* families is that she may end the child's fantasies of reconciliation and hopes of the mother's return.

> The stepmother's presence may act as a constant reminder to the child that the loss of her mother is final. . . . It may be that these children displace their anger, hurt and disappointment toward their [noncustodial] mothers, and even their fathers, onto their stepmothers. (p. 291)

This description, while discussing a different type of mother-loss, is relevant to the daughters in our sample, who did not express anger toward their mothers for abandoning them, but whose rage at the father and the stepmother was often vitriolic.

In summary, the young daughters experienced catastrophic changes following their mothers' deaths. In most (but not all) cases, a "Cinderella" family pattern developed. These girls lost not only their mothers but the security of their homes and families. Fathers became distant and preoccupied with replacing the lost wife, while daughters struggled to maintain their identity and loyalty to their mothers. They also sought escape from their new home situations either through surrogate families, school activities, or friends.

Survival

This is the second theme identified in the period following mother's death for the youngest group of daughters. Carol's statement ("Maslow's hierarchy of needs was there. You have to survive! So, forget your grief . . .") clearly demonstrates this theme. After her mother's death, Rita delighted in her strength. Free to be a tomboy, she enjoyed playing football and was proud that she didn't cry when stung by a bee. Most mothers' main goal is to prepare their children for adulthood—to be able to protect and nurture them until they are able to fend for themselves. In the animal kingdom, death of a mother usually means death of the children, who become easy prey. In modern American society, death of a mother is relatively rare, but women instinctively know that their children might be in jeopardy if they are not able to protect and nurture them. Children also seem to know this.

Loss of the mother shatters a child's core sense of safety (Harris, 1995). The literature suggests that "bereaved children may worry that their basic physical needs for survival will not be satisfied" (Krupnick and Solomon, 1987, p. 353). "The child often experiences the event as overwhelming and feels powerless and helpless in the same way as does a trauma survivor" (Pill and Zabin, 1997, p. 182). The grieving process may not begin until the child feels his or her survival is ensured. "Children may not be able to grieve until they feel secure that they will be cared for physically and emotionally" (Pill and Zabin, 1997, p. 181).

The young girls in the current study hid their feelings and tried to "act tough." This strategy is common in animals; a false bravado often can scare off a stronger, threatening predator. The focus on survival left little time or energy for grieving. Regardless of whether the children attended mothers' funerals, there did not seem to be adequate meaningful grief periods for any of them. With little communication, the children were left to figure things out for themselves. Nora describes how she sat in the funeral home, looking for clues on how to behave so as not to appear "dumb." Rita was relieved she did not have to attend the funeral because she thought she would be embarrassed by the attention. In the years following the death, daughters rarely were given an opportunity to mourn their mothers. They were not given pictures of their mothers or objects that might stimulate memories, nor were they told stories that keep memories alive. In some homes, it seemed to the daughters that the mother's memory was banished. Sometimes this was attributed to stepmother's discomfort with mention of the previous wife (see Marci, Appendix III), to her discomfort with the children's grief (Carol), or to the father's inability to grieve (Marci, Nora, Carol). When they *were* performed, rituals of mourning did not comfort these children.

None of the young daughters had a father, an aunt, grandmother, or sibling who helped her to mourn. Nor did these girls know any other children in their situation. Instead of dealing with their grief, the daughters were acutely aware of their new, stigmatized status, and often tried to hide the fact that their mothers had died. Rita didn't want to "mess up," because people would attribute any problems to her mother's death: "I didn't want there to be anything wrong with me." Some of these young daughters took on the function of nurturer to other family members. Marci (Appendix III) talks about how she, at the young age of three, took care of her father's emotional needs after mother died. Some daughters felt that it was *their* job to make the new family work (Marci, Carol).

Extensive literature exists on the nature of children's grief, controversy about whether children grieve at all, and if their grief is similar to that of adults. Because this issue goes to the core of modern psychological ideas about human growth and development, it has received extensive attention. Freud's classic model of grief (1917) differentiated a healthy grieving process, "mourning," from a pathological process, "melancholia," in which the grief is not resolved and the process of "letting go" does not happen. According to this theory, grief in children is impossible because children lack the cognitive capacity to understand what death means. Studies based on observations of children who have experienced a loss show a different pattern than what typically happens in adults. Children seem to grieve intermittently, and switch quickly from sadness or anger to oblivious playfulness (Worden, 1996; Christ, 2000).

Freud's view was challenged by Bowlby's (1980) work on childhood separation from the mother, which concluded that grieving is essentially similar for children and for adults. Bowlby identified three stages that children go through upon separation from their mothers: protest, then despair, and finally, detachment. "Children who suffer loss of mother show intense efforts to restore the bond and, when this proves unsuccessful, the attempts wane but do not entirely cease" (Bowlby, 1980, p. 181). Bowlby emphasized that once the stage of object constancy is reached, around three or four years, healthy adjustment can take place following loss of a mother if a child receives consistent care from another caregiver, and has opportunities to express feelings. (Krupnick and Solomon, 1987). "Feelings of loss and a longing for reconnection are normal aspects of mourning that continue throughout life, even after the period of acute grief passes" (Bowlby, 1980, p. 181). Even though children are capable of grief, according to Bowlby, grieving often is inhibited because children are too young to understand and process the loss, and they often are surrounded by denial and the silence of grief-stricken adults.

More recent theorists who have studied children's grief emphasize the child's developmental level (Christ, 2000). Recent research (Silverman and Worden, 1992; VanEerdewegh et al., 1982; Worden, 1996; Christ, 2000) on children who experience parental loss contends that most parentally bereaved children cope well, and do not show pathologic effects. Some researchers do allow the possibility that "children who appear well-adjusted in the short term may remain at risk for later emotional problems" (Siegel, Karus, and Raveis, 1996, p. 442). Siegel, Karus, and Raveis argue that the period of terminal illness is more traumatic for children than the bereavement period. Other authors have noted that bereaved children use coping skills such as denial, idealization of the dead parent, or identification with the deceased (Krupnick and Solomon, 1987).

In contrast to the major emphasis grief receives in the clinical literature on bereaved children, when asked about their grieving, our informants usually replied that it did not exist. According to the women, this resulted from, the general mistreatment they received from their stepmothers and fathers, which led to abuse or neglect. The daughter was cut off from the loving (deceased) mother and therefore

not allowed to properly mourn her. This supports the idea that secondary stresses can greatly impact bereaved children. For our respondents, the loss of the family and home was at least as devastating (if
not more) as was the loss of the mother.

Our findings suggest that children may not be ready for grieving
after the loss of their mothers, not because they do not have the capacity for grief, but because they are more worried about whether they
will survive. If children are not able to grieve until they feel secure,
the disruption in the family after mother's death may mean grieving
may not take place until many years after the death (Edelman, 1994;
Rando, 1984; Worden, 1996). Implications for these findings are discussed in Chapter 11.

Long-Term Impact

Women whose mothers died when they were children identified
the early loss of the mother as the single-most important event of their
lives. They uniformly felt that their lives would have been completely
different if the mother had lived, suggesting a tendency to idealize
their mothers and the relationships that they lost. Four themes are
identified in this period for this group: seeking information, delayed
grieving, mental health impact, and strong independent personality.

Seeking Information

A common theme among women whose mothers died when they
were children results from the extreme lack of information provided
them about their mothers' illness. As adults, they try to learn as much
as possible about their mothers' lives and illness (Nora, Carol). They
have a strong desire for information about their maternal roots (Edelman, 1994). This is especially true in families that did not openly discuss the mother (e.g., stepparent families where the stepmother did
not know the mother). Also, daughters whose contact with the mother's
family was curtailed after the death are unlikely to have much information. In adulthood, these women often engage in a search involving recovering the mother's medical records, and making contact
with her family or those who knew her when she was young. These
women also seek mementos of their mothers, such as clothing, jewelry, photographs, even recipes. If most of the mother's possessions

were discarded after her death, any item that remains is very precious to the daughters. (Bettina, Chapter 5, uses her mother's old dishes.)

Delayed Grieving

The women in our study were able to find support and to mourn their mothers only after they became adults. Carol did not allow herself to grieve until she was a young adult and had left home. ("One night I just had this horrible sense of missing my mother.") In therapy, she recognized her need to grieve for her mother. Many of these women were seeing therapists. In the course of therapy, they would recognize their need to explore their mothers' lives and deaths, and they would belatedly grieve. All women in this age group entered mental health professions, perhaps so that they could work indirectly on resolving their own early losses.

Mental Health Impact

Similar to the literature on childhood grief, the literature on the long term impact of parental loss is extensive. According to Freudian theory, because children are unable to grieve, they cannot come to a state of resolution. Therefore, libido is not available to invest in new relationships. On the basis of this theory, one would predict long-term problems in forming new relationships, and in investing in normal adult activities. While Bowlby's research suggests that although children above age three are capable of adultlike grief, they often do not grieve. In "Disordered Variants and Some Conditions Contributing" (1980), Bowlby identified specific problems in adult survivors, such as persistent anxiety, desire to die, persistent blame and guilt, compulsive self-reliance, and aggressive outbursts (Dilworth and Hildreth, 1998). A classic study (Brown, Harris, and Copeland, 1977) identified the loss of the mother before age seventeen as a key vulnerability factor for adult depression in women (with the highest rates in those who lose their mothers before age six). Studies of those with psychological problems in adulthood, especially depression in women, find higher rates of parental death than in normal populations. (Although these classic studies suggest a connection between early mother death and mental health problems, they do not prove any causal relationship.)

Common mental health problems among the women studied included insomnia, anxiety, depression, and low self-esteem. Carol, for example, has panic attacks and insomnia, especially at times of transition. Nora has had several bouts of depression. Marci also has severe insomnia, low self-esteem, and depression. The frequent identification of mental health problems does not prove a causal connection; however, it is consistent with theories and research on the long-term impact of maternal loss mentioned previously.

Strong, Independent Personality

Losing their mothers early and their own subsequent survival has led these women to feel strong and independent. Although they sometimes recognized that this may make close relationships difficult for them, they also take pride in this aspect of their personalities. Nora, for example, says, "I'm much more independent." Rita also takes pride in her strength and independence.

An important component in the long-term impact on young daughters whose mothers die may be found in feminist analysis of how young women develop connections. The conceptual frameworks developed by Chodorow (1999) and Gilligan (1982b) show how girls' attachment to and identification with their mothers contribute to an emerging sense of self. Women's approach to relationships evolves from the mother-daughter relationship. These theories emphasize the centrality of connectedness to women's lives. Although feminist literature has not studied maternal bereavement, one can speculate that the loss of a mother would leave a woman feeling disconnected, and might make the formation of close relationships difficult. The woman whose primary attachment figure became ill and died may fear abandonment in all subsequent relationships. The resulting lack of connectedness might result in the woman feeling different from other women, and could explain the ongoing yearning for a mother that many of the women in our sample experience. "For a daughter, the yearning for the mother continues throughout the life course, and the loss is frequently reactivated at transitional moments in life" (Edelman, 1994, p. 181).

SUMMARY

This chapter has identified themes that describe the experience of women who, as young children, lose their mothers to breast cancer (see Box 4.1). Three case studies (Rita, Carol, and Nora) were presented, and were supplemented in the analysis by additional cases. The themes identified for these youngest "breast cancer survivors" during the period of the mother's illness and treatment were lack of communication, am I still safe?, and independence. These young girls were aware that something was wrong, but were told very little about the mothers' illness. This created anxiety, and discouraged the children from inquiring or seeking reassurance. In addition, young daughters were particularly upset by separation from their mothers, and by changes in their routines. They were less upset by the symptoms of the disease and treatment than were older daughters. Lastly, the daughters spoke of an awareness of their mothers' attempts to make them more independent, something they may have recognized only after mother died. The period after the mother's death was traumatic for these daughters and involved major changes within the family situation. Most had to adjust to life in a stepfamily, with a stepmother and possibly new stepsiblings, a new home and a different, more conflictual relationship with father. They focused on their survival, a very basic need level, and did not grieve until much later. Many were numb. However, they were devastated by their mothers' loss, even if their strong demeanor did not show it. The long-term impact on these daughters includes a search for information about the mother, delayed grieving (often as a result of therapy for another problem), and strong and independent personalities as adults. Because of their young age at the time of their trauma, this group needs special attention in all of the phases: during the illness and treatments, after mother's death, and in the long term.

Implications from these findings are discussed in Chapter 11.

Chapter 5

Experience of Young Adolescent Daughters When Mothers Die from Breast Cancer

In this chapter, four cases are presented: Bettina, Kara, Cathy, and Gloria. All were young adolescents at the time of their mothers' deaths from breast cancer. In the discussion section following the case studies, themes relevant to each of three critical time periods are discussed.

CASE STUDY #1: BETTINA

Age at Her Mother's Breast Cancer Diagnosis: 9;
Age at Time of Her Mother's Death: 11

Background

Bettina was the oldest child and only girl in a family of four children. Her parents moved to a farm in New England when she was about four years old. While her father was busy with farmwork, which included raising pigs, her mother, who had a master's degree in home economics, managed the household and did the bookkeeping for the farm. There was a lot of work, in part because there was no hot running water in the home.

> She had a garden in the summertime, and she did housework kind of from scratch. My father took care of getting wood for the stove, but she did all the cooking, and she always had a little boy in diapers. I mean, she was busy.

Bettina was jealous of one of her younger brothers:

> I do remember once, being jealous when she took my brother for a walk, because I recognized that was something that she didn't do with me. Long after my mother died, my grandmother told me that that brother was my mother's favorite child.

Bettina's mother taught her to read well before she entered school, and later taught her arithmetic and French. "Now, she didn't teach me any housework skills whatsoever." Bettina thinks her mother was not happy.

> She wasn't a talkative person. We were not close at the time. My grandmother told me that it would have been better if she had taken us to a baby-sitter and gone to work, because she wasn't made to stay home. She wasn't happy being a housewife and just taking care of kids; that's for sure. Somehow, she thought that it was okay to cuddle babies, but beyond that, children weren't to be touched. She was of German background. I have a picture of her holding me when I was a baby, and it surprises me because she was looking like she enjoyed it, and she is giving me so much attention. I just accepted that my brothers got most of the attention because they were smaller. I look at that picture, and I'm startled to see her attention focused on me.

Bettina has only a few happy memories. Once her mother saved up orange juice labels and sent them away in exchange for a necklace that she gave to Bettina. "This was the only frivolous gift I remember my mother giving to me. I remember I was happy about it at the time, and my mother smiled because she was pleased that I liked this gift."

Bettina's mother had two sisters who lived far away. She did not have friends in New England, but Bettina's maternal grandmother was an important figure in Bettina's life.

Experience of Her Mother's Illness

When Bettina was nine, her family took her mother to the doctor. After the visit, her mother told them that she had an infected breast. "My mother talked about it in the car coming back. It wasn't hidden from me that way, you know." Life went back to normal, but several months later her mother was diagnosed with breast cancer and had a radical mastectomy. Bettina remembers her grandmother coming to stay with the children when her mother was in the hospital. One aspect of this she liked was that her grandmother was not as strict as her mother: "We were not [usually] allowed to watch very much television, only the news, and the Encyclopedia Britannica films that were shown very early in the morning. Grandma allowed more TV viewing. We could watch *The Lone Ranger* and *Zorro.*"

When her mother became ill, Bettina's relationship with her father changed.

> From right around that time, I started to become like an adult to my father. He [had] leaned on my mother to meet certain emotional needs, and so he started to lean on me. I was probably more informed than I needed to be about her progress because my father started treating me as some kind of substitute for her. There were things that he didn't tell me about, like financial difficulties and paying for her cancer treatment, which I'm glad he didn't.

After Bettina's mother came home from the hospital, the family was hopeful that she would recover. "I remember seeing my mother's mastectomy, and I guess I thought she was going to recover from it. I mean, we all did." The following spring,

> Mother was doing spring cleaning of my summer bedroom (four of us shared one bedroom during the winter) and her back went bad. The cancer ate away at a vertebra or something like that. She couldn't walk well after that, although there were some periods when she could walk with a back brace. Then one day she woke up and she couldn't get out of bed. And she was very angry at my father, not because of anything he did. I was nearby because I was needed to do things. My mother was talking to me that day about the difficulty she was having with my father, which was just due to the fact that all of a sudden she was a cripple and in terrible pain, you know, overnight. She was just taking it out on him. She was so angry. There were times when he was out of the bedroom because he couldn't do anything, but I was in the bedroom, because my mother wasn't angry at me [tearfully].

During the next few months, Bettina became a caregiver for her mother.

> One time I offered to read to my mother from the Bible, thinking that would make her feel better. That summer, I spent quite a bit of time in the bedroom. I was either sitting in the bedroom or I had to be somewhere in the downstairs of the house, so that she could ring a bell or call out to me. She would ask me to make a milk shake. (I had instructions on how to make them.) I'd make the milk shake and take it in to her. Then, not much later, she'd vomit the thing up. I mean, fill a plastic basin with vomit. And I'd carry it out. I don't know; it just seemed so futile to me.

Bettina also remembers that a public health nurse taught her to give her mother a back rub. While her mother was ill, Bettina's father took on much of the housework.

> It wasn't as if my father was failing to do things. I mean, he had several hundred pigs to take care of. And he was having to take on a lot of housework and cooking. He still talks about how happy he was that he took a course in college, something like "Cooking for Lumber Camp Management." It was a special course to teach men to cook. So he was able to take on the cooking and not be fazed by it.

At some point along the way, Bettina's mother had a hysterectomy. "I remember her saying that it just didn't bother her one bit, because relative to everything else, it was nothing to her." Eventually, her mother was placed in a nursing home.

> During the last few months, my mother's consciousness of the world around her was not good. She had metastases to the brain. The last time I saw her alive, she did not recognize us children. I'm not even sure she recognized my father. I remember him looking at her. I remember her looking at him. I think it was my grandmother who told me my mother was going to die [tearfully]. One morning, the woman who lived across the street came walking over. We didn't have a telephone, so I knew that the hospital must have called her and she was coming to tell my father [that she had died].

Experience Following Her Mother's Death

Bettina did not talk about her mother's funeral, but she did remember not wanting to go back to school after her mother died.

> I was very worried about returning to school after my mother's death. I thought I would be treated as an outcast, you know, as an oddball, by both students and teachers. There weren't any other children that I knew at that time who had lost a parent.

Bettina did not feel particularly sad after her mother's death.

> Maybe it had some sort of numbing effect on me, but I didn't feel much loss. I wasn't close to my mother. I didn't want her around before she got sick because I was just independent. I think she and I were too much alike to get along well at that age. And I'm relieved that she wasn't around when I was a teenager. I think we would have had a bad time together that way.

Reflecting on this lack of strong feeling, Bettina remembers how stoic her mother had been about her mastectomy.

> She did those reach-for-recovery exercises. She showed no emotion whatsoever about the loss of her breast. It makes me feel like I could go and have a breast off and wouldn't let myself be very upset about it.

In contrast, her father was very emotional after his wife died. "He cried and cried and cried. Some people cry easily, and he was inclined to cry at the dinner table." Bettina says her father was not able to help her with her grief, "I had to help him with his grief." Bettina's relationship with her father continued to be confusing. He continued to share his feelings with her. "This thing about my father confiding in me, that continued after she died. Like he asked my permission to join Parents Without Partners." On the other hand, she says,

> After my mother died, my father kind of dispensed with me at some level by saying, "I didn't have any sisters so I don't know what to do with you." He thought that the fact that he didn't have sisters relieved him of any responsibility for looking out for me.

Bettina's father started going to Parents Without Partners about a year after mother died, and began dating women he met there. When Bettina was twelve, her father remarried. "When he was going to marry her, after I got to know her a little bit, I was like, 'How could he marry somebody so different from my mother?'" When her stepmother moved into the home with her children, life became complicated for Bettina.

> She was drunk, and she didn't like me. We had a fight about something to do with religion. I wasn't her religion, or I wasn't religious enough. Well, this is as old as Cinderella. She beat me up. I had big welts and bruises on my back. I don't remember the pain, but I'm sure it hurt.

It especially hurt Bettina to see her stepmother pick on her little brothers, but she felt helpless to stop it.

> My stepmother turned to picking on my middle brother. I remember him crying after taking some kind of verbal abuse from her. My youngest brother was scared to death by the whole situation. At the dinner table, my stepmother would sit at my father's left, and my youngest brother would sit at my father's right. He would be practically trembling with fear. He would have been about six when my father remarried. And he was just speechless with fear at the dinner table.

Bettina's father continued to confide in her after his marriage.

> He just continued in that mode of giving me information about the development of his relationship with my stepmother, and I was somehow in no position to question it. My job was to listen to him. He said he was going to leave her, but he never did. I believed him when he told it to me, but somehow I never felt angry at him for not leaving her.

When Bettina was thirteen, her stepmother beat her in front of her father. He decided to send Bettina to live with an aunt.

> I was put on a bus and sent from New England to the Midwest. I had never ridden the bus before. It was like the big event of my life. It was a very big bus station, with many gates and levels. I didn't know I was supposed to move my suitcases from one bus to another, so they all got lost. I remember getting in line for one of the information counters, and the guy slammed the window closed when I got up to the counter. I didn't fall apart. I just got in another line. That experience had a great impact on me, and I think of it often.

Bettina lived with her aunt for two years.

> They made me do a lot of work. I washed, ironed, and did all kinds of heavy farmwork. I could never do enough work, because when I got everything else finished, I was sent down into this huge raspberry patch to pull crabgrass. It was just an exercise. There were so many mosquitoes that all I could do was stand and fight off the mosquitoes. I couldn't really get any work done. I wasn't allowed to have any time to play.

Conflict about religion posed problems between Bettina and her aunt. "She was a born-again Christian, and I never wanted to convert to my aunt's religion. I never came forward to be saved, and I think that was a problem for my aunt." Money also was an issue. "My father sent my aunt money for taking me. Some of the money was supposed to be for my clothes, but she may have spent some of the money because I didn't have very many outfits." Bettina remains bitter about her father's abandoning her. "He took no responsibility for seeing how this money was spent. He never called up long distance, and he never came out and visited."

Two years after moving to her aunt's home, Bettina returned to her family. At this point, she was fifteen years old. "I was very strong from working on the farm, and so I was no longer afraid of being beat up by my stepmother. I think she [Bettina's aunt] told me to write a letter to my father, saying that I had been bad or something, but I wrote to him saying I was ready to come back home. I outsmarted my aunt on this, somehow, and wound up back in New England." By this time, one of her stepsisters had moved out. Bettina worked hard to get the second stepsister out of the house.

> I knew I had to make that stepsister's life bad enough so she would go somewhere else. And I did. It was only a short time before she decided to move in with her father. I really don't remember what I did, but I felt completely justified in doing it.

However, living at home wasn't comfortable for Bettina, and she soon moved out, first to an alternative high school and then to a rented room.

Although Bettina was not able to protect her brothers from their stepmother, she did try to offer them support.

> I was a strong leader in their lives when they were small. I was somebody they looked up to. I was some antistepmother person there. I wasn't able to protect them from her, but . . . I was somebody. I was so numbed by everything that it's hard to say. I think of myself as being nurturing toward them. I helped them get through it. I couldn't do very much, because I wasn't even physically there, most of the time. But I played some positive role for them in living through that.

Once Bettina came home to visit her brothers when neither her father nor stepmother was home.

> I remember I made my brothers milk toast. I don't know if my youngest brother remembered my mother making that. There were no adults around that day. It was just the four of us kids sitting at the table. And he (youngest brother) started talking and he just chattered the whole meal. He just talked and talked. He was really happy. And he'd never talked like that [tearful].

Bettina helped her brothers leave home when they were teens, inviting one to stay with her when she was in college.

Long-Term Impact

One impact of losing her mother so young on Bettina was losing a guide to womanhood.

I just didn't learn how to behave as a woman. I was clueless on dealing with boyfriends. I wonder if my mother had lived, she may have helped me learn some dating skills, and maybe she would have helped me avoid marrying my ex-husband. You know, maybe she would have steered me away from that. That's what I see as the biggest impact on my life. I might have been more successful in marriage if I had help from her.

Lacking adult supervision in her late teens, Bettina learned to be very self-sufficient.

I didn't get into any real trouble, but I got into some dangerous situations. I did some hitchhiking, and I got into an incident I don't want to talk about. But I came out of it unscathed, and without the emotional trauma most other women would have suffered. I just came through. When I was seventeen, I got into a situation with some people in their twenties. They introduced me to marijuana, but I never took to it. It was just a social thing.

Bettina was able to salvage some pictures of her mother.

Now, there were a couple of photo albums. I don't think my father so much gave them to me as he kind of waved them around and I knew I had to grab them. There are photographs of my mother when she was a child.

Bettina now treasures the few items of her mother's that she has. Bettina did not have any of these things when she went to the Midwest.

There were a lot of things of hers that my stepmother disposed of while I was [away]. But, later in life, I was given a number of her things. Like every day I eat off of dishes that were the dishes of my parents' marriage. I have a few pieces of jewelry. They are very meaningful to me.

Although Bettina sees herself as very independent, she sometimes suffers from social unease and depression. She does not attribute these characteristics to her mother's death. She feels that these are characteristics of her family; her mother was the same way.

Risk

Bettina had her first cancer scare shortly after her mother's death. "My right nipple was developing, and I immediately went to my father and asked if it was cancer. And he said, 'No, I think it's just starting to grow.' So it [her mother's experience] has certainly made me afraid of cancer."

For some years, Bettina had regular clinical breast exams.

> I did regular breast self-exams when I was younger. I found a lump when I was twenty-six. I had a baseline mammogram on my own at age twenty-five, so when this happened, I had already had a baseline mammogram. This lump was neither biopsied nor removed but it went away after a few years. I found another lump after that, which was some big, tender cyst. I detected it myself. It was terrifying, because I was forty, a year younger than my mother [was when she was diagnosed]. They couldn't aspirate it, so I had that one biopsied. It was a benign fibroid. I was relieved. I was kind of surprised to be alive and free of cancer at age forty-two, when at this point my mother was crippled by metastases. As I approached and then passed the age at which Mother's cancer was diagnosed, I became a little more nonchalant about it. And at this point, I'm barely able to remember to do any breast self-examination. When I get to be forty-three, the age at which my mother died, or maybe when I get to forty-four, it's like, "What do I do?" I have this life that I didn't expect to have. You know, most people have trouble setting aside money for retirement, and it's still hard for me to believe that I'm ever going to retire and need to put money aside for that. I still have to figure out what this means. How do I get the most enjoyment out of my friends, my nieces and nephews, my brothers, my job? You know, it's just all uncharted territory.

Current Situation

Bettina was forty-two at the time of the study. She was divorced and lived alone. She worked as a computer programmer. She continues to maintain ties with her brothers, although they are not close. Her youngest brother has a family, and she tries to stay connected to him and her nieces and nephews.

Recently, Bettina has become more comfortable with her femininity.

> I'm a little better connected socially than when I was younger. I used to think that *Cosmopolitan* magazine was just some female nonsense, and then a few years ago I started reading it and thinking, you know, that this is a whole part of life that didn't happen to me because I didn't get connected to other women in that way.

CASE STUDY #2: KARA

Age at Her Mother's Breast Cancer Diagnosis: 9;
Age at Time of Her Mother's Death: 12

Background

Kara lived with her mother and father, both professionals, and older brother in a large, close African-American family. Kara's maternal aunt lived nearby, and her maternal grandmother was also close. Her father also had family in the area, as well as in the West Indies. Kara's parents had many close friends both in the area and in the Midwest. Kara was extremely close to her mother and very dependent upon her. She admired her mother for her beauty, for her cooking, and for being a wonderful mom. Her mother worked as a professional social worker.

Experience of Her Mother's Illness

Kara was nine at the time of her mother's diagnosis.

> My mother called my brother and I into the bedroom, and she told us that the doctor found a lump in her breast, and that she would have to go to the hospital to have it removed because otherwise it might make her very sick. She said they would have to be safe and they would be removing her breast. My mother was a very honest person. She was always explaining everything, and if I went to ask her a question, she would always tell me the truth. Like, she wouldn't sugarcoat anything. Now we're both looking at her like, "What are you talking about? What the hell are you talking about?" Even though she was describing everything and telling us what was going to happen, I remember not really knowing what to think. It was still confusing to me.

Kara went to visit her mother in the hospital but was not allowed to see her.

> They wouldn't let us up to see her, and I was so mad. I was so upset. I was crying. And then, when it was time for her to come home, she had to stay one day longer, and I remember that I was hysterical at home. I was sitting on my father's lap, and I was crying so hard, because I wanted her to come home, and I didn't understand why she wasn't coming home.

Kara remembers the recovery process after her mother came home.

> Her left breast was removed, and I remember looking at the crater in her chest. It was very strange. She was in lots of pain. I remember her doing exercises with her arm, just regaining movement. I went with her to get her prosthesis. She kept me very much a part of her whole experience. She wasn't hiding. She talked to me about her feelings.

Shortly thereafter, her mother returned to work and "everything was back to normal again." Kara remembers how her mother's prosthesis would "float all over the place"; the family would often laugh about this. Kara never talked with her friends about her mother's illness. "I think they knew my mother had cancer, and you know, we didn't talk about it."

When her mother's cancer was in remission she told Kara about menstruation.

> She had me put on a [sanitary napkin] and wear it. And I remember thinking that my brother and father would be able to see it. But she wanted me to wear it so that I would know what to do. She was preparing me.

She goes on to say,

> My mother had us making our lunches for school. I remember our friends, their mothers made their lunches. But my mother was preparing us all along. It was as if she knew, even before they told her. She was preparing us and we didn't even know it. I think that's one of the legacies she leaves behind. It's just amazing the things she was talking to us about, teaching us about, that most parents aren't doing at that age. She was preparing us for her to leave. She did it with grace, and she wasn't upset. She never let us see that. I mean, there was incredible bravery and endurance. It's just one of those incredible things that women do.

About three years later, when Kara was twelve, her grandmother had a stroke and died. Shortly after that, her mother began to have pain in her leg.

> She went back to the doctor and that's when they said that the cancer had come back and that it was terminal. They told her she was going to die, and she would not tell us. She would not tell [Kara's brother] and myself. She would not tell us, and wouldn't allow anyone else to tell us. My mother never let on that she was going to be leaving me.

Kara remembers that her mother was cold all the time.

> When she would get off from work, she'd come in and get in bed. She had an electric blanket, she had electric gloves. She was always cold. Always trying to keep herself cozy. I didn't understand that this was connected to the cancer.

Her mother went into the hospital again, and when she came home, moved into a separate bedroom.

> She bought herself this beautiful antique bed (she loved antique furniture). She placed the bed where she could look out. I knew she was sick, but I still wasn't understanding what cancer was. But what did cross my mind was, "Do mommies die?" I didn't ever have this discussion with anybody, but I thought, *No, it doesn't happen. I don't know anybody that it happened to, I've never seen anything like that on TV, so mommies must not die. So she's not gonna die. She's just ill and she'll get better like she did before.*

Kara began to notice physical changes in her mother. "It was scary. It was just eerie watching her lose a lot of weight and be very ill." Chemotherapy began and

> it started making her hair fall out. That was very difficult. Her hair was thinning, and her lip was hanging. She lost movement on her left side. She had always been very shapely, very pretty. She always dressed well—she was very beautiful.

During this period, Kara spent a lot of time in her mother's room, talking, bringing tea, sitting on her bed, and drawing her pictures. "I was up underneath my mother most of the time."

That summer, Kara's brother went to sleepaway camp, and Kara was sent to stay with family members in the Midwest where she had previously spent the summer. She went home briefly to visit to her mother, and was shocked to see how she had deteriorated.

> Her left eye was closed, she didn't have any hair, and she was maybe eighty to ninety pounds. People kept visiting her, but she just kept looking at me. Like everybody's talking to her, and she's turning her head and looking at me. It made me feel very uncomfortable. I was like, "Why is she looking at me? Do I have on makeup?" I remember feeling really eerie and strange.

Back in the Midwest, Kara was relieved to be away from the stress at home.

I was happy to be away because I think all along I was just very stressed and everyone was moving me around because they were stressed. I was away and playing with my friends. I drew pictures for her every day, and I sent her cards. I missed her. One day my aunt said to me, "Your mother is taking a turn for the worse,.and we're going home." I didn't understand what that meant, and I left in a daze. The next morning, we drove back home, a seven-hour drive.

This time, Kara was even more distressed when she saw her mother in the hospital.

My mother just kept looking at me, and she looked worse than she did the last time. It was frightening, and I hated the hospital. My mother was just a very beautiful woman. Now, she was so little. She was just like a skeleton. To look at her just deteriorating, I just didn't know what to make of it.

Two days later, Kara's mother died in the hospital. Kara was at home, watching one of her favorite programs on television, when she heard her aunt calling her name.

I was just annoyed that she was interrupting *The Smurfs.* When I came upstairs, she hugged me so hard, I couldn't breathe! She said, "Oh, baby, your mother has passed." I was like, *What the heck is she talking about? Passed? Passed where?* I didn't know what she was saying to me. She said it three times, slowly, and then I understood. Then she walked me into my father's room. My father was sitting on the bed and he put his arms around me. I think my father began to cry. I'm still not sure what to make of all this. I'm just kind of sitting there, like in shock. After that, everything is a blur.

Kara has very little memory of what happened next. "I don't even remember. I was in a daze." At her mother's funeral, Kara sat with her brother and maternal aunt, who had been picked up at camp by a family friend. "I remember I was cool as long as I was holding her [aunt]. People were coming up and saying all types of shit to me and I was like, 'Well, whatever.'" When the pallbearers were carrying the casket out of the church, Kara's aunt began to scream, "Get me out of here! Get me out of here!"

Then I lost it 'cause I didn't know what to do. I was crying and she was holding me. After that, I was just in a daze. You know, you're walking down the church and everybody's looking at you. Then we were in the limousine, and people kept sticking their heads in and saying some mess. I didn't know what was going on.

That night, the family came back to Kara's house. She remembers that various friends and family members offered to have her live with them.

> I was like, "Who are you talking about? You aren't talking about me, because I'm not going anywhere. I am staying right in my house!" I guess my father wouldn't let them take me. Mind you, I didn't have much of a relationship with my dad. I was underneath my mother most of the time, and she took care of most of our basic needs. So all of a sudden, we were all looking at each other like, "Okay, now what are we gonna do? How are we going to make it through? What are we going to do without our mother?"

Experience Following Her Mother's Death

The period after Kara's mother died is vague.

> I remember feeling a little strange going back to school. I got cards, and everybody was real nice to me and everything. But really, I was in shock for three years. And I was kind of numb. I didn't start mourning until four years after she died 'cause I just didn't know what to make of any of this. I just kind of went into survival mode.

Kara's father assumed what had been her mother's role: "He would come home and [he] did exactly what my mother did, you know. He would come home, take his [work] clothes off and cook dinner for us." To her surprise, Kara's father knew how to cook.

Kara's aunt also became a substitute mother for her. " I'm thankful that my aunt [mother's sister] is still living, because she became my mother, really." Kara went each summer to spend time with different family members or friends.

> After that, I just kind of went all over the place. I think people started moving me around because they didn't know what to do with me. I had lots of great experiences, a lot of exposure to lots of different things.

Kara's father began to date about six months after her mother's death.

> He dated about four women before he dated [her stepmother]. And I was real clear that there is no other mother [for me]. Any woman he would date, I made it very clear that, "Your biggest mistake is gonna be coming in here trying to talk to me like you're my mother. My mother is dead. I had one. That's it." I was a hard child. Not too many of them wanted to mess with me. He started dating and then he got married

and that was very difficult on all of us. It was just very difficult for me to think about my father marrying somebody else."

Kara's new stepmother was someone she and her mother had known. Kara can even remember hearing her cry at her mother's funeral. When her stepmother had a baby girl, Kara's hostility softened. "I'm so glad my new sister is here. That was very helpful in our healing process. It is still very painful for me, and we are still healing." Kara said this during the interview, about fifteen years after her mother's death.

Kara feels that her mother's death, and his new marriage, changed her father.

He was cool. He's very intelligent, very aggressive, and very driven. But I didn't really know him. I didn't spend a lot of time with him. But what I do know is that he has grown tremendously since my mother died. He was not very expressive. He was emotionally detached, or didn't know how to express his emotional side. He could communicate intellectually but just not with his feelings. I always knew that my father loved me [because] he would spend time with me, and he would always tell his friends how proud he was of me. But it's not like he would run around telling me "I love you." After her death, he began to do that. He became a different man. He got a second chance and he started doing things very differently. He has another daughter, and he is much more involved with her than he was in my brother and my lives, prior to my mother's death.

Kara is also now aware that she was extremely angry when her mother died. "I was very angry, but it took me almost ten years to realize how angry I was, because I felt like she left me." Kara directed her anger at God.

My mother dying probably screwed up my faith. When she died, people were telling me that God took her to a better place. And I really didn't understand that. What better place could there be than right here with me? I was very angry. I was angry with God. I think I'm a spiritual person, but it's just very hard for me to conceptualize a God who could take someone's mother away from them. I've just been angry about that for many years. That whole experience has really screwed me up. I've never really had a place to put my anger. I haven't figured this out, and I have talked to lots of people from lots of different denominations, but no one could tell me why people die of AIDS, why people are dying of cancer, why innocent people get slain in cold blood. You know, like, explain it to me!

Long-Term Impact

When Kara finished college, she experienced some depression and sought counseling.

> The woman that I went to see reminded me of my mother. She even had the same name as my mother. I went to see her, and I just sat in her office and started to cry. She asked me why did I want to come to talk to her. I just cried. I think I just needed to cry. And I talked with her. It was good for me.

After the counseling, Kara began to talk with her brother about their mother's death.

> My brother and I didn't talk very much about what we were experiencing until a few years ago. We always talked about her, like, "Oh, Mom used to do that," thinking about things that were pleasant. We didn't talk about pain. This time, I asked him what was he thinking. And his response was, "When Mom died, I kind of looked at it like this: I had more time with Mom, so I was luckier [than you]. I was worried about you, because you had less time with her." I remember looking at him, thinking, *It must be such a burden to be worrying about me.*

Kara and her brother talked about the family friend who had picked him up at camp after their mother died, and realized how difficult this must have been for the friend. "My brother later went to his office to thank him. And they cried about it again, you know, years later. They are still close today."

The first anniversary of her mother's death was extremely difficult for Kara. She has actively mourned her mother, starting with visits and long talks with her mother at her grave. "I have many pictures of my mother all around, and I usually am very candid about talking about her, but it's taken a lot of years to be able to do that." Kara now realizes that she has a hard time around the anniversary of her mother's death and birthday. "I am usually real pissy, and it isn't until I look at the calendar that I realize why. I will usually talk with [her aunt], and we will say happy birthday to my mom and talk about her around those dates." Kara has learned to focus on the positives.

> It was a very traumatizing time, but I am very fortunate also to have had her in my life and to have had the love and lessons of an extraordinary woman. I'm thankful for that. I am blessed to have had her. There were so many things that she shared with me. She gave me so much in so little time.

Reflecting on how her mother's death affected her, Kara says,

It will affect the rest of my life. It affects me every day, because I think about her. I realize how cancer just changed my life forever. It destroyed some things that were there, but it also made me grow up a lot faster. I had a lot more responsibility.

Risk

Kara is very fearful about getting cancer herself. She had her first scare when she was only fourteen, two years after her mother's death. "I remember I was so afraid. I thought to myself, *I'm going to die! Because this happened to my mother, this is going to happen to me.*" Fortunately, the lump went down after Kara was given an antibiotic. Her fear was again heightened when her mother's first cousin died of breast cancer.

Kara is aware that genetics might be involved, but she also thinks her mother's smoking could have contributed. Kara resents the fact that every time she visits a new doctor, he or she lectures her about her risk, even though she is not yet thirty and is too young for mammograms. She does regular breast self-exams, but does not feel confident that she can tell the difference between normal tissue and a dangerous lump. Recently, she took a "risk for breast cancer" quiz and learned that if she didn't have children before age thirty, she would have an even higher risk. "I didn't realize that not having had children by thirty was another risk factor. I realized that I needed to have a baby, not at thirty, but I needed to push one out before then."

Kara also tries to reduce her risk by watching her diet ("I just lost fifty pounds"), although she is not sure that this necessarily prevents cancer.

I have an uncle who got colon cancer. He was telling me how my aunt made him eat broccoli because it had cancer-fighting nutrients. He was so angry when he got cancer anyway. And I'm thinking, *Wow, sometimes that doesn't even make a difference.*

Although Kara is now actively trying to prevent or detect breast cancer early, this was not always the case. When she was a teenager, she started smoking.

> I remember part of those destructive years, I smoked cigarettes. I didn't care. My father and I got into a big fight about that. He said, "These are death sticks, Kara. Why would you do this?" And I was like, "Why? I don't care. I figure I'm gonna die anyway. I'm gonna die of this cancer." That was not rational. I was a teenager. But I stopped smoking.

Kara expressed interest in genetic testing, and discussed this with her uncle, who is a surgeon. After the interviews, she sought out genetic counseling. She told us this turned out to be a "waste of my money." The genetic counselor told her no pattern of cancer existed in her family. Kara was upset that the counselor was not alarmed by the cancer in her family, especially by her mother's early death.

Current Situation

Kara was twenty-seven at time of interview. She decided to become a social worker, her mother's profession, and had recently completed her master's degree. When completing our questionnaire, Kara said that she misses her mother at important life events and is still angry that she's gone. She wonders if she will ever be able to get past this anger. She says she is superindependent and is sometimes depressed. She agrees that her mother's death changed her outlook on life. However, she does not feel isolated or alone; she does not have difficulty with intimate relationships ("My mother taught me intimacy and the importance of being loved and loving people"); and she does not suffer from low self-esteem or separation anxiety. Kara was recently married and hopes to become pregnant soon.

CASE STUDY #3: CATHY

Age at Her Mother's Breast Cancer Diagnosis: 5;
Age at Time of Her Mother's Death: 13

Background

Cathy is the youngest child in a Jewish family with three children. Her mother stayed home to care for the children after retiring from her job as an elementary school teacher. "We had a close family. Mother was just unconditional love. She was very focused on my life and building my self-esteem. I would tell her everything. We had a very, very good relationship."

Experience of Her Mother's Illness

When Cathy was five, her mother went into the hospital. She knew her mother was sick, but didn't think too much about it. Later she learned that her mother had a mastectomy and that the doctor had told her father that the cancer had spread to the lymph nodes. Cathy's mother was not told this. Cathy assumed that her mother was better. Her mother did tell her about the cancer but not until much later. Cathy remembers that, "The way she described it to me, it was like she had one [abnormal] cell, and they took it out, and she was all better." She goes on to say, "I had a normal upbringing. It was not like I had a sick mother or anything."

When Cathy was in the sixth grade, her mother began to have trouble with her eyes. When she came back from the doctor's office, Cathy's mother told her that the cancer had spread to her eyes, and that she needed chemotherapy. Cathy sensed the seriousness of this talk. "She tried to prepare me. She told me many things. I went upstairs and I remember I wrote them down." One of the things her mother told her was that

> if she dies, that I should want my father to remarry. That the person he remarries would not be my mother in any way, but would be a friend to me. That that's something I should welcome because it would make my father happy, and I needed to remember that.

Cathy's mother also told her that she'd always love her.

Cathy was concerned that she needed to remember everything that was happening because her time with her mother was limited.

> I was terribly aware of the fact that I was young and that I would not remember everything. I was trying to take mental notes all of the time. I was writing in my journal. I thought, *This is the last time I'm going to have my mother and I'm very young. I'm going to look back the rest of my life and will want to remember so many things.*

Because of this sense of impending loss, Cathy was not completely unhappy when she was injured in an automobile accident and had to stay at home for six months. "I look back on that time and I think that in a way I was lucky because I got that much time [with her mother]."

Cathy feels that her adolescent way of treating situations, which she now describes as "selfish," was inappropriate when her mother was so ill. At one point, she was upset about having a blemish on her face and then thought, "*Wow. I have a zit on my cheek. That's so terrible. But my mother has no hair!* It made worrying about the little things seem very trivial."

During the following two years, the cancer spread to her mother's lungs, bones, and liver.

> It is very difficult to see someone you love suffer. I knew what she was going through. It was terrible. We had some situations that I'll never forget between us in that time that she was dying. What was physically happening to her—her hair falling out, watching her cry, watching her suffer. It was horrible.

Cathy has vivid memories of this period. "There are some things that she went through toward the end which I don't want to share out of respect for her."

Cathy's mother tried to prepare her for her death by telling her that the most difficult thing she would have to face was that "No matter where I looked on Earth, I would never be able to find her. I wouldn't be able to make her feel better by stroking her face. That losing somebody physically would be very difficult, and she was right." After her mother died, Cathy felt relief. She recalls thinking, "Thank God she's not in pain anymore."

Experience Following Her Mother's Death

Cathy describes the period after her mother died as follows: "My father was wonderful. I could confide in him. He never stifled me. He let me talk about my mother as much as I wanted." In reflecting on this period, Cathy now feels guilty that she did not do more to help her father.

> One of the things my mother told me before she died was, "I don't want you to become a replacement mother when I leave. I don't want you to be doing all the wash and the cooking and taking over this role. You're a teenager and you should be doing teenager things."

After her mother's death, Cathy never volunteered to help her father as he struggled to learn to cook, clean, and do laundry. "I didn't lift a finger. He would come home after commuting an hour and a half, and

I would not have made dinner." Cathy later apologized to her father for her behavior, but he was not angry. "He's very easygoing. He never laid any guilt on me for not helping him."

Cathy felt isolated from other children her age after her mother died; she yearned to have others with whom she could share her experience. "I wanted to talk about it with other kids, and there were no other kids whose parents were dying or had died." Cathy's father tried to convince her to get counseling.

> I mean, he tried so hard, but I ran screaming from the counselor's office. He knew that I was in need of some kind of help, but I couldn't handle it. I'm not against counseling, but it brings out too many [things]. . . . I probably can't go to counseling without crying. It's very difficult to talk about this stuff without losing one's cool. All those memories just come rushing out, and I don't want that. I guess it gave me a sense of losing control. I actually felt that there was a stigma attached to it, because none of my friends went to counseling.

Cathy's aunt attempted to become closer to her after her mother's death, but Cathy pushed her away. "I wasn't very close with her [before], and I rejected the idea of having her get close to me just because my mother died."

When Cathy started menstruating, she made an arrangement with her best friend. The friend would ask her mother any questions Cathy had, pretending they were her own questions. Then, she would pass the answers on to Cathy. It was difficult for Cathy to watch her own breasts develop. "My breasts were just developing at the time, and I'm thinking about breast cancer. It was a strange time—adolescence—because my body was developing and I was just looking at the grim aspect of it."

Cathy channeled her energy into school. She got the best grades she ever had, joined every extracurricular activity, and became captain of the cheerleading squad. She was trying not to be home alone after school. When she did come home after school, she would binge. "I would eat and eat and eat. I was probably eating to satisfy the need of comfort of having my mother at home, because I had never binged like that before in my life."

Cathy's father remarried eight years later, when Cathy was in college. She is grateful that this happened after she moved out of the home, because she does not like her stepmother. She describes how her stepmother wanted a close relationship with her. She began to send her care packages at college and tried to talk with her about sex. Cathy rejected what she perceived as forced intimacy, but she tried to respect her mother's wishes and accept her stepmother. Eventually, the strain of acting as if she liked her stepmother was just too much, and Cathy told her father that she didn't want to have anything to do with her. She did, however, want to stay close to her father. Given all of this conflict, Cathy is grateful to her father that he did not remarry until she had left home. "It would have been horrendous because then there's no way out. At least I could get in my car and go back to college. But if I had to live there, that would have been terrible."

Long-Term Impact

Cathy says,

> I have a wealth of problems in my life as a result of losing my mother. I can't think of anything positive that happened from my mother's death. It just kind of ruined my life. That probably sounds very melodramatic, but it just definitely killed part of my life which will never be the same.

One area in which Cathy has special problems is intimate relationships. She fears the potential pain should a relationship end. "When I'm getting out of a relationship with a man, it really throws me into quite a depression. It is almost like experiencing a death. I don't think it's like that for other people." Because of her fear of the pain of loss, Cathy holds back from getting into relationships. Cathy also has trouble with sexual relationships, because she finds herself thinking, "The breast is such a sexual organ. If I'm with a man, and I get compliments on my breasts, the first thing I think about is, *Will he still love me if I don't have them?*"

Even common separations, such as when she returns home after visits to her brothers, are very difficult for Cathy. She anticipates the pain of losing her father, feeling that her mother's death will make future losses even harder.

Risk

Cathy worries about her risk for breast cancer.

> I'm approaching thirty and my mother was diagnosed when she was in her thirties. I try to be vigilant with my eating habits, eating fruits and

vegetables, and I don't drink any alcohol and I try to exercise. But sometimes I get lax about my exercise, or I'll eat more fats than I should and more artificial colors, which I know are carcinogenic.

Cathy has trouble doing breast self-examinations.

I do them, but you would think that I would do it every month, but there must be some psychological reason why I'm not. But I just can't. I guess I sometimes get discouraged 'cause I feel like I don't know if, when I feel a lump, if it's a cyst or not, and the process makes me a little bit nervous. But I do it, but just not the way that you should.

Cathy has a physician do a clinical breast exam two to three times a year.

It's kind of contradictory, that somebody's scared to do a breast exam, which everyone knows is the first line of defense against this. This is the number-one thing I can do for myself, and yet I drop the ball way too often. I'm not exactly sure why, but I'm trying to be better about it [laughs].

Cathy found a lump several years ago. "I have fibrocystic breasts and I had quite a scare about four years ago, because I found a lump and I was terrified." She was in graduate school at the time, and the clinician at her university recommended that she see a surgeon immediately, because of her mother's history.

Thankfully, I called my father, and he said, "You should come home right away. We can take you in for a sonogram." So I did and it was a pretty easy procedure. They told me that it was a cyst. It was non-invasive. Had I gone to a surgeon to have it removed, it would have just been terrible and I'm sure it would have conjured up these terrible images in my mind.

Cathy has seriously considered having genetic testing.

I would like to know if I have the gene or not, not that I would have a radical mastectomy or anything, but I would be more vigilant. I recently went to find out about genetic testing, and when the oncologist was doing my family tree, she made me aware of the fact that there was a great deal of information that I just don't have. I don't have much of a genetic tree to look at in terms of breast cancer, because I don't have sisters and my mother didn't have sisters. My mother's mother's sister had breast cancer, so that is one link, I guess. I felt very strongly that I want to know. I definitely want to know. But I went into counseling and they did a great job. After hearing more about it, I wasn't so sure whether I wanted to get the test. It seems that the information I want isn't available yet. Then, there's the issue of locating my mother's tissue. They'll know a little more in a few years, so I figured I would wait and then get tested. Even though I want to know personally for me, I'm having a hard time understanding what I would do in terms of insurance. That's really worrisome for me because I want to know, because I feel like the more information I have, the better my quality of life will be. But I can imagine that the quality of my life would be significantly diminished if I couldn't get insurance. I'm also worried emotionally how I would deal with that, how it would affect my life if I have that gene. I figure that, like dealing with her illness, knowing in advance and working through things was better than not knowing. I have to wait and see, but I suspect that I would be someone who would go for the genetic testing in a few years. I'm not sure.

Current Situation

At the time of the study, Cathy was twenty-eight and had a job teaching at a university. She was single. The family still experiences ramifications of her mother's death and father's later remarriage. For example, when Cathy and her father get together, her stepmother does not come. She feels hurt by Cathy's rejection. Also, when her brothers had children, Cathy got upset because her stepmother wanted the children to call her their "grandmother." Cathy insisted that they not do so, and she prevailed. She has tried to convince her father to agree to be buried beside her mother instead of her stepmother. When her father refused, Cathy yelled angrily at him, "I hope I die first! Then you can bury me next to Mom so she won't be alone."

CASE STUDY #4: GLORIA

Age at Her Mother's Breast Cancer Diagnosis: 13; Age at Time of Her Mother's Death: 14

Background

Gloria is the third of four children in a middle-class African-American family. She has an older brother and sister, and a younger brother. Her parents had to overcome many racial barriers. Her father was one of the first black detectives on the police force of a large city. Her mother started a day care center, then while her children were small got her PhD and became the principal of a school. The children went to parochial schools, and both parents had high expectations for them. Mother hoped that Gloria would be an opera singer. Gloria's father was not nearly as involved with his children as was her mother. "He had a very busy schedule. And he was a womanizer, really. He opted to have this family but he really kind of, like, took us for granted. The majority of time he wasn't around." Gloria also felt that her father may have been an alcoholic, as well as abusive to her mother. "Now, women [in her position] would leave. She was making good money. She could have left him. But it wasn't the thing to do, you know, in the mid-1960s. You just didn't do that with four kids."

Gloria had a large extended family, who all lived in the same large brownstone home. Her paternal grandmother and great aunt were especially active in helping to raise the children. But it was her mother who was the peacemaker.

> Being a principal and a teacher, she was very soothing. If my sister had booster practice, and my brother had a swim meet, she just knew how to get all of us in her car and disseminate us to different places without everybody, you know, cutting each other's throats.

Gloria's relationship with her mother was "very warm and loving." She describes mother as "almost like my best friend," and talks about how she

> did not want to separate. I mean, most kids don't even want to be seen with their mother, but when I think back on it, all of us wanted to do everything with our mother. We always wanted to be, like, solo. . . . It was like you could just never get [enough]. She was just one of those kind of people where you just wanted to be around her all the time.

Experience of Her Mother's Illness

Gloria first remembers her mother being ill about a year before her death. She thought this was due to sciatica; her mother had been seeing a chiropractor for the condition. The following summer, her mother became very ill, but no one told Gloria anything about it. "She kept going back and forth to the hospital. I believe I overheard my grandmother speaking to another relative saying that it was the breast." It wasn't until after her mother's death, when her sister saw the death certificate, that Gloria learned that her mother had breast cancer.

Gloria can't understand why it took so long to diagnose her mother's cancer.

> We had some of the best hospitals in the city. My mother had very good insurance. I just wish it had been detected [earlier]. I mean, coming from an educated family . . . I don't know if it was because of my mother's busy schedule and raising four kids, or if it was just one of those things that you just didn't talk about. It just amazes me.

In August, after Gloria's thirteenth birthday, her maternal grandmother came up from her home to help care for the children. She remembers that her aunt had to alter her school uniforms because her mother was in the hospital and school was about to start. Her aunt gave her permission to cut her hair. "I was starting my freshman year of high school." When she went to visit her mother in the hospital, Gloria wore makeup so she would look old enough to visit. When her mother saw her, she started crying, saying, "She's all grown up." Another time, Gloria's older sorority sisters from high school signed her in, while she sneaked up the hospital stairs.

Gloria knows little about her mother's treatment.

> I don't ever recall knowing if she had a mastectomy even. I think it was too far gone when they finally did admit her to the hospital. They immediately started giving her, I think, radiation therapy. I don't know back then if they had chemo or not. But I believe she had radiation therapy because her skin was real dark.

Gloria saw

> old glass jars that sat on the floor. There was a whole lot of mucus. I don't know if it was in the lungs or what. But it was one of those old green jars with the little machine going.

Gloria also remembers seeing her mother deteriorate.

> I mean, my mother was like five feet, and she probably weighed about a hundred thirty-five pounds. She was plump, and you know, she had a head full of hair. I just remember my mother dwindling to nothing. And losing all this hair.

On her mother's birthday, Gloria went to the hospital with a cake. She was told that her mother had fallen into a coma. "It just seemed like it just went on and on and on. That [next] Thursday, my cousin sent me up there, and just seeing her lying there, just so fragile, with patches of her hair missing." Even then, Gloria did not realize that her mother was dying. "Nobody was giving me straight answers, especially those grandmothers. They aren't gonna tell you anything. 'Child, mind your business!' Something like that." Gloria thought that her mother would be coming home.

> They said they were letting her come home for some reason or another. So I thought maybe, you know, [like with a sick plant] you poured some water on it and it bloomed today whereas yesterday, it looked, you know, [terrible]. Because they were letting her come home, there was this great belief that she was gonna be okay.

The following Sunday morning, Gloria's mother died. The next morning, Gloria remembers coming downstairs in her pajamas, "thinking she was gonna come home and all these flowers [were] in the kitchen, and my two grandmothers, just, you know. And we ran into the bedroom and there was my mommy [mother's body]." Gloria had a good friend whose mother had died suddenly of spinal meningitis the previous spring.

> I took off in my pajamas. My girlfriend lived about eight to ten blocks away. I ran in the rain with no shoes to [my friend's house]. I couldn't wait for the elevator to come and I ran up the stairs. When she opened the door, I remember boo-hooing and saying, "I'm just like you. I'm just like you." You know, it was devastating. It was devastating.

Experience Following Her Mother's Death

Gloria attended two funerals for her mother—one held locally and one later at her maternal family's home in the South, where her mother was buried. The first was "packed with teachers from all different nationalities" and because "my mother's father has a lot of people [family]," many attended the second funeral as well. Gloria describes it as draining. "It just went on and on. You know, masses and masses of people. And to be in your forties and die back then, and then what was so sad, to leave four children."

After her mother's death, Gloria no longer enjoyed being at home.

> I hated to come home. I used to join everything [at school] so I wouldn't have to come home. The house just seemed so different. You knew she was never coming home. It was just something very hard to comprehend at thirteen. Very hard.

Gloria's paternal grandmother cared for the children. "It's a blessing that his mother lived nearby, because I believe that if she wasn't there to hold us together, we probably would have gone into foster care." However, Gloria's grandmother was "quite different [from my mother]. She was much sterner. They [father's family] were just sort of like real stern. Not southern. They had the rough edges of [the big city]. My mother's family was a lot more loving and caring and close-knit." Her father's drinking got worse.

> I really think that all of us lost a lot. 'Cause we never really were rooted in my dad anyway. It was basically my mother. My father always had an alcohol problem, but it increased. I think my father buried his sorrows in alcohol. I think he took my mother for granted a lot and he probably had a lot of pain and anguish with that, and being left with these four kids to raise.

Gloria had two close friends in high school—one was the young girl who had also lost her mother. These friends were her main source of support. Her other friend's mother "became like my second mother too." She also had a strong group of friends through the black student union; many of these girls attended her mother's funeral.

Without their mother to hold the family together, the children began to leave. "We all sort of went in different directions. My mother just expected so much of us and wanted so much for us, and after she passed away we just kind of gave up." Gloria's older brother was the first to leave.

> My older brother, he was very rebellious. My mother was the mediator between him and my dad. So after my mother died, my brother was having a really rough time. His report card went terrible. We were really close, and I remember him telling me that he was running away. "Yeah, cause Daddy and I will never make it. He threatened to kill me." He ran down here to my mother's people.

Gloria's older sister finished high school that year, and started college, where she "met a guy and ended up marrying him at a young age" (nineteen). Shortly after that, Gloria also left home.

> I didn't get along with my father. He was drinking and he was bringing women over, and they were nothing like my mother. I didn't want any part of it. I ran away and went to live with my sister. Her address was secret [from my father] because he was belligerent. I lived with my sister my senior year of high school. My grandmother's congregation got the money up for me and paid my tuition that year.

After graduating from high school, Gloria moved to the city where her mother's family lived. Here she started college but soon dropped out. Her uncle encouraged her to take up a degree in X-ray technology, which she completed successfully. When their paternal grandmother died three years after their mother's death, Gloria's younger brother left home, and he too went to live with his mother's family. "After I left, my younger brother came down here and my aunt [mother's sister], she raised him."

Although the children no longer lived together, they stayed close, and Gloria's older sister began to take on some of her mother's roles.

> She took the mothering role. I think we all kind of, like, owe her stuff. My brother spoils her and sends her music now. She had to grow up fast. I started her with a teddy bear collection about ten years ago, because she had to grow up so fast—she never got a chance to really, like, be a kid.

Gloria met the man she would marry several years later when she was fifteen. She now regrets marrying so young. "I didn't give myself time to work, or get a new car. None of those things. It was just like, 'Hurry up and get married.' He was like my knight in shining armor."

Long-Term Impact

Gloria and her brothers and sister often speculate on how different life would have been if their mother had lived.

> We talk about how nice it would have been for her to be here to see this and that, and how our lives would have taken different turns. I think we would have been doing other things. My mother always believed that each generation should have been better [than the previous one]. [Had she lived], I think we would have excelled. She wanted me to be an opera singer. I didn't do that. I didn't have the gumption.

The children's career choices illustrate their mother's impact. Her older sister is a teacher (in their mother's field), and her older brother now owns a business that was named for their mother. Gloria's career eventually led her into mammography: "I do it with zest. I do it with all my heart. I'm like a breast detective. I do it as a memorial to my mother." She feels she has a special obligation to detect breast cancer early in African-American women.

Gloria feels that her mother's death led her to a different philosophy of life.

> I live each day at a time. I give as much love as I can. I don't think it made me bitter or anything like that. It made me live each day to the fullest. I mean, we just take so much for granted. I don't like to deal with a whole lot of aggravation. I used to be really a people person, and I had to learn to take some time for me. Now I do what makes Gloria happy. I mean, I'm just living life. You can't go back. You can only do the best that you can do for now. Sometimes you think about it and you only get depressed.

Gloria is no longer married, and she attributes her failed marriage to her mother's early death.

> I was in a troubled marriage, and my sister has been married for twenty-five years and she's in a troubled marriage. My sister and my best friend and I talk about that all the time. I think my mother's death left many scars on all of us because I think it led to us picking the wrong men. You know, wanting to be taken care of so early and losing our aspirations. You know, we married these big men that we thought were gonna save us from the world, and they [turned out to be] insensitive. They were not family oriented. My mother went through the same thing with my dad.

Gloria finds herself getting sad around the anniversary of her mother's death.

> In the fall, I hate to see the leaves fall. She died October fifth, so it's real emotional around that time. Last year, I did Race for the Cure [charity event], and it was real [deep breath] momentous, because it was on the twenty-seventh anniversary [of her death].

Risk

Gloria found a lump in her breast when she was only seventeen.

> I kept, like, willing myself to die. It just got bigger and bigger and bigger. It was almost the size of a cherry tomato, or almost the size of an egg, when I think about it. It was the craziest thing. I was being a martyr, like wanting to die. I didn't want to tell anybody.

Eventually (about a year after finding the lump) she had surgery, and the lump was diagnosed as a benign fibro adenoma. She has had two other lumps removed; both were benign. When asked about breast self-exams, Gloria says she does them "monthly . . . weekly, daily sometimes. It's like constant. I mean, I do this for a living."

Because her mother neither smoked nor drank, Gloria attributes her breast cancer to marital problems. "He [father] was abusive to my mother and, looking at it now, they say that blows and things can cause reactions within your bloodstream and cause you to have cancer. I mean, even stress."

She has thought about taking tamoxifen as a preventative, but decided against it. "More and more I thought about the side effects, and the possibility of me not getting it [even without the tamoxifen], and I thought, 'this is really going to the extreme.' So I just left it alone."

Gloria is now thinking about having genetic testing: "As long as it's not something that's really painful, I wouldn't mind seeing if I'm a carrier for the next generation." Gloria's maternal aunt was recently diagnosed with breast cancer and has been doing well since treatment. Gloria is concerned about many causes of breast cancer other than genetics.

> There's so many cases that have never ever had it in their families. Just being a female, and living in these toxic areas, and drinking this water. I mean you could really become paranoid. What are you going to do about it? Because at this point, nobody can really tell you where it's coming from. I thank God that there's treatments. There's early detection. I have a slight fear, but I think the attitude of how you would handle it [is more important], seeing so many other women survive it.

Current Situation

Gloria was forty-one at the time of the study interviews. She maintains close ties to her high school best friends, and was about to attend her twenty-fifth high school reunion when we interviewed her. In addition to her work at a mammography center, Gloria supports a family choir at the church her mother's family attends. She attends special events twice a year and she always visits her mother's grave during these trips. She also hopes to locate her mother's medical records and do some research on how many women died from breast cancer in the area where her mother lived at the time of her death.

DISCUSSION

This discussion identifies major themes for girls who were young adolescents at the time of the mother's death for three important time periods: the period of the illness itself, the period after the mother's death, and the long-term impact. Two themes are identified for these young adolescents during the period of mother's illness. One describes the daughters' focus on mother's physical deterioration, and the other addresses the conflict that develops between the adolescent's need for separation from the family and the demands of the home when mother is too ill to function. During the period after the mother's death, two themes are identified for young adolescent daughters. One is the difficult relationship between young adolescent girls and their fathers, who become so important after the mother's death. The other emphasizes the importance of the peer group, which becomes a potential source of support during bereavement for these girls. In the section on long-term impact, two issues are identified. Excessive anxiety is identified as a possible long-term consequence, including a form of post-traumatic stress disorder (PTSD). Another long-term consequence is difficulty forming intimate attachments.

Although the discussion section focuses primarily on the four case studies presented in this chapter, the section also refers to one case in Appendix III (Mary). Also, three women in this age group whose mothers survived breast cancer are referred to (Lisa, Jane, and Mandy, Chapter 8). Finally, two cases in the "late adolescent" chapter (Chapter 6), Alicia and Janice, are included in this discussion, because some aspects of their stories demonstrate some themes of this chapter. As discussed earlier, the lines between the age categories used in this book are somewhat arbitrary. Sometimes, a mother's illness spans several age categories (e.g., Janice's mother was diagnosed when Janice was thirteen but did not die until she reached twenty-one).

Daughter's Experience of Her Mother's Illness

Two themes for young adolescent girls during mother's illness are mother's bodily deterioration and conflict between separate and added responsibilities.

Mother's Bodily Deterioration

Young adolescent girls in this sample focused on the observable changes in their mothers' physical appearance. For example, Kara states how beautiful her mother was, and how this beauty was destroyed by breast cancer. "It was eerie watching her lose a lot of weight . . . her hair was thinning, and her lip was hanging." She says she was not sure how to react to her mother's deterioration, which included weight loss and thinning hair. Cathy felt so strongly about her mother's final symptoms that she would not comment on them, "out of respect for [her mother]." She does, however, talk about watching her mother's hair fall out, and watching her suffer. Gloria vividly describes the mucus being pumped out of her mother's lungs, and, again, her hair loss. Her mother's fragility left a lasting impression: "I just remember my mother dwindling to nothing." Mary (Appendix III) describes her mother's "thinness of skin, sunken-in face, weight loss."

Lisa, whose mother survived (see Chapter 8), describes how her mother looked "almost blue" and tells us how frightened she was to see the roomful of cancer patients when she accompanied her mother to chemotherapy. "When I walked in there and saw all these cancer survivors, with their hair gone and everyone so sick, I was just like, 'Why is my mom here?' I mean it was really really scary." Later, when her mother had a recurrence, Lisa focused on the hair loss: "So now my mom's gonna be bald in front of all my friends!" Jane, whose mother also survived (see Chapter 8), describes her mother's chemotherapy, "All [of] her hair fell out and she was just very sick . . . she was so at the mercy of those chemicals." Later, Jane attributes her problems with weight to her mother's illness.

Although almost all daughters took note of their mothers' symptoms, those who were young adolescents seemed to remember physical symptoms most vividly. For them, these symptoms symbolized the mother's deterioration. To understand this, it is important to consider what is occuring in these girls developmentally. Girls' bodies begin to mature earlier than boys', and often well before the girls are psychologically prepared. They may be thinking and acting like little girls, and suddenly their bodies are behaving like those of women. In U.S. culture, tremendous emphasis is placed on women's bodies. As adolescents, girls may not feel they have changed, but the way others react to them has. Suddenly, people are staring at these girls' chests. They realize that they are being evaluated according to a different set of standards than was the case in the past. It may seem to them that their bodies have become the only part of them that is important. Popularity at younger ages may have been based on intelligence, athletic skill, leadership, and personality. Suddenly, for some girls, how their bodies look becomes practically the one and only source of social status. Researchers have focused attention on the plummet of self-confidence that commonly occurs in girls at this age. Although they may have had high self-esteem at ten, by thirteen, it has fallen so low that they actually hate their bodies and themselves (American Association of University Women, 1991; Gilligan, Lyons, and Hammer, 1990).

When a mother has breast cancer, her young adolescent daughter may see her mother's body deteriorating; these physical changes are paramount. Wellisch, a researcher who has studied daughters of women with breast cancer, suggests that this may be because the young girls may be envied by their mothers because of their own intact body, creating a rivalry between them (Wellisch, 1979). In a later paper, which found that adolescent daughters have more long-term problems than do younger or older daughters, Wellisch et al. (1992) state,

> At the representational level, the image of a sick and potentially dying mother must be integrated by the daughter into her own sense of self, along with the preexisting image of an intact and well mother. These contrasting views of the mother, when fused with the daughter's nascent self-concept, form the basis for the daughter's ultimate self-representation that is carried into adult life. (p. 177)

Related to their focus on the mother's physical deterioration is the young adolescent daughters' connection between mother's illness and their own breast development. Certainly, Cathy made this connection. Mandy (Chapter 8), who was fourteen when her mother was diagnosed, states, "I thought, *I'm just starting to get these now, and they're gonna have to go soon.* . . . It scared me to think that now that I'm getting breasts, I can get cancer." Alicia (Chapter 6) had a particularly strong focus on breast development as a young adolescent. Alicia's grandmother had died of breast cancer, and her mother was sure she would die of the same disease at the same age. Alicia's mother connected her entire womanhood with her breasts, and after she had a mastectomy, she told Alicia, "I am no longer your mother."

Wellisch et al. (1992) discusses the connection between mother's breast cancer and the adolescent's breast development: The daughter connects "development and maturity with illness, body-image trauma and even death. Thus the experience of the mother's disease becomes a heightened threat to the daughter's emotional growth, self-esteem and identity" (p. 178).

In addition to the strain adolescent girls are feeling under normal circumstances (watching breasts develop and fearing that they are too early, too late, too small, too large), they also are learning that these breasts can lead to a terrible disease that can cause removal, loss of beauty, and even death. Some adolescents respond with eating disorders. Eating disorders are fairly common in adolescent girls, even without maternal breast cancer. Some girls want to take control of a body that seems out of control. Some may see anorexia as a way to stop their breasts from developing. In a study of adolescent daughters whose mothers had breast cancer, Spira and Kenemore (2000) identified six themes. One of these themes was "fears associated with physical/sexual development." Discussing a case, they state,

> On some level she harbored the fantasy that if she did not develop fully as a woman she might avoid getting breast cancer. She also experienced a sense of control through limitation of her food intake. This was important to her since she had no control over the cancer. (Spira and Kenemore, 2000, p. 190)

Oktay and Walter (1991) also found that some adolescent daughters of women with breast cancer developed eating disorders.

It also is important to note that some of the young adolescent daughters thought that they might have cancer when their breasts started to develop. Gloria went so far as to wish she had breast cancer, so that she could die and join her mother.

Conflict Between Separation and Added Responsibilities

Another theme identified in the cases of young adolescent girls was the conflict many experienced between the demands placed on them due to the mother's illness and the normal activities of adolescence. Bettina, for example, talks about how when her mother became ill, her relationship with both parents changed. Her father began to lean on her emotionally. Her mother also leaned on her and talked to her about "the difficulty she was having with my father." Thus the illness takes Bettina out of the role of an adolescent, establishing a separate identity, and involves her in unnatural relationships with both parents. After her mother dies, separation comes prematurely and suddenly when Bettina is sent halfway across the country to live with an aunt.

Mary (see Appendix III) was thirteen when she began to take on many of her mother's roles after mother's death. "I am the one that took over and made everybody's lunches and picked up most of the household chores." Janice (Chapter 6) provides another strong example of the conflict between the normal teen role and the role of the young adolescent girls whose mothers had breast cancer.

Alicia, fifteen when her mother was diagnosed, provides an example of a teen who moved out of the family and separated in spite of her mother's illness. Alicia didn't listen to her mother's dire predictions about breast cancer, describing her mother as "crazy." Later, however, when she was nineteen, Alicia returned home to care for her dying mother and stayed to care for her father after mother's death.

Mandy (Chapter 8), whose mother survived, discusses how she took on her mother's household responsibilities as well as cared for her during the illness. She illustrates the conflict of the adolescent weighing her own needs with those of her family. She also seems to regress from adolescence into childhood when she begins to sleep with her mother. "It made me feel better to listen to her sleep at night." Lisa (Chapter 8) also found herself taking on new roles while her mother was in the hospital and ill from chemotherapy.

Traditional theories of adolescence have emphasized the task of separation of the adolescent from the family, thus leading to development of the adolescent's identity. Erikson's (1963) very influential theory presents the psychosocial conflict of the adolescent stage of development as "identity versus role confusion." In Erikson's model, the adolescent must search for his or her own identity outside of the family. If an adolescent does not struggle with and resolve the question "Who am I?" a "foreclosed" identity may result. Theories of family life cycles show adolescence as a time of "centrifugal" force, where family ties are loosened, so that the young adult can be "launched" into the adult world (Carter and McGoldrick, 1989; Rolland, 1994). To apply this idea to the young adolescents in our study, two further considerations are necessary. First, to what extent are these theories appropriate to women? Second, what happens to families when a parent is ill or dies?

Apter (1990) has studied relationships between mothers and their adolescent daughters in England. She points out that the classical oedipal models of psychosexual development do not work with women, because they are based on castration fears; these do not apply to the relationship between girls and their mothers. She points out that feminist authors, especially Chodorow (1999), show that girls stay connected to their mothers through adolescence. Her qualitative research, based on interviews and observations of adolescent girls, emphasizes how important the mother remains in the adolescent girls' development of their new identities. These adolescents struggle against enmeshment with their mothers, but at the same time, want the mother's recognition and support for their new selves (Apter, 1990). Gilligan's work on adolescent development suggests that the relationship with the mother "provides girls with the context for development of identity, autonomy and connection" (Gilligan, 1982b, p. 187). During normal adolescence, a shift occurs from a relationship of dependence to one of interdependence.

What happens in families with young adolescent girls when the mother gets breast cancer? Lewis and Hammond (1996) studied seventy families with adolescents. Although the sample differs considerably from the women in this study, one finding is relevant here. One of the strongest predictors of self-esteem in the adolescents was a positive parent-child relationship. The authors conclude, "Clearly, adolescents highly benefited from parental attentiveness as they dealt with the centripetal pull of the mother's illness and the centrifugal pressures of their own evolving independence" (p. 464).

Christ and colleagues (1994) found that girls had more problems than boys.

> Emotionally overwhelmed parents responded with anger and resentment toward the increased aggressiveness of their daughters, who in turn became more angry, fearful and depressed, experienced lowered self-esteem, and often acted out their anger. In addition, early adolescent girls often felt profoundly wounded,

rejected and abandoned by the withdrawal of parental attention caused by the medical crisis. (p. 606)

Further, she finds, "When the mother was ill, girls tended to change the quality of their involvement with her, resulting in a different type of closeness between them" (Jordan, Kaplan, Miller, Striver, and Surry, 1991). Most had more household responsibilities, some were "drawn into providing the patient with nursing care," and "most found it extremely difficult and stressful." Most were resentful, particularly if this interfered with activities they wanted to do (p. 608).

Christ et al. (1994) report that adolescents tended to feel guilty about "developmentally normal anger toward parents" (p. 609). Christ's (2000) book on children's grief includes a discussion of Gilligan's (1982b) work and how "for adolescent girls, a parent's death interfered profoundly with their developmental task of changing their relationship with their surviving parent rather than only withdrawing emotional investment from the relationship" (Christ, 2000, p. 193). This is in contrast to boys, who are

> usually engaged in more fully separating from both parents . . . girls were often angry because their responsibilities at home greatly exceeded those of their brothers. When guilt was present it focused on regret about their misbehavior, their anger at the patient, or their desire to separate and be independent at a time when the family needed them to be closer. (Christ, 2000, p. 198)

Note that these comments on adolescents are on those fifteen to seventeen, while Christ has an earlier section on those thirteen to fifteen, which is more relevant to this group. In attempting to explain why the adolescent group had more long-term problems, Wellisch et al. (1992) state,

> Emotionally, adolescents are undergoing a phase of ego development in which the personality is particularly vulnerable because of separation/independence issues. Such issues create intense feelings of ambivalence about involvement with the mother that are present in the adolescent daughters. (p. 178)

Spira and Kenemore (2000) also studied adolescent daughters of women with breast cancer. They use the typology of illness in the family developed by Rolland: "Dissonance between the developmental needs of adolescence and the needs of the family during illness" (p. 184). They review the literature on the effect of maternal depression on family functioning: "Some mothers feel guilty over being less available physically and emotionally to their daughters" (p. 186). They point out that, using Gilligan's theory, a shift from a relationship where the child is dependent to one where the mother is dependent is "troubling": "Also, definition of the girl's self as distinct from her mother may be blurred by the fear of getting the disease. The threat of loss of mother is likened to the fear of loss of self" (p. 188). Finally, they note that "The gradual emotional withdrawal from parents and intensification of relationships outside the family which many adolescent girls experience may be delayed or reversed during the course of mother's illness" (p. 191). Spira and Kenemore (2000) found in their sample that when household responsibilities fell on teen girls, girls were willing to help, but feared that this would change the nature of the relationship they had with their mothers.

Experience Following Her Mother's Death

Themes identified for young adolescent girls following mother's death were problems with fathers and influence of peer group.

Problems with Fathers

Many women in the sample reported changes in father-daughter relationships after the mother's death. Bettina, who was eleven when her mother's died, received two conflicting messages from her father. On one hand, she became his confidant; even after he married he continued to confide in her about marital problems. Bettina captures the nature of the relationship, recognizing that confidences are shared between equals, but she was still a child in the relationship. On the other hand, her father seemed to "dispense" with her, and he eventually sent her off to live with her aunt. In Bettina's words, "He thought that the fact that he didn't have sisters relieved him of any responsibility for looking out for me."

One role of parents is to protect their children from dangers to which they may be vulnerable. Because girls generally are considered more vulnerable than boys, especially as they begin to develop sexually, much of the conflict in adolescence between parents and adolescent daughters focuses around the parent's need to provide protection and the teen's need to separate from the family. Traditionally, the function of protection falls on the father, and in a patriarchy, it is the father's role to ensure his daughter's virginity as he "gives" her away at the time of her marriage. According to this way of thinking, fathers who relinquish the "father" or "protector" role with their daughters following the mother's death may be making their teen daughters more vulnerable to various dangers, including sexual assault. In Bettina's case, she indicates that she got into some "dangerous situations," including possible sexual assault and marijuana use. This is not surprising considering the lack of parental supervision in her adolescence. Finding the correct balance between too much and too little separation is a difficult task for all families. However, when the family is overwhelmed, a premature separation can result.

> For the adolescent who is cast out or runs away, the casualty rate due to other-inflicted or self-inflicted violence (including drug overdose) is high. Vulnerability to exploitation is also high. Underemployment, unemployment, prostitution and involvement with an abusive partner are more likely outcomes for the adolescent without family supports. (Preto, 1988, p. 265)

Gloria's father was distant, even when her mother was alive. His alcohol problem worsened after her mother's death. "He was drinking and he was bringing women over. I didn't want any part of it." Gloria's grandmother tried to assume the mother role, but she could not hold the children together and they all moved out on their own. Eventually, Gloria and her younger brother went to live near her mother's family.

In contrast, Cathy had a strong relationship with her father, and she stayed in a "child" role after mother's death. Cathy's father took on mother's roles in the family, perhaps because Cathy's mother had told her not to become "a replacement mother" when she died. Cathy says she could confide in her father. Cathy's father also recognized her need for grief counseling, showing an awareness of her emotional needs.

Although the father-daughter bond often is strong when daughters are young, many fathers become more and more distant as daughters begin to mature. Apter (1990), who studied adolescent girls and their parents, also finds that girls are less close to fathers during adolescence than during childhood. In part, this is due to embarrassment about the girls' physical changes. Classically, the explanation given is that the physical changes in the daughter reactivate oedipal desires, and fathers, disturbed by their incestuous feelings, retreat. "Fathers often become awkward about relating to their daughters as the daughters approach adolescence, fearing their budding sexuality" (Carter and McGoldrick, 1988, p. 50). Also, fathers may feel that their daughters need privacy, and retreat, leaving mothers to provide guidance and advice. Shulman and Seiffge-Krenke (1997) state that "the adolescent's physical maturation is a secret which cannot be shared with the father" (p. 40). Physical contact between fathers and daughters is greatly reduced from that which took place in childhood. In a book titled *Fathers and Daughters,* Sharpe (1994) places some typical reactions into an understanding of women's role in a patriarchal society. "A father's perception of a daughter is complicated by several related factors, such as possessiveness, a desire to preserve her innocence, and the implicit threat presented by male competition for the daughter's affection and attention" (p. 85). Sharpe also raises the issue of control of the potential power of women's sexuality, which is threatening to men:

> The incest taboo generally distances sexual desire and replaces it with a distaste for such unacceptable feelings. The point when fathers become aware of their daughters growing more physically mature, and essentially more sexual, often coincides with a process of withdrawal. (p. 92)

Pipher (1994), in her popular book on adolescent girls, *Reviving Ophelia,* posits that fathers have been socialized into misogyny, so that when the little girl they loved (sugar and spice) turns into something they devalue (a woman), they emotionally distance themselves. At the same time, as girls mature, fathers are aware of daughters' sexual vulnerability, and this may lead to increased restrictions. Some fathers become overprotective of vulnerable daughters and "may interfere with the adolescent's striving for independence and consolidation of a differentiated and mature ego identity" (Shulman and Seiffge-Krenke, 1997, p. 105). In some cases, father-daughter relationships become sexualized, presenting a danger of sexual abuse for the teen daughter. Perhaps Bettina's father sent her to her aunt's in part because his relationship with her had crossed a boundary and he feared the development of a sexual relationship. Sometimes a remarriage is seen as a solution to this type of attraction.

In general, parenting by fathers differs from that of mothers. Mothers tend to have more difficulty controlling their children, while fathers have more difficulties in communication and monitoring (Hetherington and Stanley-Hagan, 1999). Apter also found that fathers are often insensitive to feelings when communicating with teen daughters. They often are "too quick to offer a solution," rather than to listen as the daughter mulls over her options and sorts through her feelings. Daughters tended to consult their mothers about relationships, sex, or their bodies, even if they were living with their fathers after a divorce (Apter, 1993). Fathers may focus on their traditional responsibilities to their daughters, such as providing a home, food, and clothing, rather than focusing on the relationship itself.

Most research on fathers' relationships with adolescent daughters is done in the context of an intact family, where girls have both mothers and fathers. Somewhat more similar to the situation of breast cancer families in which the mother has died are studies of those in which the father has custody. Shulman and Seiffge-Krenke (1997) note that fathers can change their relationship with daughters in this situation, and may develop a "sudden closeness" with them. These authors question the ability of a father alone, or a father and stepmother to help a daughter resolve oedipal conflicts and achieve identification with the same sex parent. They conclude, "Adults in a newly formed family are not always adequately prepared for dealing with the sexual development of a growing girl" (p. 103). DeMaris and Greif (1992), who have extensively studied single-father households, have found that fathers with adolescent girls have more problems than fathers raising preadolescent girls, and that fathers generally feel unprepared for childrearing responsibilities. In some households, fathers develop a relationship with the child that is more like that of a peer than a parent. Sometimes a role reversal takes place, and the child becomes the parent. For example, when Bettina was asked if her father helped her with her grief, she responded, "No. I had to help him with his grief."

Gray (1989), in a study of adolescents after the death of a parent, makes an important point. "Frequently, adolescents wanted but failed to obtain support from the surviving parent. Some parents appeared to have been so overwhelmed by their own grief that they could not reach out to their children" (p. 141). Although this study included adolescents whose fathers died as well as those whose mothers died, an understanding of male grieving would suggest that this problem would be especially likely in girls whose mothers died. In most families, feelings tend to be in the female realm. Men often rely on their wives for social support and connections. When the wife is ill or after she dies, they find themselves isolated and lacking the support they need to deal with their grief. When Hilton, Crawford, and Tarko (2000) studied men whose wives were undergoing chemotherapy, they found that they tended to respond within the parameters of traditional gender roles, focusing on "identifying the threat," "engaging in the fight," and "becoming a veteran." The men tended to keep their feelings at bay and focus their energies for the "battle." With regard to their children, the men tried to "protect" children (and wives), which often led to "protective talking" that can interfere with effective communication and lead to misperceptions, as well as utilize energy (p. 453).

Rates of mortality and even suicide are especially high for men in the first six months after a wife's death (Tudiver, 1991). None of the men in our study died or committed suicide; however, we do see clear patterns of withdrawal from their young adolescent daughters. In those who did not "desert," fathers physically were there to "do their duty," whether this meant keeping the household going or providing financial support. Some also were there intellectually for their daughters but generally could not provide the type of emotional support their daughters needed. Kara expresses this well: "He [father] was emotionally detached, or didn't know how to express his emotional side. He could communicate intellectually but just not with his feelings." (This pattern of daughters caring for their fathers also was evident in some of the cases discussed in Chapter 4, especially as the girls moved into adolescence after the mother's death. For example, Carol described a similar pattern in her father, who held extensive theological and philosophical discussions with her in her adolescence but failed to address emotional issues.)

Influence of Peer Group

It is well known that as children move into adolescence, the influence of the peer group grows. Although younger children in our study were concerned about being perceived as different by their peers, this fear was much stronger in the adolescents. Some of the young adolescents were able to get support from friends after their mothers died.

Bettina was afraid she would be treated as an oddball by both students and teachers. When Lisa (see Chapter 8) was ten and her mother was diagnosed, her concern was about whether Mommy would be there; when she was twelve and the cancer recurred, her response was, "Now my mom's gonna be bald in front of all my friends!" Cathy speaks poignantly about her need for peers with whom to share her experiences. "I wanted to talk about it with other kids, and there were no other kids whose parents were dying or had died." Cathy also refused to go to the counseling her father suggested, in part because none of her friends went to counseling. Mary (Appendix III) did not mention peers in her interview, but commented on the final questionnaire that she sometimes felt alone.

Gloria was able to get valuable support from a friend whose mother had died only six months before. It is significant that the first thing Gloria did when she learned of her mother's death was to run over to her friend's house, not even taking the time to get dressed first. The two girls cried together, as she said to her friend, "I'm just like you. I'm just like you." Alicia (Chapter 6), whose relationship with her mother was not good before the cancer, also turned to her friends for support during her mother's illness.

Even when mothers survived, young adolescents worried about how their mothers' illness affected their relationships with peers. Mandy (Chapter 8) says her friends felt "really awkward." She thinks they were afraid to say the wrong thing, so instead, they didn't say anything. Whether friends ostracized the young adolescent, or provided support, their importance should not be minimized.

Studies of bereaved adolescents show that they generally turn to peers rather than to parents after a loss (Gray, 1989). Gray's own study of adolescents showed that 40 percent rated their peers "most helpful," compared to 26 percent who found parents helpful. Gray (1989) also found that teens didn't want to be different from their peers and were willing to forego support to appear the same as their friends: "Being one of the crowd, then, seemed to be healthy and necessary for adolescents who were dealing with a difficult loss and may have contributed toward reassuring them that life could go on despite the loss" (p. 141). Although support groups were very helpful for some, others, such as Cathy, felt stigmatized. "A bereaved teenager may be so sensitive to the perceptions of peers that the fear of being singled out as different may override the need for their support" (Elkind, 1968, as cited in Gray, 1989, p. 129).

It also is important to consider the unique issues that girls experience with peer relationships in order to best understand adolescent daughters. Study of girls' adolescence is fairly recent, and our understanding is quite limited. However, fiction (Atwood, 1996) and popular literature (Pipher, 1994) have illustrated a phenomenon called "shunning." Adolescent girls form friendship groups which enforce their codes of behavior and appearance by excluding girls from the group. "Scapegoats are shunned, teased, bullied and harassed in a hundred different ways" (Pipher, 1994, p. 69). Pipher primarily describes scapegoating as enforcement of standards of "femininity"; it is not difficult to see why a young adolescent girl would not want to risk being different from those in her peer group.

Long-Term Impact

Fear/PTSD

Several studies on the long-term impact of breast cancer suggest that adolescent daughters are more vulnerable than are children of other age groups. Wellisch's study (Wellisch et al., 1992) based on retrospective interviews of breast cancer daughters found that when compared to women who were children or adults at the time of mother's diagnosis, women who were adolescents were the most likely to experience adjustment problems. Compas et al. (1999) also found that adolescent daughters were the most distressed among all groups of children. Christ (2000) notes that although severe reactions in adolescents were unusual, she did find that symptoms of depression were common. In our study, the long-term reactions were connected to the themes during the illness and after mother's death. For example, in the section on illness experience, we discussed the emphasis the adolescent daughters placed on the changes in mother's physical appearance. A number of these adolescents had problems when they developed breasts, and many of them have excessive fears of breast cancer as adults. Another long-term problem related to body image is the development of eating disorders.

The women who were adolescents at the time of the mother's illness had strong and vivid memories of mother's physical symptoms.

The PTSD-like symptoms, such as intrusive thoughts in the daughter, are probably related to specific symptoms in the mother. For example, the loss of hair, which accompanies chemotherapy, seems to be very traumatic, as does weight loss, weakness, and "wasting." In fact, the strength of these images, combined with the strong emotions accompanying the memories, suggested a subclinical form of PTSD. Originally, PTSD as a diagnosis was reserved for those who had suffered trauma, such as rape, battle, or a natural disaster. However, in 1995, the diagnosis was broadened to include severe physical illness. In recent years, PTSD has been found not only in people who have suffered a severe illness but in family members as well. For example, studies have found evidence for PTSD in parents of children with cancer, and spouses of cancer patients (Smith, Redd, and Peyser, 1999). A recent study (Boyer et al., 2002) found that rates of PTSD were as high in daughters of women with breast cancer as they were in the patients themselves. Some research suggests that the loss of a parent through illness can be more traumatic for children and adolescents than is violence or child abuse (McCloskey and Walker, 2000; Stoppelbein and Greening, 2000). The findings of this study would predict high levels of PTSD in young adolescent daughters who have lost mothers to breast cancer.

Problems in Intimate Relationships

One long-term impact on daughters who were young adolescents at the time of the mother's diagnosis relates to their ability as women to form stable and meaningful relationships with others, particularly men. For example, Bettina says,

> I just didn't learn how to behave as a woman. I was clueless on dealing with boyfriends. I wonder if my mother had lived, she may have helped me learn some dating skills, and maybe she would have helped me avoid marrying my ex-husband. . . . I might have been more successful in marriage if I had help from her.

Cathy has problems making commitments because she fears the pain (comparable to bereavement) that she will feel when the relationship ends. Cathy also has a difficult time separating from her father and her brother after visits. Mary (Appendix III) tells how her low self-esteem, which she attributes to her mother's death, affected her relationships with men. "Relating it to guys, I didn't think I was good enough for anybody, so I'd let them walk all over me." Mary's first marriage was abusive. As with Cathy, Mary focuses on separations, even small daily ones, such as when she says good night to her children. She makes sure to say "I love you" at each separation, so that if something happens, she won't repeat her failure to say "good-bye" to her mother. Gloria, who is no longer married, says that her mother's death led her and her sister to seek the "wrong" men.

Janice (Chapter 6) feels that she has a difficult time convincing herself that she doesn't have to be a martyr in relationships. However, when men are kind and try to support her, she rejects them. Janice also sees this pattern in her sister.

In order to understand this issue, it is important to think about what happens between mothers and daughters during a "normal" adolescence. Although some views of the sexual development in adolescent girls create conflict between mothers and daughters, either because mothers are jealous of the girl's developing body or because they are afraid of the consequences of their daughter's sexuality (e.g., pregnancy), more recent research on mothers and adolescent daughters suggests a much more complex picture. Studies by the American Association of University Women have shown a precipitous loss of self-esteem in adolescent girls (AAUW, 1991). Work by Gilligan and her colleagues (e.g., Brown and Gilligan, 1992) demonstrates how adolescent girls lose their "voices," finding that they cannot both stay connected to others, be well liked, and also speak their minds. They give up opinions that might make them unpopular, and become the "nice girl," who "doesn't know" anything. In their work at a private girls school in Cleveland, Ohio, Brown and Gilligan found that the girls who remained strong and true to themselves had strong mothers who didn't fit the "perfect woman" stereotype. Pipher (1994) emphasizes the important role mothers can play to counter the girl's loss of self-esteem. Her clinical work shows mothers trying to protect daughters from the dangers of growing up:

> Mothers want their daughters to date, but are terrified of date rape, teen pregnancy, AIDS and other diseases. They want their daughters to be independent, but are aware of how dangerous the world is for women. They want their daughters to be relaxed about their appearance, but know that girls suffer socially if they aren't attractive. Daughters struggle to individuate, but also need

their mothers' guidance and love. They resist their mothers' protection even as they move into dangerous waters. And they are angry when their mothers warn them of dangers that they understand even better than their mothers. (p. 105)

While some mothers emphasize the "being nice" and "fitting in" aspects of womanhood, others help their daughters to feel confident, smart, and loved for who they really are. Loss of a mother can mean a loss of support to resist the social pressures of the peer environment, loss of a role model who is not "perfect" and is comfortable with herself, and loss of protection.

Bettina mentions getting into some "dangerous situations." Nora (Chapter 4), who was a child at the time of her mother's death, experienced a sexual assault when she was a young teen. Mothers can play an important role in helping teen daughters negotiate a sometimes dangerous world. Mothers and daughters fight about clothing, and this is often about how much of the (developing) body to show. While daughters may fight to wear the low-cut dress or the tight pants, mothers object so that daughters will be protected from possible sexual harassment or assault. When daughters do not have mothers, they may not learn the cultural meanings surrounding women's clothing and makeup. Mothers also try to steer daughters toward men who are "safe" and "protective," and away from those who may be dangerous or damaging. Although daughters often fight with mothers over these issues, increasing research shows that daughters often adopt mothers' values and goals.

Women's choice of abusive or dominant husbands also may be related to an adolescent version of the escape theme discussed in Chapter 4. Adolescents who seek to escape from the home and replace parents with "pseudoparents" have an option that younger girls do not have. They can turn to relationships with men for protection (e.g., Gloria and her sister, who sought "big men" to protect them) or support, to replace the lost relationship with mother. Alicia (Chapter 6) established this pattern early in her adolescence, and married a very protective husband soon after her mother died. However, while these relationships may have seemed appealing to the adolescent girls, they didn't necessarily work out that way. Alicia is the only one of the adolescent cases who is still married. Bettina, Mary, and Gloria all are separated or divorced.

SUMMARY

This chapter focused on the experience of young adolescents whose mothers died from breast cancer. Four case studies were used to identify and illustrate major themes in three important time periods: the period of the illness itself, the period after mother's death, and the long-term impact (see Box 5.1). During the period of the mother's illness, young adolescents seem to focus on the mother's physical deterioration, and they are very disturbed by it. In addition, during this period, a conflict develops between the young adolescent daughter's need for separation from the family and the demands of the home when the mother is too ill to function. After the mother's death, relationships between these girls and their fathers can become problematic. The peer group is important for these girls as a potential source of support. Excessive anxiety, including a form of PTSD, is identified as a possible long-term consequence. Another long-term effect is difficulty forming intimate attachments.

Implications of these results are discussed in more detail in Chapter 11.

BOX 5.1. Themes Found in Daughters Whose Mothers Died When They Were Young Adolescents

Phase I: Mother's Illness and Treatments

1. Mother's bodily deterioration
2. Conflict between separation and added responsibilities

Phase II: Following Mother's Death

1. Problems with fathers
2. Influence of peer group

Phase III: Long-Term Impact

1. Fear/PTSD
2. Problems in intimate relationships

Chapter 6

Experience of Late Adolescent Daughters When Mothers Die from Breast Cancer

This chapter discusses the experience of daughters who were late adolescents when their mothers died from breast cancer. The four women presented were between ages eighteen and twenty-two at the time of mother's death: Janice (thirteen at mother's diagnosis), Trisha (fourteen at mother's diagnosis), Alicia (fifteen at mother's diagnosis), and Veronica (sixteen at mother's diagnosis). As in the previous chapters, the case studies are divided into six parts: background, mother's illness and treatment, after mother's death, long-term impact, risk, and current situation. Following the case studies, the late adolescent daughters' experiences are discussed and themes are developed for each of three phases: during the illness, following the mother's death, and long-term impact.

CASE STUDY #1: JANICE

Age at Her Mother's Breast Cancer Diagnosis: 13; Age at Time of Her Mother's Death: 21

Background

Janice was the middle sister in a middle-class Catholic family with three girls. Her father worked and her mother did part-time substitute teaching. Of the three sisters, Janice was the closest to her mother and the most like her. "People would say I was a carbon copy of my mother. And I got along with Mother very well. We just had a lot of things in common. She is probably the only person that really understood me." As a young teen, Janice was sometimes embarrassed by her mother. Once her mother picked her up at school in their old station-wagon ("It was a piece of junk"). Another time, her mother gave a talk in Janice's class about a painter, and Janice wished she could have stayed home from school that day. For the most part, though, she was proud that her mother was very involved in her activities. Janice says that her parents were very happy together. Janice never knew her maternal grandmother, who died from breast cancer when Janice's mother was seventeen.

Experience of Her Mother's Illness

The summer that Janice was thirteen, the family took a road trip to California.

> Somewhere past the halfway point of the trip, she [mother] discovered a tumor. At that point, there was tension, and we [children] didn't know what it was. We thought maybe my parents got into a fight, or maybe there was a problem with money.

After they returned home, Janice's mother did not go to the community swimming pool as she usually did. When her friends asked about her, Janice said, "She's turning forty so I guess it's just routine check-ups." Once, Janice overheard someone use the word *mastectomy* and looked it up in the dictionary. Soon after, Janice and her sister were sent away to camp, with no discussion of their mother's illness.

> Before I knew it, I was going to YMCA camp. So I had to go to camp for two weeks while this was going on. I just remember being there when my mother had the surgery, and I didn't receive any letters. I couldn't call home. My sister was there too, but we didn't discuss it. I remember being really, really frustrated that I didn't know what was happening and being left out in the dark.

When camp was over, their mother came to pick them up. "I noticed right away that one of her breasts was removed. That seemed a little strange."

Janice returned home and started school, more concerned about whether she would make the soccer team than about her mother's illness. Her mother went into the hospital to have lymph nodes removed, and then started chemotherapy. Janice's mother told her that this was due to an infection, never mentioning breast cancer. "I began to understand these things more, so I felt like I wasn't being left out in the dark so much. But I didn't know why it was going on, or what happened." During the time her mother was in the hospital, Janice's step-grandmother came to take care of the household. "That was strange that my mother wasn't there, and she wasn't doing the laundry and cooking the meals. There definitely was an emptiness in the house. Her absence was definitely noticed and she was missed." While on chemotherapy, her mother lost her hair; Janice remembers that her mother hated her wig and wore scarves around the house instead. When the family went skiing at Christmas, Janice's mother was the only person in the ski lodge who kept her hat on during lunch. "That was scary. And when it [mother's hair] grew back, I was really happy. It was sort of, 'She's getting better! She's getting better!'" Janice's mother wouldn't let her see her naked anymore. "I remember after the surgeries, meandering in there and the door was closed. I couldn't do that anymore." Janice's mother's illness affected her by limiting any rebellion.

> When your mother is sick, home in bed, it's so hard to try to be a normal teenager. To do the things a person of your age should be doing. I didn't rebel when I was thirteen. I didn't. I sort of stayed home more and took care of things for her. How could I have a good time when she's suffering so much? In those crucial teenage years when you're trying to be confident and discover who you are and who your friends are, I think I lost a lot of confidence. When she was doing well, I would be doing well too. And when she was not doing well, I thought it was the end of the world. I couldn't do anything.

By spring, her mother was better, and life for Janice went back to normal. Even though it was never directly discussed, Janice remembers feeling,

> "It's gone! It's gone!" Four years of high school. Nothing. Absolutely nothing. It was always on the back of our minds, you know, *Will it come back?* Whatever "it" was. I think we knew that my mother had breast cancer, but it was never discussed as breast cancer.

Mother returned to her active life, worked on a master's degree, and took a full-time job when her youngest daughter entered school. Janice noticed that the family began to spend more money, going on trips and building a summerhouse instead of always saving for the future.

Janice graduated from high school and left for a trip to Spain. "I was really excited. I knew I liked Spanish literature and language." While Janice was in Spain, her mother's doctor found some cancerous cells in her lungs. "The first time that my mother called me and used the words *breast cancer* was when I was in Spain. So this is when I knew it was serious." Shortly after learning this, Janice met a Spanish man on a train and told him about her mother's illness.

> He was the first person that I really talked to about it. When I left Spain, I wrote to him, and he wrote to me. I could write to him and tell him about it, because it was safe. I didn't have to talk about it to anybody in my family or any of my friends. They didn't know what to say to me. It was much safer to write to this guy who I barely knew.

Back in the United States, Janice started her first year of college. One day, she went to a Christian fellowship meeting. When everyone bowed their heads, "I didn't know what was happening. I just started, you know, just crying, crying, crying."

Janice often went home on weekends. Her mother was put on tamoxifen. One day, her father called and told her that her mother would be having an operation. On the ride to the hospital, her father told her that her mother had had a hysterectomy.

> I didn't know what that was. I'm like, "Hyster . . . what?" When we were waiting to see her, I pulled out a dictionary of medical terms and, standing in the lobby, I read what it was. I remember that I felt very faint. I was so upset because I finally realized what happened. I had to sit down, and then I fainted. I was trying to be sort of myself, you know, be a support for her. [in a cheerful voice] "How you doing? What's going on? Yeah, school's fine." Talk about myself [so that] she only had to tell me what was going on with her if she wanted to. Just to take the pressure off of her. I couldn't, though. I fainted. And that was really scary.

Her mother recovered quickly from the surgery, and "right away, she wanted to be back on track. She always had a really good spirit. Real strong will to survive." The rest of that year was postive for Janice. She made plans to spend a semester in Spain. Just before she left, the family took a vacation to Aruba. There, they had the best time ever.

> Everything was good. If she [mother] was sick, she had it under control. My sisters and I got along really well. That was the last time I remember her being in really good shape. She was happy, talkative. I think for that trip, we forgot that she had cancer.

While Janice was in Spain, her mother's cancer got worse.

> It felt like I was back in YMCA camp, because I didn't know what was going on. I remember for my birthday no one called me. [I was] not hearing anything. They didn't want me to worry. [They wanted me to] have a good time. At this point she almost died. She was waiting for me to say, "Can I come home?" And I was waiting for her to say, "Janice, come home!" My father said, "Oh yeah, we had a tough time. We were down at the hospital the whole weekend." I knew he couldn't talk about it. It was tough. But I wanted answers.

When Janice came home at the end of her semester, her mother met her at the airport.

> When she saw me, she cried. My mother doesn't cry very much. And she said to me that she didn't think she was going to see me again. And I didn't know how to respond to that. I didn't know how bad things had gotten.

Janice began her third year of college, once again coming home frequently on the weekends. "I would call her and she wouldn't [answer]. I knew she was there, but she had the answering machine pick up. She was too sick. I knew things were getting bad." On Thanksgiving,

> She did a turkey. She woke up that morning, prepared everything, and went back to bed. When the doorbell rang, she threw her clothes on, went downstairs, and put a show on. She fooled them all. Then afterward, she went back to bed. I think she slept for three days straight after that.

In spite of her illness, Janice's mother wanted the family to have another vacation in the Caribbean.

> She wanted a trip like Aruba. She was back on chemo and she lost her hair. She put weight on. She really couldn't move. But she still wanted to go. She wanted to be revitalized. We thought, "This is a bad idea. She's too sick."

But when her mother insisted, the family went on another cruise.

> We got there on the boat. She didn't leave her room very much. She was so sick. So it was hard for us to have a good time. Things got so bad that they had to have her removed from the boat by helicopter. My father told me at that point that he didn't think my mother would be

around for much longer. The ship's doctor told him probably three months. And that's when I realized that my mother was dying.

Her mother was flown directly from Florida to the hospital near her home.

Janice, then twenty-one, spent many hours in the hospital by her mother's bedside. "My sisters didn't go in as much. I think they were in denial." Around this time, Janice began to see a therapist, who told her to "tell her [mother] everything."

> I brought all these pictures in. I thanked her for everything. Told her how much she meant to me [sobbing]. She [therapist] gave me tips, things to do, suggestions. So I had a chance to say good-bye. I was really fortunate to be hooked up with this woman [therapist]. I was able to talk to her that whole week that she was dying. I thanked her for being my Girl Scouts leader, and for teaching my class about Edward Hopper. And it really helped me a lot.

Several days before her death, Janice's mother had a stroke and became incoherent. One evening, even though she couldn't speak, her mother managed to communicate that she wanted her husband to walk Janice to her car. "She's in all this pain, but she could tell my father that I could possibly be in danger. She wanted me to be safe." Her father began to rely on Janice to communicate with her sisters. "One time, my father told me to go tell my sisters—the week before my mother died—'Janice, tell your sisters that Mom is dying.' And I had to do that."

In the end, Janice held her mother's hand, while a family friend held Janice's other hand.

> It was very nice. She was sort of giving me support while I was with my mother. Mother said, "Janice, Janice, Janice" and "Janice, I love you." My father and I were in the room, and my sisters were out in the hallway. She took her last breath, and I remember I said, "Oh, God, Mom is dead" [sobbing]. I remember I was just incredibly, just incredibly so sad.

Janice also felt some relief after her mother died.

> The hour after she died, I remember thinking, *Well, this wasn't as bad as I thought.* The worst was the anticipation, the waiting. After she died, it was just peace. No more pain. Then, we could sort of move on. Seeing her in pain was the hardest thing. And then our own pain—the physical pain and the emotional pain.

Janice went out and told her sisters their mother had died. Then, Janice's father asked her to call the relatives and to make the funeral arrangements. "I think my father didn't know how to deal with these things. The whole thing with the funeral, the limo. Everything. I sort of took care of that, because no one would do it except me."

Experience Following Her Mother's Death

After her mother's death, Janice took a semester off from college.

> I stayed home and went to the [local university] to be at home. I cooked. I was the surrogate mother. I filled her place for six months. It was really tough. I didn't know how to deal with myself, so what I did with the pain was take care of other people. Not myself. Took care of my father. Took care of my [younger] sister.

This was a demanding period. Janice had a difficult time dealing with her younger sister.

> She was fifteen and very rebellious. She treated my mother badly before she died, and that was sort of superimposed onto me. All of a sudden, I was being treated badly. I didn't put up with that. She really resented that. She liked the fact that I was home and helping out, but she didn't like the fact that I wouldn't put up with her.

During this period, Janice and her boyfriend of five years broke up.

> I ended up breaking up with my boyfriend in that six-month period, because he couldn't help me. He was just very needy. He needed me to be there. I was like, "Hey, I can't be there for you. I need someone to be here for me."

She also had problems in her relationship with her best friend.

> I said, "You know why I'm not talking to you right now? You know what it is? I'm just so mad at you! Because you have a mature relationship with your mother and I can't. I'll never have that. So I don't want to be your friend. I don't want to be anybody's friend." You know, you're working on getting past that stage in a mother-daughter relationship. I remember we just started that. We just crossed over. A few talks we had, my mother opened up to me and that was rare. She was very private, and she became even more private after she became sick.

Janice and her friend later made up. "She said, 'Janice, come on. I've known you for so many years. I know this is tough for you. I'm not going to abandon you.'"

Although staying home was difficult for Janice, it also gave her some satisfaction.

> Part of me wanted to stay home. I didn't want to go back to school. I didn't want to leave home. That was still a sacred place. That was the home that [her mother] created. I sort of kept things in order, the way she kept things. I sort of kept the spirit of the house alive. Kept things intact, as my father said. My father really appreciated me staying home.

Janice also took on some of her mother's peacemaking roles. "I never had a rebellion. I wanted to keep the peace in the family between my sisters and my father. They were both very rebellious. I was the responsible one."

Later, when her father began to date, Janice was resentful.

> When I wanted to go to see my boyfriend one weekend, my Dad said, "Don't go." He wanted me to stay home with him. I immediately cancelled my plans with my boyfriend and stayed home. Then, when he started dating women, it was, "See you guys later." That really hurt.

In the period following her mother's death, Janice suffered a number of other losses. Her grandfather died a year later. Her father started dating and soon remarried. "That set me back too." Then her father sold the house. "Selling the house, that took me back." Janice looked for support from boyfriends and from organized groups.

> I have made some mistakes in the past looking for support. Dating somebody who's been a real jerk. Getting involved in a religious group in college that was bordering on a cult. I'm always looking for a support group. Trying these different groups. I have many, many friends, but there's still something missing.

Initially, Janice had a difficult time with her father's remarriage.

> I was so mad at my father for getting married to her. I think that I was almost a substitute [wife]. I was like a surrogate mother to my sister and I was like a wife to my father. My sister and I had the emotional closeness with my father that my mother did, and we loved it. And now he has a wife, so it's just like, that's it. He can't just spread his emotion out to all of us. It's just one person at a time.

She didn't want to attend the wedding.

> I almost didn't go. I called my relatives and said, "I don't want to go."
> And they said, "Just do it. You'll regret it if you don't. And they'll never
> forgive you either." So I'm glad I went through it. I put on a pretty face at
> the wedding. [Like] "Everything's wonderful!"

However, Janice decided not to spend the next Christmas with her
family, and went to visit a close friend instead.

> I didn't want to go home for Christmas. I didn't want to see her [step-
> mother]. Also, they sold our house. We'd be having Christmas dinner in
> a hotel. My father was really upset [that Janice did not come home for
> Christmas]. My sisters were too. But I had to do it. I needed to relax. I
> needed somebody to take care of me. My friend's family, both her par-
> ents are alive, and her parents treat me like I'm a daughter, so I was
> completely pampered there. I was part of the family.

Later, Janice's new stepmother reached out to her, and tried to re-
unite Jance and her father. "She's the one who remembered my birthday. She's the one who made a real effort to keep in contact with me.
She helped my father. I thought, *Hey, this isn't a bad deal*." One reason Janice can accept her stepmother is that she does not try to take
Janice's mother's place.

> She's my father's wife. She's not a mother. She was my father's new
> wife, and then she was a friend. She never tried to mother us. She's a
> caring person. I don't need her mothering. My mother died. Now I'm
> glad my father married her. She does all she can and I realize that I
> don't see her as a threat anymore.

When Janice returned to college, she buried herself in her studies,
working as hard as she could. She felt elated when she was accepted
into a prestigious graduate school. Her father purchased a condominium for her as a "thank-you" gift for her staying home after her
mother's death.

Long-Term Impact

Janice feels that her mother's illness has affected her relationships
with others, especially men. In talking about one relationship, she
says,

I dated somebody that I really loved. I liked him more than he liked me. I was putting up with so much, and I realized that part of my problem is that I put up with things. I mean, my mother was sick for eight years of my life. I just had to put up with things, had to bear things. [I realized] that things were out of my control and I put up with them. He told me that he cheated on me, and I realized that I didn't have to put up with anybody. I think I still fight with it now. I think about it every day, but the pain isn't as overwhelming as it used to be. What I struggle with now is knowing that I don't have to put up with shit. I don't have to be the martyr.

However, Janice finds herself feeling suspicious when men try to provide support. "I almost reject boyfriends who want to take me under their wing and be like a father figure. I think that they're gonna deceive me along the way." What is difficult for her now is "knowing how to distinguish what is healthy and what is not." Janice notices that her sisters also have issues with relationships. "My younger sister just dates men that treat her like dirt." Janice realizes that she is attracted to men who have intact families.

The guy that I'm sort of dating now comes from a traditional family. I love his parents. They're wonderful. So I wonder, *Are you with him because his family's so great or because you like him?* I have a lot of problems when someone gets too close to me. My immediate reaction is to try to protect myself and I sometimes may become very angry and yell and scream. Sometimes my rage just comes out and it's uncontrollable. When my mother was sick, I was thirteen. I don't know when women first learn to be very angry or to protect themselves. But for me it didn't happen till last year. Sometimes I have so much pain and hurt. I finally realized I was not going to bear it any longer. I think sometimes I'm still experimenting with that, and I just lash out at the people closest to me.

Janice still grieves actively for her mother. "It still hits me every year with a vengeance. It's always tough the day she died. That whole week I sort of go into a depression. I don't know I'm in it until I get out of it." Five years after her mother's death, Janice decided to take control. "I was not going to be depressed [on the anniversary of mother's death]. I tried to do something life-affirming this year." Janice arranged a memorial service. "It was my way of celebrating instead of being depressed and mourning her. I just have to celebrate life. I don't think I could have coped with it any time earlier. I don't think I was ready for it." On Mother's Day, Janice sends cards to women who are important to her. "Mother-like figures. I appreciate them very much. I still need them in my life, but I'm not as close with them anymore."

Janice continues to miss her mother's love and support.

> Other people I grew up with have mothers alive, and they always have that mother's support, which I don't have. When I'm having a tough time in my life, I have no one. No, the maternal unconditional love is not there.

Risk

Initially, Janice was sure she would die from breast cancer, but now she doesn't think about it.

> I thought about it a lot when my mother died. A lot. "I'm gonna die. We're gonna die. We're all gonna die of it. It happened twice. Why not me? At least one of us." I was very, very afraid right after it happened. I was convinced I was gonna die at age forty-eight. I think I thought of it so much for such a long period of time and was obsessed with death, my own death. Now, I'm taking a break from it. Now, I feel like it's possible. But now I haven't thought about it. When I'm thirty I'll think about it. They told me that when I'm thirty I should have my first mammogram. My cousin asked me, "Well, do you do self-breast exams?" And I said no. "Well, why not?" "I just can't. I've never done it."

Janice buys books and gathers literature about breast cancer but doesn't read it. "I'll read it someday. Now, I work more on prevention. I try to eat an organic diet. I do try to reduce caffeine." She exercises, drinks filtered water, and feels she should eat less fat. She avoids alcohol, "not just because of breast cancer, but other things." She also does not take birth control pills. "I had thought about getting on the pill, but I opted not to do that. Unless they come up with a landmark study and say, 'It will not affect you.'"

Janice has considered genetic testing. "Oh, I should do that sometime. But I never make an effort to do it." However, she remains hopeful about the illness. "I hope in the next fifteen years they find a cure for breast cancer."

Current Situation

At the time of our interviews, Janice was deciding to leave her graduate program after her master's degree, and not seek her PhD, although she knew her father would be disappointed. She was proud that she was able to take some rebellious actions, such as violating the rules of the condominium association by keeping two cats. "I'm still rebelling. I'm making up for lost time."

Janice met with her counselor recently, and they celebrated her progress, such as "How my voice was sort of finding itself. It was freed again—no longer muted." After this meeting, Janice walked into a church and sat there for a long time. "I realized that I've been mad at God for a long time. I have a lot of anger, and now I'm not afraid to show it." She found the church experience calming, and she lit candles for people who died. "I'm still spiritual, but not religious. I can't go to church. Not yet. But I think I'll get there eventually."

Janice enjoys running in the Race for the Cure, sponsored by the Susan G. Komen Breast Cancer Foundation, in honor of her mother and grandmother. She enjoyed participating in our study, with the hope that others would be helped. "It helps me deal with the loss." She feels that she would like to meet other women who lost mothers at a similar age. Her family does not discuss her mother, or share remembrances.

> At Christmas, we didn't remember her. I mean, she was in our hearts. When you're through the muck of the grieving process, how do you hold onto the person? My father can't say, "Oh, remember the time when your mother did this?" I can. My father to this day can't deal with his emotions.

Janice thinks she has gained strength as a result of her experience. "I see myself as someone that does very well with emotional stress."

CASE STUDY #2: TRISHA

Age at Her Mother's Breast Cancer Diagnosis: 14; Age at Time of Her Mother's Death: 18

Background

Trisha, who is African American, was raised by her parents in the Northeast. She had four brothers who were substantially older and a twin sister. Trisha's parents were divorced when she was nine. After that, her father lived nearby but was not involved in the children's lives. Mother worked as an electronics technician, assembling personal computer (PC) boards. Trisha was very close to her mother and sister. Trisha loved just lying around with her mother or reading with her. They used to laugh a lot. Her mother would say, "You girls are just crazy!" "She used to laugh a lot because we used to laugh a lot. Me and my sister were just nuts when we were at home."

Her mother's sister lived close by. Trisha's uncle died of cancer when Trisha was about eleven.

Experience with Her Mother's Illness

When Trisha was fourteen, her mother told the girls that she had a lump in her breast.

> We were so young. We were like, "Well, okay, fine." So she went to the doctor and they told her, "Now we're going to do a biopsy." I remember her going back and forth to the doctor a lot. It was serious but we could laugh about it in some ways."

Trisha was never told her mother's diagnosis. "It was, 'This is what we're going to do.' We really didn't talk about it too much at all." When her mother went to the hospital for her surgery, Trisha remembers her mother told the girls not to visit her. "So we went to go see her, and she was like, 'I told you guys not to bring the girls.'"

When mother came home from the hospital,

> She had to wear a little cup under her breast to carry the fluid when you're draining it. Then when they took it out, it was okay. I remember she had to do some exercises. They didn't do a complete removal of the breast. They did breast reconstruction of some sort. That was about all that we really saw. We didn't really do any real talking about it.

Trisha didn't tell her friends at school about her mother's illness.

> It was something that you just don't hear about. I remember that I didn't tell any of my friends though. It's like, "Oh, my mom had to go to the hospital." They are like, "Well, okay!" I was more interested [then] in how things looked.

While her mother was ill, one of Trisha's older brothers and her aunt took on the caretaking duties. "We would do the laundry. My aunt was there and she came over a lot." After the treatment, her mother went in for tests every six months. "After the operation, she still had to go get radiation every six months." Sometimes, Trisha and her sister had to drive her mother places. "We did a lot of driving, because she didn't always drive with her arm. We had to drive her back and forth. Something like that."

Four years later, her mother developed a cough.

> She just thought it was a cold that wasn't ending. So she went to the doctor's, and the doctor said, "Oh, I want to run some tests." And they ran their little tests. So they were like, "The cancer is back again, and there is not really anything we can do this time." So they told her, basically, "You're gonna die. We'll start chemo but we can't promise you anything." They really didn't know [what happened]. They said, "It must have just come out of nowhere." It was like growing so fast and they said it was just everywhere. So we were just like, "Wow." They gave her two months. She lived for five.

During chemo, her mother lost all of her hair, but she was able to return to work.

Mother's recurrence came just as Trisha and her sister were supposed to start college.

> So me and my sister, we're like, "School? Should we go to school? Should we not go to school?" And my brothers were like, "Well, what are you going to do around here? You know, this is what your mom wanted." And so, we went to school. It was crazy! We tried to see if we could go to school later, but my mom would not have been having that. She was like, "I don't think so. Y'all best go to school." So we went to school. She came down with us. So she saw where we went to school.

Trisha's adjustment to college was extremely difficult. She and her twin were at different schools in neighboring states.

> We wrote and we talked every now and then. We did a lot of talking on the phone. I think maybe my family might have been keeping some stuff from me, because they didn't want us to worry. But we were worrying anyway. I think she [mother] was going into remissions [recurrences] and stuff. So when she went into one, we didn't hear from her for a while. If we called her at work and she wasn't there, then we figured maybe that she was at home and she wasn't feeling good. Every now and then that would happen and my brother would give me a call and say, "Okay, this is what's going on."

Trisha did not tell her roommates at college about her mother's illness.

> I didn't really tell anyone. 'Cause it's really hard. You're going to a new school, new environment. You're not really close to anybody. And I

didn't know my roommates before I got there, so they were new people. So they were always worried. They were like, "What's wrong?" After a while I told them, because I was getting phone calls in the middle of the night. If I told them anything, they would always run and get the RA [residential advisor]. "Are you all right?" I was like, "Man, you know, I was just talking." So they would always get nervous. People didn't know how to handle the situation. I mean, they're not even losing their grandparents yet and my mother is dying. They really didn't know what to do. It just made them uncomfortable. It was so pathetic because the RA would say, "Oh, you should reach out to your teachers." And none of my teachers and I were close. It's the first two months of my college career. I'm not close enough to anyone to be pouring out my life!

One time, Trisha's mother asked if she and her sister would like to go to counseling.

My mom said, "The doctor asked today if you guys wanted to go to counseling." And we were just, "What are you talking about, counseling?" I think we just never thought she was going to die. It just didn't occur to us.

Shortly before Thanksgiving, Trisha's brother called.

He was like, "They don't think Mom is going to make it for the next two weeks." And I was like, "Well, I will be home next week." And then he called the next [day] and he's like, "You'd better talk to your mom now, 'cause they don't know if she'll make it through the night." So we talked to her. She wasn't really responding to anything I was saying. So the next morning, I got home. My little sister [cousin] came up to me and she said, "Do you know Mommy died?" I didn't see her before she died.

The funeral was particularly difficult for Trisha's brothers, who do not easily express emotions.

Everybody thought we were the ones they were going to have to worry about, me and my sister. But my brothers were, like, falling on the floor. None of them really made it through the funeral. They took it really hard.

Experience Following Her Mother's Death

After the funeral, Trisha and her sister had to decide where to live.

We decided to live with our brother, 'cause he was the only one who had enough room. My [other] brothers are married and have their own kids and stuff. I go home for Christmas now, but "home" doesn't have the same sense of feeling that it did when my mom was alive. I'm kind of in limbo 'cause I don't have this home that I knew as a home. My brother has his own family. So it's me and my sister. That's all it is.

Trisha returned to school to complete her semester.

We had that week off for Thanksgiving and then I took one more week off. Then I went back to school. My teachers were so nasty. Not all of them were good about it. It was just a lot to deal [with]. It was just a mess.

She contacted the counseling center, and learned of a bereavement group that would be starting the next semester.

So I went to that, and that was pretty good. It was a loss support group, so different people had different losses. It wasn't like everybody could relate, 'cause people lost like a sister or brother. But it was good to know other people around my age had lost people. I didn't do that much talking. I just listened a lot of the time, but it made me feel better to listen.

Trisha and her twin sister became very close during this period.

I talked to my sister a lot. That's about it. My sister went through this whole thing. She wasn't eating and she wasn't doing anything. My brother was there for financial support, but we really haven't talked that much about it. My twin—there was instant role reversal. When my mom died, my sister was my mommy. She was the one that's always got to know about the guys. She's the one that always calls if my grades are screwing up. And, it's the same way with her. She will call me. So, we're "mommy." After my mom died, we talked daily. That daily thing. But now, we go a couple of days without talking.

Trisha visited her sister a couple of times a month.

"After I came back to school, I didn't do anything. I spent a lot of time by myself. I'm pretty much an extrovert. I had to go to work. I like my job. Then I went home." It took Trisha some time to get caught up at school.

I think I really didn't get myself out of my hole until, God, until maybe like sophomore or junior year. Finally, like junior year, I was like, "Look, you'd better get yourself together if you're ever going to go to grad school."

One problem for Trisha was dealing with the reactions of others.

> I didn't talk about it a lot. Some of my friends still don't know. I think I was uncomfortable. I didn't want people to focus on the fact that "Oh, her mother died." I don't like people to be all sympathetic. I'd rather they like me for who I am. I had this big thing with "Oh, I feel so sorry for you." I can't stand that. I felt like everybody was looking at me: "That's the girl whose mother died." I'm sure my roommates had their own little group discussions about me while I was gone. "We don't know what to say to you. We don't know what to do." And I really didn't know how to handle that. One time I was like, "All right, I'm gonna share with them." So I started telling them that I miss my mom, and this is what Mom used to do and, oh my God, you would think that I just said I was having a heart attack! They took it the wrong way. They were so worried. They thought something was wrong, wrong. And I don't know how to handle "You are so strong." Still to this day I really have a hard time with people saying things like that. And some people, when they find out, they're horrified, 'cause people make silly comments. Then they feel worse when they find out. But I can't get mad with them because I'm not sharing. If someone asks me if I live with my parents, I just say, "No. I live with my brother." I don't say, "Well, my mom died." 'Cause that's when this sympathy thing comes in. And I'm like, "Oh man, I done got myself into this one again." I hate that to be the first thing that people know about me.

Trisha sometimes thinks about how things could have been had she stayed home from college the fall her mother died.

> One thing I'll always be, not jealous, but I'll feel like, man, he [brother] had something with her that I'll never have because he was home with her that whole month and a half. He was there. That's one thing I fuss with myself, too. Why didn't I just go home? You know, she only had a week left. But I don't regret it or anything. I just wonder, why didn't I just go home?

Trisha's family gathers every Thanksgiving, which is the anniversary of her mother's death. "Thanksgiving, the whole family gets together at home. We always sit around and talk. It always gets back to my mother somehow. We don't sit around and mourn. It's happy."

Another special thing that Trisha did was take her mother's ashes on a trip with her.

> She wanted to be cremated. We never got to travel when we were little and she always wanted us to travel. When I took this trip abroad, I took the ashes with me. So I put them everywhere we went. So that was nice.

Also, on her mother's birthday, Trisha tries to do something special. "I'll do something, like I'll buy flowers. She always liked things like flower pots. Or, I'll get up early. She used to get up in the morning. Something that I remember about her." Trisha and her sister still talk about their mom. "If I feel depressed, I'll call her up and be like, you know, 'I miss Mom.' Then she'll say, 'Okay.' We might just talk about her for a little while. That's what we do."

Long-Term Impact

Trisha says one result of her mother's death is that she had to grow up fast.

> Like the independent thing. I have to take care of myself. I pay my own bills. I don't have anybody to say, "Send me some money." I got a whole lot more responsibilities. 'Cause I'm on my own. Sometimes I get frustrated. Sometimes I just want somebody to do something for me. You learn to deal with it, I guess.

Risk

> I get nervous getting close to people, being that it [cancer] runs in my family. 'Cause my grandmother had [bone] cancer and my mom had cancer. So I think it makes me nervous sometimes when I get close to someone. I'm like, "Oh, man!" When I do my breast exam myself, it makes me nervous. I think, "God!" It's so crazy. Why should I be so nervous every time I go to touch my own breast? I'm like, "Oh, man! I've got to do a breast exam." Just going through that whole thing, I would be so scared if I woke tomorrow and had a lump in my breast.

Current Situation

At the time of the interview, Trisha had completed college and had her first job working in a bank. She planned to return to school for a master's degree. Shortly after the interview, Trisha and her sister enrolled in the volunteer program AmeriCorps. She was assigned out of the area and so no further interviews were possible.

CASE STUDY #3: ALICIA

Age at Her Mother's Breast Cancer Diagnosis: 15; Age at Time of Her Mother's Death: 19

Background

Alicia, who is from a Jewish family, lived with her mother, father, and older brother. Alicia's grandmother had died of breast cancer when she was fifty-three, and Alicia's mother was

> crazed about breast cancer. She worried about it all the time. She told us that she was going to die of breast cancer when she reached fifty-three. Whenever we were bad, she would say, "You can treat me miserably, but I'm going to die when I'm fifty-three." I didn't believe her.

Alicia's mother was brilliant, but didn't really enjoy being a mother. "She was very emotionally abusive to me. I was quite different than she, educationally, built differently, and I was very popular and friends were important to me, and dating." When Alicia began to enjoy her adolescence, her relationship with her mother deteriorated.

> She had these ideas in her head that I was a wild girl, which I really wasn't. I was very developed at a young age and she had a hard time dealing with the acceptance of my body maturing. She was convinced I was wearing falsies. She just had a hard time with anything dealing with bodies. When those breasts grew, she just went crazy. It all had to do with this disease, I'm convinced. We had a very strained mother-daughter relationship. I think that she really didn't feel good about herself as a woman, and didn't enjoy being a mother.

Alicia's mother had two aunts whom Alicia used to visit on her vacations.

Experience of Her Mother's Illness

When Alicia was fifteen, her mother detected a lump in her breast, but didn't seek medical attention for about six months. During this period, Alicia remembers that

> She was crazy. She really went off when she found the lump. I think she was in a great deal of pain at that point. She started drinking prior to disclosing the lump [to me]. It was kind of abnormal behavior. She

predicted she was going to be dead soon, and she did a lot of drinking and was just very, very unhappy.

Her mother had a radical mastectomy.

By the time they did do the surgery, it was pretty advanced. It had gone into the other breast and I guess at that time they didn't want to tell her how severe it was and they didn't remove both breasts. They did a radical [mastectomy]. And she was so upset. She had this thing in her head about death. Her first words to me in her [hospital] room when I went to see her were, "I'm no longer a woman. I can no longer be your mother." She felt dismembered, like the funny lady in the circus. She felt she was peculiar and weird and disfigured. And from the age of about sixteen, she was really never my mother.

Alicia never saw her mother's scar. "She never wanted to show it to me. I sort of got a glimpse one time, but I didn't see the whole thing." During the period from the surgery until her death,

she became more and more detached from me emotionally. Wanting me to grow up and become more independent. She would go about her chores, you know, the traditional housewife, cooking and having meals ready, but she really was no longer a mother. She did a lot of drinking and she would drink so much [that] right after dinner she would go to sleep. She was just very depressed. She kept seeing the cancer go through her body and she suffered painfully. Emotionally painfully. It could be one hundred degrees and she'd be complaining and yelling. I'm sure she felt miserable and tired and weak from the radiation and everything else, and he [father] still expected dinner to be made and on the table at six o'clock. The demands on her were great, and I was no support. I really wasn't. I didn't volunteer to do anything. I just went about my life. I would just seek salvation in my friends and in the guys I was dating. I did a lot of crying in those days, and talking to my friends. And I would talk a great deal to my brother. He was a very big support.

During this period, Alicia's father never talked about her mother's illness.

He does not do well with anybody that's ill. We don't talk about illnesses. He called it "the condition." He didn't want to deal with it. In those days they didn't have any counseling or anything, so they copped her on to lithium, and she was having a hard time balancing all these medications. She was just really miserable. I just tried to be away from home as much as possible. When I did come home, we used to have big battles. I couldn't understand her not understanding me. Being a teenager and self-centered, I didn't want to deal with her. I didn't really want to know what she was going through. She would always say, "Oh, I'm gonna die. I'm gonna die." It was almost as if she was playing on my sympathies to manipulate me to do what she wanted me to do. Sometimes I wished she would die because she was so abusive to me.

During this period, Alicia tried to form relationships with other mother figures.

I guess I was seeking out this mother. I had a really good friend [who] lived across the street. Her mother got involved because when I called the hospital to find out how my mother was after surgery, they said, "Your mother has breast cancer." And I ran across the street to my friend's house and I told her mother and I was hysterical. I kept trying to find it [mothering] in friendships and in my friends' mothers and guys.

Alicia went off to college. At the end of her freshman year, her father came to pick her up and said,

"Your mother's home sick. She has a virus and you may have to take care of her." So I came home and I took care of her up until the day before she died, eventually giving her bedpans and suctioning straws so that she could get a bit of liquid in. He never told me she was dying, and I was young and naive and kept thinking she had a virus. She just stayed up in the room, and I would cook for my father and became in charge of the household, which I never did [before].

During this period, Alicia had some positive interactions with her mother.

She and I had some time together. That was sort of important bonding time for me with her. It was the first time ever that we had shared even to say "I love you." We could just share. The bedpans smelled and she would apologize and say, "I'm gonna get well, and I'll make it up to you." She was apologizing for all kinds of horrible things she did to me as a parent. It was an amazing time, and I was very lucky to have that. In the end, I really felt remorse. I started keeping a journal and becoming very religious and praying to God or some spiritual being that was going to take it [the illness] away from her and make her well.

Alicia recalls her mother's final hours with detail:

One night the doctor came over. He told my father that she was going to die in twenty-four hours. I called my brother and told him, "You need to come home. Mom's really sick." And he didn't believe me. He said, "Aw, you're being emotional." So my aunt called him and said, "You really need to come home. This is serious." So he came home. She [mother] was very bonded to my brother. They were very, very, very close. But she just told him to get out. At that moment she just wanted me. We had a nurse then, and she [mother] kept throwing up, and I kept throwing up, 'cause whenever I got stressed, I would throw up, and the nurse would be running back and forth between the two rooms. I just kept praying with all my might, *Don't die. Don't leave me. Don't die.* It was awful. The next morning, the nurse said we needed to go to the drugstore to get some syringes. Mother was going back and forth with her head. Talking incoherently. In just miserable pain. So we went, and when we came back, my brother came outside and he said, "I've got to tell you something." And I said, "No way are you telling me anything." I ran down the street. And he ran after me and said, "You've got to hear me. You've got to face facts. Your mother died." And I kept saying, "She didn't die. She didn't die." And they wouldn't let me go up-stairs and see her. I saw my father was on the phone in the den crying. My father would never cry. And finally my uncle said, "Let her come up-stairs." And they brought me upstairs. She was lying there but her eyes were sort of open, and I said, "She's just sleeping." And they said, "No. She's dead." And they made me touch her, and it was this dank cold-ness that [stayed in] my hands and arms for weeks. I was afraid to touch anybody. It was just awful. They put her in a bag, and then they came down the stairs. They were, like, bumping her [on the stairs]. It was really bad.

Alicia remembers that her aunt bought her a dress.

They bought me this brown dress that I still have hanging in my father's house. [I remember] picking out flowers to put on the coffin. [They] made me part of the whole funeral process. I liked the support of hav-ing other people around me. We sat shiva and people were in and out. High school friends came in and out. That was really helpful.

Experience Following Her Mother's Death

Shortly before her mother's death, Alicia had fallen "madly in love" with a young man her mother didn't approve of. Because of her mother's opposition, Alicia broke off her relationship with this boy-friend. "My mother died in June, and he [boyfriend] left in July, and my brother left [to study abroad] in August. And I was running the house, cooking for my father. I filled in my mother's role, cooking and cleaning." Describing her father during this period, Alicia says, "He was really painfully lonely. I just felt responsible for him. He never showed any real emotion. He would always talk her up, even though their marriage was lousy." That fall, Alicia transferred to a college closer to home.

> I would come home weekends and cook for him, and freeze meals and do his laundry. I just took on the responsibility of caring for Dad. My father would call me every night at college 'cause he was lonely. He used to call every night. The remaining three years of college were horrible. I just had a horrible, horrible time. I think I was lost. I was just a lost soul. I felt like I was so needy and nobody understood me. Everyone would be going home for Christmas vacation, and everybody was all geared up and excited. Their mothers were going to bake them their favorite meals and go shopping with them and see a show together. I'd go home and the house would be empty. Dad would be at work. I'd walk in and the house would talk to me. I'd see my mother dead on the bed, and the memories were just . . . I'd go home to nothing and it was real hard having to go to the store and start to cook the dinner. Life was just very empty.

Alicia often visited her mother's grave while in college. "I would come home and swing by and just sit there and cry and cry. I was so miserable. Nothing made me happy and I spent a lot of time there."

After graduating from college, Alicia moved back with her father. At this point, he had remarried.

> I was happy that he had somebody, because it took a lot of stress off of me. But my relationship with him changed from being like his equal to back to being his daughter. I had a very hard time with that. I was no longer his confidante. I disliked her immensely. They bought a house together, which I was very angry about. We were packing up our house, and we all were going to move into another house. It was very bad. My father was put in the middle many, many times between me and this other woman and it was not nice. It was not good.

At about the same time, Alicia's brother got married. "I was pretty angered about that and felt that he abandoned and left me too."

Fairly soon after her father and brother were each married, Alicia fell in love with and married a young lawyer. At her wedding, Alicia says,

> I was standing outside the sanctuary, and I was crying because I felt the loss of my mother. It was very weird. We had a florist, an old man who looked like a fisherman, with a long beard and the most sensitive eyes. He just sort of appeared to me and said, "You look beautiful! When you walk down the aisle, hold your head high and kick your foot and take your strides slowly." I didn't know where he came from. I believe that there are miracles and messages that are sent. I looked at

my father and said, "That was Mom! She wanted me to know that she was here." It's happened so many significant times in my life to let me know that she's there. It's just been amazing.

Alicia also feels that her mother's spirit helped her find her husband.

I never found Mother until I got married. I really lucked out. Everybody that knows me knows that I believe my mother had part to do with it. I always believe that. That he [husband] serves all these important roles in my life. In emotional needs, he got me to who I am today.

Long-Term Impact

Alicia believes her mother's death impacted her personality.

Because of my experience with my mother, I'm happiest when I'm really more programmed. And my time is so precious. The older I get, the more selective I am with friends. And I create islands to be with just my family. I run during the day with my activities. I enjoy the work that I do. I see I make a difference in people's lives. I love being a social worker. It's definitely who I am.

Alicia is aware that her children seem to watch out for her.

My daughter was going to go to [a school far from home] and she freaked out and said, "I don't want to go that far away from home." And I said, "Well, why not?" And she said, "Well, what if something happens to you? Something happened to your mother when you went away to college and you told me you were too far from home." And I keep saying, "I'm not my mother." But inside I'm thinking, *Well, how do I know?* My son also feels very nurturing toward me. He doesn't like to see me upset. I don't want them to take care of me. I want them to be normal kids. They don't have to worry about Mom. Mom's emotionally strong and can handle it. And if I can't, I've got a great husband who can; I've got friends who understand. My brother's great and my sister-in-law's great. I have support systems. And when I feel that I can't handle it, I always go back for counseling.

Alicia continues to fear abandonment. This affects her relationships with friends.

Even today, I think it affects the way I relate to people. I know that I'm very needy. I need friends. I need people around but yet, I don't do a lot of sharing, because I don't want to take advantage of friendships. Fear of abandonment is very hard for me, obviously. Even with my daughter leaving to go to college, I take it as almost an abandonment thing. I have to be really careful when I deal with her. And I think it all has to do with this initial loss. It has intensified the feeling that this is the end of the family time. The kids are growing and, when we all [Alicia and her brother] started to be at this age, it was really the end of our family time.

Risk

Alicia is very anxious about getting breast cancer at the age her mother and grandmother died.

> I worry tremendously about my own health. All the time. I've worried about breast cancer since the time she died. I just felt there was a genetic link, and I'm just scared. I do mammograms once a year, and I go to a breast specialist three times a year. So every three months I'm being checked. I have a hard time doing breast self-exams myself. I don't do them.

Alicia had a breast cancer scare at thirty-five.

> They thought they found something. I just remember shutting down. I could not eat. Could not sleep. I had to wait two days before I could go see the surgeon. Fortunately he thought it was nothing. But that forty-eight-hour period was pure hell.

Getting her annual mammogram is very stressful for Alicia. "Getting ready to go, the whole day before, I have diarrhea, I can't sleep, I can't eat. The minute they just mention my name, I burst into tears. I'm a mess!"

Alicia is starting to go through menopause.

> I struggle now with going on estrogen or not going on estrogen. I should be on estrogen. I desperately need it. The doctors want to put me on it. They are very insensitive. [They say] "If you get breast cancer, we'll monitor you closely. We'll get it [early]." But to me, breast cancer still signals a little bit of a death sentence. I don't believe you can get rid of it and be healthy, even though I have seen many women get over it. For me, there's too much [of a] leap of faith in that.

Alicia is very fearful of being fifty-three years old—the age at which both her mother and grandmother died.

> Every birthday that comes, I get more and more depressed, because it's getting closer to fifty-three, and fifty-three is the big number. Every day of my life, fifty-three comes up. I get fifty-three cents change, or I'll turn on TV and its fifty-three degrees outside. And my kids look at me. They all know that number. I've told all my friends, "I'm going to have a big party at fifty-four, and if you don't know why, you can't come in the door."

Alicia recognizes many differences between her behavior and her mother's regarding risk factors.

> She smoked. I've never smoked. She was heavy, didn't exercise. I exercise a lot. I eat a healthier diet. I do everything I can do that I know. And that gives me some kind of false hope, I guess. I keep thinking, *Well, I'm not her. I don't live her life. I'm totally different.* Emotionally, I'm a lot healthier. I'm happy. I don't think she was happy. I love being a mother. I love being a woman. I'm not my mother. Hopefully I have my father's genes.

Alicia has followed the discovery of breast cancer genes with interest.

> I was thinking of doing the testing. I'm scared to do it. At first, I thought that if it came back positive I would go in and have mastectomies with implants. Then I decided that would be too radical for who I really am. I would just want to know genetically if I'm predisposed to it, for the estrogen purpose, and for my daughter. For my peace of mind. If it turned out yes, then I would just monitor myself even closer. If it was not, I wouldn't decrease what I was doing, but I might live my life a little freer. I would go on estrogen. And I think I would loosen up with my daughter. I would feel better about her own sexuality. So I'm leaning toward it, but I'm scared. I'm so afraid of medical confidentiality. If I did it, I would pay cash, and use somebody else's Social Security number. To find out I'm not [genetically predisposed] would be the greatest liberation for me, but I don't know if I can handle finding out that I could be.

Current Situation

Alicia was forty-six at the time of the interviews. Alicia has a number of her mother's things, and these are precious to her, especially her mother's wedding ring, which carries special significance. "I wear the ring every day." Alicia always remembers her mother on her birthday and her parents' anniversary. "I still remember their anniversary date, and think, *What would I have brought? What would I have done?*" Mother's Day is "not as bad 'cause now I have my own children. My own family. And I have a mother-in-law."

Now that Alicia has her own children, she does not actively mourn for her mother.

> I don't go there [mother's grave] often [anymore]. If I do go, I have my children and I don't want them to see it as something so sad, so that they don't feel that if it happens to me that it's such a terrible thing. It's just what happens in life. I don't want them to feel the way I do.

During the study, Alicia's daughter decided to have breast-reduction surgery.

> We went through a big trauma because she's built a lot like my mother. She's tiny, with very big breasts. She has been wanting a breast reduction. And I just couldn't deal with it. The thought of anybody tampering with my daughter's breasts, and her coming home bandaged up. It just freaked me out and I could not stop crying. Finally, she [daughter] said, "You've lived your life. Why can't I live mine? Why do you have to keep bringing up your mother and what happened to you? Why don't you see me? I'm not you and I'm not your mother!"

Alicia's daughter had the surgery, and when she was in the hospital, Alicia had a vision.

> It's like my mother came to me and said, "I lived fifty-three years hating my body. [Daughter's name] should live out her days being as happy as she can be and if this is gonna give her the sense of happiness, you have to support that." All of a sudden, it clicked in me and I felt good about it. It was weird, the whole experience.

CASE STUDY #4: VERONICA

Age at Her Mother's Breast Cancer Diagnosis: 16; Age at Time of Her Mother's Death: 19

Background

Veronica, the oldest of three girls, was raised in a professional African-American family. Her father was a physician and her mother taught in an elementary school. Veronica described her mother as kind, gentle, and very supportive, while her father played the role of a stern but supportive disciplinarian who pushed Veronica to achieve. Her father always expected Veronica to become a doctor. "He sort of, like, guided me to become a doctor, exposed me to science. If he was going to a conference, he would bring me along." Veronica had an unusual relationship with her father.

> We had developed a friendship aside from a father and daughter. We could talk. I could call him about anything, even relationships I was having with guys. When I got my period, I told him about it. You know, most daughters wouldn't tell their father. This meant a lot to him, that I felt comfortable sharing something that normally would have been just

the domain of females. I think he trusted me and gave me more latitude than what you would expect. Just to contrast, I couldn't tell my mother everything because I had the sense that my mother was a prude. This was at the time of the "sexual revolution," and my mother wasn't for that sort of thing. My father would at least discuss it. The relationship with my mother, I think she counted on me as the oldest daughter that was gonna do well in school, not give her much trouble. When I became an adolescent, some of the sexual development issues that I was dealing with really worried her and became a source of conflict for us. Because my father was more permissive, I almost feel like I was closer to my father than I was to my mother. But then my mother was like a buffer or a balance against my father's intenseness and controlling. There was a softness and a gentleness to her approach that I think I really appreciated.

Experience of Her Mother's Illness

At sixteen, Veronica was preparing to leave for college at a very prestigious university. The family was on vacation when her mother discovered a lump.

[Mother said] "Oh, Veronica, I found this lump in my breast." And I was like, "Oh, Mommy, don't worry. It'll be okay. It's probably nothing. Just get it checked out." Of course, I had just wanted it to be a benign thing.

Veronica had hardly gotten settled at college when her father arrived unexpectedly at her dorm.

When my father came up, he told me that she had had the surgery to look at what the tumor was, and when they discovered right then and there that it was malignant, they removed her breast and lymph nodes. I remember being really angry that there wasn't some other way that they could have dealt with it without removing her breast.

Veronica saw her mother later that fall.

She was fine. I mean, she looked really good. I know I was going through some changes, not so much about her breast cancer but just being out on my own finally and sort of feeling my oats, feeling independent and probably being sort of frisky. My mother noticed that I was behaving differently. I remember she said, "You're sort of snappy." So I think what overshadowed my concerns about my mother was that I was getting into a new life, and it was exciting. Making new friends, my courses, and having my own place. It was like being emancipated. And there was a guy that I met who was in love with me and just started showering me with all this attention. So I was all wrapped up in that too.

That probably distracted me from really dwelling on my mother at that time. After I saw her at Thanksgiving, she just looked so good. She looked like she'd been on vacation. She didn't look like she'd been through a really major operation. And she was just herself. So that gave me a false sense of security that everything was all right. The cancer was gone. Okay. They took her breast. That was a shame. But she looks great and she seems fine.

Veronica remembers seeing her mother's scar.

I mean, in a sense, I was horrified, because it seemed like mutilation. But the fact that I was planning to be a doctor, and had been exposed to medical stuff, I was trained not to look at something and go, "Oh, my God!" But to look at it from a scientific standpoint. But it was just such a shame. She was really a beautiful person and to have to lose a body part that is so symbolic of female attractiveness . . .

For the next two years, Veronica's mother was healthy. "I think throughout my college years it was always in the back of my mind that she had had cancer. That hopefully it was all gone. The way she looked helped reassure me." When Veronica was a junior, she came home for Christmas, and noticed that

something didn't seem right. I think my mother might have been coughing a little bit, and she wasn't as meticulous about her dress as she had always been. She was a shopper and she always looked really nice. I think she started getting depressed and she was forgetting things and maybe having shortness of breath.

Shortly after Veronica returned to school, her mother was diagnosed with metastases to the brain and lung. When Veronica heard that her mother would have to begin chemotherapy, she volunteered to take a semester off and return home to help out.

It was weird because I felt like it was my responsibility to help her because I just didn't know who else was gonna be there to take her. I took a lot of weight off my father because I could drive her to her appointments and so forth.

Veronica arranged with her advisor to stay in school, but to do the work from home, returning only for exams. Thinking about why her father agreed to this, Veronica says,

Either because he thought that I should do it—it made sense to him— or it was a way for him to save money. But maybe having somebody who was a stranger didn't seem like a good idea. By having me do it, I knew my mother and there was that closeness and it was a way for her to maintain her dignity without dragging in some stranger—sort of just like keeping her care as much within the family as possible.

Life at home was difficult for Veronica during this period.

I can remember taking my mother back and forth to these chemotherapy appointments, and she would just be so sick after them. I could never understand. *Why does she have to go through all this? This is terrible.* And then she started losing her hair. In my family, and I guess in most black families, hair was, like, a big deal. She always prided herself on looking nice. Not only was her hair nice, she was always well groomed and very tastefully dressed. So when she started losing her hair, that was a nightmare for both of us. I remember it was just sort of coming out in clumps. She did a good job not to show that she was freaking out about it. I mean, you could tell she was sad, but she didn't really lose it. I remember we went to this wig shop and she was trying them on. "Well, how does this one look? Which is the best one?" I've always felt bad about this because the wig that we ended up choosing, I really didn't like. I think I said it looked good just to reassure her. In the end, she started going without the wig, wearing her hair bald. I remember one of her close friends took her shopping, and the people who saw her were saying how striking she was. I was really proud of her. She was very humble about it. It's just sort of like, "Well, this is me and this is what I'm going through and you people can take it or leave it."

One of Veronica's most precious memories from this period was a simple hug from her mother.

I think I had come home from school, and . . . we embraced at the door when I came in. She just gave me a really long hug, and it was a really nice hug. She said something like, "I really love you!" It just really always stuck with me.

During her mother's illness, Veronica began to question whether medicine was the right career for her.

I had been premed all along, and as I saw her suffering, saw what a disease like cancer could do to somebody, I started questioning whether I wanted to pursue medicine as a career. I was like, "Wait a minute. If I'm going to have to be dealing with people who are sick like this, and suffering, I don't know if I can deal with it. I don't know that I want to deal with it." I remember getting this bright idea that I would go into advertising, and get a master's in business administration. I talked to my mother about it, and she was encouraging me. She was saying, "If that's what you want to do, you should do it." And my father went ballistic. He said, "You'll never survive in the business world. You're too sensitive for that. And besides, I can't help you in business."

Veronica goes on: "It got really hard when she started being really sick. Weak and vomiting and just not wanting to get up. Just not being herself. She was really weary from the whole process." Veronica has one disturbing memory from this period.

> I was going to get the car after her chemotherapy treatment and she was standing in front of the office. Before I could get the car up to the front steps of the building, she fell. I think she was hurt and embarrassed, and she was crying. I blamed myself that I wasn't there for her, but the truth is I couldn't be in two places at the same time.

Another time, Veronica remembered

> her [mother] calling out to me to help her shower. And I had feelings like, "I wish she could do this by herself!" I just wanted her to be okay and not need me as much as she did. I had some guilt feeling because of being a little impatient. I tried not to show those feelings. I mean, I came to her aid, but I had that attitude. I was maybe a little bit short and irritable. I don't like that about myself, that I had those feelings.

Veronica admits that at times she

> felt overwhelmed by it. I guess I felt helpless because there really wasn't anything I could do. At times, I felt angry and resentful that I had to be the one to do this. I think in some ways we were spoiled growing up. We had chores and responsibilities, but I don't think we were ever prepared to be in a primary nurturing role. I know my mother and I know that she knew that I was doing that. I know that that may have made her feel bad because she was depending on me to help her and I don't think she wanted to feel like she was a burden to me.

In addition to Veronica, the family had help from a housekeeper and one of her mother's friends. By fall, when Veronica returned to college "she [mother] had lost a whole lot of weight and her abdomen was very swollen from the liver metastasis. She had cognitive losses, so she couldn't think well. Her memory wasn't good and she was depressed." Still, Veronica remained hopeful—until her mother lost consciousness. "She was not exactly in a coma, but she became unresponsive. She was just there, breathing, basically. So I think I knew at that point that unless a miracle occurred, there was no turning back." Veronica and her mother never talked openly about death.

> I remember her saying something like, "Well, I don't care what your father does as long as he just takes care of my children." So sort of underneath that was that, "I [mother] know that I'm gonna die and that's all I really care about—just take care of my children."

Veronica remembers that at this point, her father "pretty much hid his feelings. He was really attentive to her, and really aggressive about making sure she had the best care. In the hospital, he arranged to get some nurses to take care of her around the clock."

Veronica was home when her mother died.

> We were in the living room, and Daddy said, "I want you all to come downstairs. I need to tell you something." And he told us that Mommy died in the hospital. I don't know if I cried or was numb. I don't think I really cried until the funeral. We chose the dress that she would wear and we went to the funeral home to make sure that she looked all right. I touched her and she was cold, and it was just so, so . . . deep. I think it was just so unbelievable to me. Like, "How could this be happening? This is just so weird." I just didn't think this was going to happen. It seemed unreal, like a strange dream.

Veronica remembers that she "held it together" until after the funeral, when she hugged a family friend that was her grandmother's age. "Maybe just the way that she hugged me, or just seeing her, sort of released all of the emotions that I had, and the floodgates opened." Her aunt [mother's sister] came up from their home in the south for the funeral; her mother's parents did not attend. "My grandmother said it just hurt her too bad. She just couldn't deal because she was closest to my mother of all her children."

Experience Following Her Mother's Death

Shortly after her mother's death, Veronica's family went to Mexico for a vacation. "It was my father's idea. Just to allow us to be together as a family and to go someplace nice and sort of chill out. Maybe we saw this trip as a way to heal." Following the trip, Veronica returned to college.

> That was hard. It was hard for me to concentrate on my work. You know, I would have dreams about my mother. I was feeling sad and alone and thinking a lot about death. Trying to understand the spiritual aspects of death. Like, where did she go? Trying to believe that her spirit stayed with us.

Veronica's cousin attended the same college. "I basically moved in with her. She was very supportive and really got me through that tough time." Veronica failed her physics course and had to spend the summer at school to retake it. A school friend's family took her in and she stayed with them.

Both of Veronica's younger sisters had difficulty after their mother's death.

> My youngest sister wasn't really doing well in school. She couldn't play the piano anymore. She said she just "couldn't even hear the music" and refused to play. She stopped grooming herself, and her hair was matted. My father sent my sisters up to stay with me for a week or something. It was like she hadn't combed [her hair] since my mother died. I realized, "Oh, my God. Here's my little sister, and Mommy died, and Mommy was the one who would have looked after these things." This is a part of our upbringing that my father just wasn't involved in. It just brought it home, like, "What do you expect?" When I saw the condition her hair was in, I made her get a haircut. That was one of the first motherly decisions that I made. I think she hated me for a while after that, because she ended up getting, like, a short natural [style], which was sort of avant-garde then.

Veronica became a kind of surrogate mother to her younger sister.

> I think in some ways it sort of came naturally. I remember her when she was a little baby. I actually had a role in changing diapers and she and I always had a really close relationship. My middle sister was sort of in charge of my younger sister. To this day my younger sister talks about how mean and neglectful she was. I think my father put her in charge, and she was not responsible. My father was traveling a lot, and I remember talking with him about, "Something is gonna have to change. This isn't right." And that was the point where he looked into finding a boarding school for my youngest sister to go to.

Veronica's middle sister was "running wild in the streets" at this point. "That was just part of her personality, but after my mother died, she probably ran harder because suddenly the whole family structure was gone. At least when my mother was there, she could exert some discipline." Veronica didn't feel comfortable disciplining her middle sister because,

> when I was a teenager, almost anything my mother told me was just not right, or I wasn't going to go along with, and if I did, it would be with an attitude. So she was that way with me. Like, "What can you say to

me?" Maybe I was doing some of the same things that she was. I probably really couldn't say anything because it would be like the pot calling the kettle black.

Veronica recently learned that her maternal relatives had offered to have the girls move in with them, but their father had said no.

He said he could take care of his own children. When you think about what happened, he sent my younger sister to boarding school and my other sister was almost ready for college but she was just basically running wild, so maybe he was in denial about how much supervision and attention my sisters really needed.

Veronica's middle sister left college after one year and went to stay with her grandmother in the South. "She wasn't getting along with my father, and I think she had some unresolved issues around mothering. So she went to be with my grandmother. I think they became very close during that time." Veronica's sisters felt somewhat disposed of. "My father was not meeting his responsibilities," says Veronica.

Veronica was at the time trying to decide on a graduate school.

I had a dilemma about whether I should apply to medical school near home, so that I could be with my sisters, or apply away so that I could separate myself and not be saddled with those responsibilities. I knew that medical school was going to be hard, and I wasn't ready for all these additional responsibilities. If I had wanted to stay home and go to medical school locally, it would have relieved my father of some stuff. I remember talking to our next-door neighbor, who was sort of extended family. The mother sort of took an interest in me and was just psychologically very supportive. She encouraged me to go away.

Veronica was accepted to Howard University; she decided to enroll there. This meant leaving home, but she was eager to attend a black school.

I had always gone to white schools all my life, and both my parents had gone to historically black colleges and they had always told me just what a positive experience that had been for them. How they found so much encouragement and dedication from the teachers who took a special interest. That turned out to be a very good experience and very nurturing at a time when I probably needed it.

Even though Veronica decided to go away to school, in part an effort to escape the responsibility of caring for her sisters, it seemed like my sisters found me. My middle sister ended up going to Howard [too], and my youngest sister went to a boarding school in Virginia. I remember the car that I had been driving was getting ready to break down, so my father wanted to buy me a [new] car. He ended up getting a station wagon so that I could get my sisters—[a car] just like a mother would have—which I really didn't like.

Veronica felt that it was normal for the sisters to become independent at this point, and she resented the added responsibility of her sisters' needs.

As the oldest and as a college student, I felt there was a silent pressure on me to rescue the family during my mother's illness and after her death. It was difficult to juggle family issues and school/career issues simultaneously. I felt like I was in a no-win situation—guilty if I didn't help out, afraid of ruining my future if I did.

Following her mother's death, Veronica and her maternal grandmother became very close.

She [grandmother] said, "You know, I'm your mother now." She didn't want me to feel like a motherless child. I used to call her all the time, like at five o'clock in the morning. I would tell her just all sorts of things, stuff about relationships or school.

When her grandmother died suddenly, it was extremely difficult for Veronica.

It was unexpected. I had a delayed grief response to her dying. I couldn't cry at her funeral or for months. Then one day, somebody reminded me of her and I was really, really devastated. The loss of her was really compounded because she was such a key person in my support system. Just being able to communicate with her on a regular basis and have her encouragement was really important.

Veronica was determined that her mother's illness and death not affect her school performance.

It was so important for me not to use my mother's illness and death as an excuse for what I didn't do or how I didn't perform. I think I was depressed for most of my college years and I don't know to what extent it was related to my mother's illness, but that played a role. It's taken me all these years of distance from that time to appreciate that I was really trying too hard to prove to other people that I wasn't going to use my mother's death as an excuse for things. That fits with the theme of being the strong one and sort of, like, just dealing with stuff and having it really not touch me.

Veronica's father began dating about a year after her mother died.

> It felt a little strange at first, but I understood that he needed companionship, and the woman he started seeing, who is still with him today, is a really nice person. I liked her. My sisters did not at first. They gave her a hard time. My father has not married her, and some people think it's because, you know, nobody could replace my mother. But she has become our surrogate mother. She's a very nurturing person, and she treats us like we are her daughters. We're very close. And she has really made a big difference, [for example, with] the womanhood sort of issues that she's helped me with over the years.

Long-Term Impact

Veronica continues to grieve her mother's death.

> November is a bad month. Fall is just a bad time. The leaves are falling and stuff is dying. It's getting dark earlier. Everything is all gloom. My mother died in November, and so it just all seems to go with that theme. When November comes, I usually feel pretty down. Everybody does. My sisters, we've talked about this. On that particular day, we usually talk to each other over the phone. That's a day that we usually reach out.

Christmas is also very difficult for Veronica.

> [In the past], my family would put on these shows. Everybody would work on a dance and stuff and it was a lot of fun. After my mother died, Christmas was just this haunting, empty thing. She [mother] was really the moving force behind those programs, and so, after she was gone, we just couldn't do it. I think at times I was just plain old depressed, and that has continued. It was really hard to get the spirit. Maybe when I have children myself, I'll be able to re-create some of the holiday magic.

Veronica especially missed her mother at her wedding. "When I got married, I did everything myself. That was definitely a time I would have liked her input. I think that my mother had a certain grace and style." Veronica had a painting of her mother placed on an easel near the altar. "It was sort of symbolic of her, and she really liked yellow roses, so I made sure there were yellow roses in the house and in my bouquet that I carried." Veronica appreciated that her girlfriend mentioned her mother in a toast and "that she had always been so kind to her. It was nice the way she did it."

Veronica has a videotape of her mother teaching music to her elementary school class. When Veronica recently saw the tape, she cried. "It was just so her." She sometimes dreams about her mother. "I had a dream maybe four or five days ago that my mother and I were together and that we went shopping. It felt really good." Sometimes in her dreams, her mother is "elusive" and she finds these dreams disturbing. "In the morning [after these dreams], I might feel sad, or frustrated, or angry that she had to die."

Risk

Veronica realized recently that she is now about the same age her mother was when she died.

> It has crossed my mind that my mother was a little older than I am now when she died, which just totally blows my mind. I guess she knew that she could die when she got this diagnosis. But to realize that you're actually going to die at a very young age, and leave your family, is just incredible! It puts me in touch with my mortality more than the average person, because I know it could happen. Hopefully it won't.

Veronica does breast self-exams and has been having mammograms. "I've been getting them since I was thirty-two. I was just nervous about it. They don't pay for it until you're thirty-five if you have a family history." In addition, Veronica has stopped smoking.

> I smoked cigarettes for a while but stopped, realizing that, "Okay, this is dumb. Your mother had breast cancer. Why do something that might increase your risk?" I didn't only stop smoking because of the risk for breast cancer, but just in general. I know that that helps, and maybe that was a factor in my mother's breast cancer.

Veronica is sometimes confused about what might be carcinogenic.

> So many things come out about what increases your risk. I'm rather confused about the most recent findings because it was revealed that some of the research findings were, like, bogus. I feel like my greatest risk factor is just my family history. No matter what I do nutritionally, if I'm going to get it, I'm going to get it.

Veronica had a "breast mass" three years ago.

> I was really freaked out and, like, my life [was] flashing before me. Like, "Oh, wow. What if this is really cancer? Are the things that happened to my mother gonna happen to me?" But I didn't fall apart. I kept my cool. When I told my family, they went crazy. Especially my youngest sister. Whenever I get sick, she gets so . . . fearful.

Veronica is aware of the genetics of breast cancer, but has not considered genetic testing. "I don't really see what the point is. I don't know why I would need it at this point. I mean, like, if I carried a breast cancer gene, would that mean I'm not gonna have children? No."

Current Situation

Veronica is a physician and works at a prestigious hospital. She became pregnant during the time of the study, and now has a lovely baby boy.

DISCUSSION

This section provides a discussion of the main themes identified in the "late adolescent" cases. During the illness period, the main themes identified are "little women" and moving toward an adult relationship with the mother. In the period after the mother's death, the two themes identified are Oedipus again?, incomplete grieving, and loneliness/isolation. The long-term impact themes focus on chronic grief/depression and loss of maternal support. In addition to the four case studies presented in this chapter, this discussion makes reference to the cases of Linda, Ruth, Betty, Sally, and Nancy, which can be found in Appendix III. Jamie, a late adolescent whose mother survived, also is discussed in the next section.

Daughter's Experience of Her Mother's Illness

Two themes are identified for the late adolescents during the period of the mother's illness: "little women" and moving toward an adult relationship with the mother.

Little Women

A typical experience of the late adolescent daughters whose mothers died from breast cancer was to return home from their first independent living situation (e.g., college), and take on heavy household responsibilities. These young women experienced a sudden role change; one day they were college students and the next they were housewives and nurses. Families relied heavily on these daughters, who often took on major responsibilities out of a sense of duty. However, they were unprepared for this sudden change, and many found themselves shopping, cooking, and cleaning for the first time in their lives.

For example, when Alicia's mother became seriously incapacitated, Alicia's father brought her home from college to care for her mother. Although Alicia had never before done housework, she began to cook for her father and served as a nurse to her mother. Veronica took a semester off from college to assist when her mother was ill. She saw this as a way of helping her father (by saving him money) and her mother (by providing family support), but at times felt angry, resentful, and overwhelmed. Jamie, whose mother survived (see Chapter 8), was a college student who came home for Christmas while her mother was in the hospital. "The whole week before Christmas, it's major chaos around my house. I thought, *I've got to clean up the house, make sure everything is presentable.*"

When her mother came home after surgery, Jamie's aunt was angry at Jamie for not taking proper care of her mother. Jamie explains that she suddenly realized that her mother couldn't perform her normal activities, and "it clicked." For months, Jamie cooked and cleaned. Linda (Appendix III) too came home from college to become the primary caregiver for her mother, and learned to give morphine shots. All of these late adolescents were attending college at the time of mother's illness, and came home at some point to take on their mothers' responsibilities and/or to care for them.

Other cases demonstrated a weaker version of the "little women" theme. For various reasons, some daughters were not as heavily involved in their mothers' care, but still took on added repsonsibilities. For example, Janice's (Chapter 6) mother's illness was long-lasting, and much of that time Janice was away at college. Although she frequently came home to visit, her father primarily provided her mother's care. The family protected Janice from bad news about her mother's health, but in the end, she was called upon to handle some very difficult tasks (telling her sisters and relatives that their mother had died and making the funeral arrangements). Ruth's case (Appendix III) also reflects this theme, but her mother died before Ruth took on major responsibilities.

Examination of other late-adolescent cases in this sample which do not reflect this theme suggests that several factors can affect whether the late adolescent daughter is pulled into a "little woman" role. Some women did not fit the pattern because they had *already* taken on the "little woman" role. An example is Holly (Appendix III), the daughter of Holocaust survivors, whose mother was diagnosed when she was sixteen. Holly describes how in many Holocaust-survivor families, young children often take on adult roles, and become very protective of their parents. When Holly's father died (long before her mother's illness), Holly developed an adultlike relationship with her mother. Also, Holly attended a college near her home, and so she did not need to move back home when her mother became ill. Despite this difference in upbringing, Holly is similar to the other girls in that she took on additional responsibilities when she became her mother's primary caregiver. "I remember . . . doing stuff I never thought I'd be doing, certainly not at that point in my life."

Another factor that may be relevant is birth order. An older daughter, or an only daughter, is more likely to be called into the "little woman" role than is a younger daughter. For example, Trisha and her twin sister were the babies in the family. They stayed at college while their mother was ill, often worrying about her, but it was their older siblings who took on the responsibility of running the household and caring for their mother. Characteristics of the mother's illness may be important here. When the mother has minimal treatment and does well, the family is more likely to carry on without the daughter's help. Also, in families where household responsibilities are shared, it might not be necessary for a college-age daughter to return home. In Betty's (Appendix III) family, for example, everyone helped when her mother was ill.

Some daughters who did not take on the mother's responsibilities were later left with regrets. For example, Janice felt very worried when she was away from home. Trisha did not get home from school in time to see her mother before she died, and she still feels sad about this. Sharon (Chapter 8), whose mother survived, still worries about how Mom is doing, and is unsure if her family is giving her accurate information.

"Role shifts" are common in families when a family member is ill. Whenever a family member needs special care, or when they cannot perform their customary roles, other family members generally provide the care needed and/or perform the functional roles of the ill member. When a mother is ill with breast cancer, the person who takes on these functions is often a late adolescent daughter. Family members likely feel that this daughter is old enough to perform adult roles and responsibilities, even though she may have had very little training for these roles. Caring for the sick is a traditional female role, as are cooking, cleaning, and child care. Walsh and McGoldrick (1991) point out that women "bear primary caretaking responsibility" and are "socialized to handle the social and emotional tasks of bereavement" (p. 23). However, very little attention in the literature has been given to how this caregiving affects the daughters, and how it affects their lives. Providing such care for a short time probably is not very disruptive for the daughter's life-course development, and may lead to a more speedy maturity. In their classic review of literature on bereavement, Osterweis, Solomon, and Green (1984) talk about a "developmental push" that propels adult children into more adult roles in their families (see following section). However, long-term care may disrupt normal life-course development and educational attainment.

Moving Toward an Adult Relationship with the Mother

Many of the young women in our study negotiated new roles with their mothers during her illness. For some, this period provided a precious opportunity to have a different and closer relationship with their mothers, one in which some of the hurts left over from adolescence could be forgiven and healed. When Janice's mother was dying, Janice was able to sit with her and thank her for all of the support she had given. Janice apologized to her mother for her adolescent behavior. Even so, after her mother died, Janice still was angry because her friend would be able to have the mature relationship with her mother that Janice wanted with her own.

Alicia and her mother did not have a good relationship during Alicia's childhood and adolescence. When she came home from college and cared for her mother, their relationship improved for the brief period before her mother died. Alicia's mom apologized for being hurtful to her; she promised to make it up to her when she got well. Alicia and her mother had a brief chance to express their love for each other and shift to a more mature relationship. Before she died, Alicia's mother chose to be with Alicia instead of her son, and they were able to reevaluate their past relationship. Veronica's relationship with her mother also changed during the illness. Veronica came home to help when her mother's health declined. She took on a more adult role, driving her mother to appointments, providing advice about her appearance (helping her mother select a wig), and trying to preserve her dignity. Although Veronica initially resented having to return to her nuclear family, she clearly remembers a warm hug from her mother, suggesting a healing of their previously tumultuous relationship. Other cases that reflect a shift to a more adult relationship with the mother include Holly and Betty (Appendix III). For example, Betty speaks of her mother confiding in her instead of her father about her illness, because "It's a woman's disease."

Birth order may be a factor in determining whether a shift in the mother-daughter relationship takes place. Trisha, who was a "baby" in the family, did not describe a change in the relationship with her mother; in fact, her mother stayed in "a mother role," insisting that Trisha and her sister start college, despite her illness. Sally (Appendix III), also a youngest child, did not experience a role shift either. The daughter being away from home also may make this type of change in the mother-daughter relationship less likely.

Little has been written on how illness in the mother of a late adolescent daughter affects the dynamics of the mother-daughter relationship. It is helpful to consider what is happening in a normal mother-daughter relationship at this life stage. Traditional life-stage theories have emphasized the increasing separation of the late adolescent from the family, and the adolescent's increasing autonomy. The focus in these theories has been on the development of an autonomous identity (Erikson, 1964, 1968).

More recent theories, based on studies of women, suggest that women's sense of self is tied to relationships, and that forming, maintaining, and managing these relationships is central to women's self-esteem. Women tend to maintain attachments, rather than to separate from them. Some attribute this to the different early developmental tasks of boys and girls, as boys need to separate from the mother to establish their gender identity, while girls do not (Chodorow, 1999). Studies of mother-daughter relationships throughout the life course suggest that late adolescence is a time of renegotiation of the relationship from that of mother-child to a more complex, articulated pattern of mutual caretaking and identification (Surrey, in Jordan et al., 1991). In late adolescence, mother-daughter relationships are not characterized by disengagement, but by "qualities of mutual empathy, understanding, acceptance and forgiveness" (Kaplan, Gleason, and Klein, 1991, p. 131). These authors consider late adolescence to be "an important period in the development of women's core relational self-structure" (p. 131). At the same time, daughters want to be able to have strong conflicts with their mothers, without having these conflicts threaten the basic connection between them.

Experience Following Her Mother's Death

The three themes most common among late adolescent daughters following mother's death were: Oedipus again?, incomplete grieving, and loneliness/isolation.

Oedipus Again?

As with the children and early adolescents in this study, the late adolescents faced major family changes after their mothers' deaths. Those who had come home from college often stayed at home after mother's death, caring for the house and their fathers. When the father remarried, and they were no longer needed, daughters often felt as if they had been summarily replaced. If the new couple moved to a different home, these late adolescent women felt abandoned for a third time, losing their homes after having lost both mother and father. Similar to the children and adolescents in this study, late adolescent women generally did not get along well with their stepmothers. Instead, competition and bitterness dominated. If the stepmothers tried to replace the mothers, hoping to discuss the daughters' intimate lives, the daughters were likely to respond with anger and rejection.

Many of these women ended up with very angry feelings toward both father and stepmother.

After her mother's death, Janice took a semester off from college, and stayed home, cooked, and took care of her father and younger sister. She tried to be the family peacemaker, and resented her father when he didn't reciprocate her sacrifices. Her father's remarriage and selling of the house in which she grew up left Janice feeling abandoned. She attended his wedding reluctantly, and spent Christmas with a friend's family.

Alicia transferred to a school closer to home so she could come help her father on weekends. Lonely, her father called her every night at school. When he remarried, Alicia had mixed emotions. She was relieved and felt less stressed, but at the same time, she felt demoted from father's confidante and equal to merely a daughter. When her father and stepmother bought a new house, Alicia felt abandoned again.

Other cases that reflect this theme include Ruth (Appendix III), whose father remarried within a year of her mother's death. "My stepmother made it very clear to me that she was not going to have a rival for my father's attention." This situation reoccurred years later when her stepmother died. Ruth immediately went to Florida to care for her father. However, when she realized that he was more interested in finding a new spouse than in spending time with her, Ruth felt rejected again. Linda (Appendix III) also took on many new roles after her mother died. For example, she did housework and made her father's lunches. She felt bitter and angry about helping her father get ready for dates, and then having to stay home while he was out having fun.

If the daughter did not take on a caretaking role for her father, she was less likely to feel rejected when the father entered a new relationship. However, there is evidence of oedipal feelings even in some of these cases. Betty (Appendix III) no longer lived at home, but tried to live with her father after her mother died (of a heart attack). The two could not get along, in part because Betty was angry at her father for having a new girlfriend.

Veronica's case was an exception. After her mother died, Veronica was eager to return to college, and medical school, but felt constrained by her father's pressure on her to care for her younger sisters. She did not, however, care for *him*. Nor did Veronica feel rejected when her father started dating. "I understood that he needed companionship." When her father got involved in a long-term relationship, Veronica was accepting. Perhaps this is in part because her father never remarried suggesting that Veronica's mother cannot be replaced. This is a thought that probably would have been affirming and comforting to many of the other late adolescent daughters in the study.

Although the literature is rich with studies of father-daughter relationships in childhood and early adolescence, little is written about relationships between late adolescent daughters and their fathers. Clearly, caring for one's father and his home is not normative for a young woman in our culture. While girls may maintain a close, although conflictual, relationship with their mother, the distance from the father that began in early adolescence only intensifies. One study of the impact of parental death from cancer (Christ, 2000) holds that one task of the bereaved adolescent is "to renegotiate a relationship with the surviving parent," and that this process can be more complicated for girls in adolescence than for boys (p. 208).

> In some situations, the surviving parent, usually the father, was unable to establish an empathic and caring relationship with his adolescent daughter. These fathers either had been emotionally distant before the death or became so in reaction to the death, and buried themselves in their work or remarried quickly. (Christ, 2000, p. 209)

Although the incest taboo is probably a factor in this pattern, another issue may lie in the nature of the relationships women have with their mothers. The section on role shift discussed how women in late adolescence are in the process of moving from an adolescent relationship with their mothers to one of "mutual mothering." Relationships among women tend to involve mutual sharing of feelings, sensitivity to the feelings of the other (empathy), and close connection. The relationship between mother and mature daughter also involves a component of supervision of the other's life and advice giving—components absent in peer relationships (Fischer, 1986). Because men tend to relate to other men on a more competitive and hierarchical basis, and because they are socialized to cover up their emotions instead of expressing them, it is not surprising to find late adolescent girls who lose mothers to breast cancer dissatisfied with the relationships they have with their fathers. Most fathers are not able to help daughters work through feelings (anger, depression), nor are they able to openly share their own feelings. Daughters may feel unappreciated, not only because their contribution to the family seems unappreciated, but because the relationships they have with their fathers lacks the mutuality, empathy, and connectedness they shared with their mothers.

It also is important to note that although it is normative in our culture for late adolescent women to voluntarily leave home and establish independent residences, some women in our study lost their homes *in*voluntarily. In some cases (Alicia, Janice) this was due to the father's remarriage, but even women who did not have fathers experienced the loss of their homes. Trisha, who did not have an involved father, now goes to her brother's home, which "isn't the same." Holly's (Appendix III) father had died much earlier, but still she lost her home when her mother died, and for a while had to live with her aunt and uncle. Describing packing up and selling her mother's home, she says, "I was putting away my former life." Perhaps in reaction to their new situations, it was not uncommon for these young women to marry soon after the father's remarriage; they then moved into their own homes.

Incomplete Grieving

The late adolescent daughters in this study did not go through a grieving process that allowed them to move past their loss. For example, Janice has not gotten past her grief. Although Janice had strong support during her mother's dying process, she had difficulty finding support (and time) for grieving after mother died. Janice did engage in some active grieving, such as visiting her mother's grave and crying, and she sought support through various groups in college. However, when she tried to engage in grieving rituals, such as remembering her mother on holidays, her father (who is remarried) resisted.

Veronica, too, did not go through a profound grieving process after her mother died. She did cry at the funeral, after trying to "hold it together"; soon afterward, her family took a vacation. Then, she immediately returned to school where she struggled to finish her degree on time and get into medical school. Veronica was sad, and mostly alone with her grief. She didn't want others to think that she was using her mother's death "as an excuse" for poor school performance; this may have led her to bury her feelings. Like Janice, Veronica was swept up in family responsibilities while she struggled to succeed in her chosen career. Veronica often dreams of her mother, indicating a lack of resolution.

Alicia engaged in traditional grieving rituals, but her grief still seems unresolved. At important times in her life, Alicia feels that her mother comes to help her, indicating an unwillingness by Alicia to "let go."

Trisha returned to college shortly after her mother's death. Trisha's college provided counseling services, and she attended a bereavement group. However, the group was comprised of students who had experienced many kinds of losses that Trisha felt were much less devastating than hers. Only closeness with her twin sister allowed her to share feelings and memories of mother. When Trisha went on vacation, she took her mother's ashes along and scattered them, because her mother had always wanted to travel.

Holly (Appendix III) did not find religious rituals helpful immediately after her mother's death. Instead, she learned to "pick up and move on," modeling how her mother coped after Holly's father's death. She felt that the only alternative was to "lose it completely." Holly now wishes that she had entered therapy earlier. "I think I carried a lot of issues around for a long time."

Linda (Appendix III) provides another example of a young woman who did not go through a healing grieving process. Even during the shiva (Jewish mourning period), she was busy preparing food and doing housework; she didn't have an opportunity to mourn. Seeking relief from her pain (often feeling that her life should have ended when her mother's did), Linda has tried psychotherapy and transactional analysis. She continues to seek a connection with her mother by consulting psychics. Linda has tried on several occasions to make contact with her mother, using séances and spiritualists.

Ruth (Appendix III) also did not go through a full grieving period. She was very angry at her mother's funeral, which hampered her healing. After her mother's death, her family did not share memories. She, her brother, and her father each "crawled into [their] shells." When Ruth tried to talk with her grandparents, they found any discussion too painful. Her father disposed of all of her mother's belongings, so Ruth had no items to help her keep her mother's memory alive. After her father remarried, Ruth wasn't allowed to talk about her mother, or to keep pictures of her; as a result, her memories have faded. Ruth's grief was complicated by the fact that she was not told that her mother was dying until the day before her death. Now, she regrets that she did not get to talk honestly with her mother before she died: "There is so much I would have told her." Ruth also feels sad that her mother died alone.

Sally (Appendix III), could not accept her mother's death. At first, she and her siblings refused to let the funeral director remove the body from the home. Because the family didn't feel comfortable talking about the death, they avoided the grief counseling Sally's oldest sister had arranged. Although Sally and her family took part in common rituals, such as visiting the cemetery and holding long conversations with her mother, she does not find this helpful. She feels sad all of the time ("still with the crying . . ."), and has no hope that things will improve: "I'll probably pretty much have the same emotions and the same feelings for the rest of my life."

Traditional theories of grieving tend to involve some type of stage model, where the initial disbelief and shock is followed by pain and depression. Finally, once this has been worked through, the bereaved person focuses less and less on the lost relationship, and invests with increasing energy in present life (Bowlby, 1980; Lindemann, 1944; Parkes, 1987). Pathology can result when this process is not followed; the bereaved person gets "stuck" in perpetual mourning or perpetual denial. Unresolved grief has long been connected with depression (Freud's concept of melancholia), and has been implicated in many mental disorders.

Age is commonly used to explain a lack of resolution of grief. Whether children and adolescents are capable of grieving has been extensively debated (see Chapter 5). However, the late adolescents we discuss in this chapter clearly have the emotional capacity to experience the loss, and the cognitive capacity to resolve the loss in constructive ways. (See Christ, 2000, whose oldest group of study participants [fifteen- to seventeen-year-olds] is even younger than this group.)

Why didn't the young women in this study go through the grieving process? Janice, Alicia, and Veronica were so overwhelmed with their responsibilities, with the sudden changes in their lives, and with the enormity of their loss, that they seemed to get stuck in a kind of chronic grieving. Trisha was the only one of the late adolescent cases who was able to access bereavement counseling after returning to college; even she reported that the services she got were not adequate.

Considering the lack of grief resolution in these cases, it is important to remember that all of the informants in our study are women, and all have lost their mothers. Although theories of grieving present models for all types of people dealing with all types of loss, it is possible that these models do not apply well to women, and most especially to women who have lost their mothers. Researchers have begun to question the assumption of classic theories that suggests that the aim of healthy grief is to "detach" from the lost object (Edelman, 1994; Rosenblatt, 1996; Silverman, 1987; Wilcox-Rittgers, 1997). Studies suggest that this idea may be a particularly Western one, and a male-focused one (Klass, Silverman, and Nickman, 1996). Western culture tends to be "death averse," and also emphasizes individualization, while other cultures are more accepting of death as an important part of life, and emphasize family over the individual. These researchers suggest that theories that emphasize detachment have pathologized normal grieving that may last long after the death.

Women often derive their sense of self through relationships, and perhaps do not separate (detach) from their mothers in the way that males do (to become identified with their fathers). This may mean that loss for women does not involve a detachment, but instead, that the connection with the deceased continues for them well past the death. This may be particularly true when a daughter loses her mother, because this relationship is so central to a young woman's identity.

Another important consideration is that particular conditions need to be met for grieving to occur. Therapists know that "creating a safe environment" is crucial for emotional release. We saw with the children and young adolescents in our study that the blow to the family caused by the mother's death was so severe that often they felt that their survival was threatened. They did not grieve, but instead worked to make themselves tough enough to survive this and other tradegies. Perhaps the late adolescent daughters were not as concerned with their own survival; they may have been worried about the survival of the family. Women with younger siblings often focused on keeping the family together, rather than on their own grieving needs. For a variety of reasons, then, the late adolescent women did not experience a classical grieving process that would have allowed them to move forward in their lives. Many were left in a chronic grieving pattern. In some, the unresolved grieving takes the form of continued seeking of a mother-like love. Like younger women in this study, the late adolescent women put the family's survival ahead of their own emotional needs.

Loneliness/Isolation

Closely related to the "unresolved grief" discussed in the previous section, many of the women who lost their mothers in late adolescence mentioned feelings of isolation or loneliness, even when surrounded by friends and family. Some sought a mother figure. The late adolescent who has interrupted her college experience to return home when her mother is ill or has died is likely to go back to school at some point. This is an especially lonely time for most. Many of these women were at college at the time of the mother's death. Colleges may not have the resources to create a supportive environment for grieving.

> When a death occurs in the family [of a college student], these individuals are usually required to experience the long-term bereavement process away from other family members and within an environment that may not validate their experiences and provide support for grieving. (Tyson-Rawson, 1996, p. 128)

Balk (1996), who has done several studies on bereavement in college students, states, "Rather than a source of nourishment and growth, the campus can become a place of loneliness, isolation , non-productivity and dread for students dealing with grief" (p. 324). Late adolescent women in our study often did not tell new friends their mothers were deceased. The daughters believed that by not disclosing this information they could avoid potentially awkward situations (e.g., friends not knowing how to respond). Some bereaved student did not want people to think they were seeking sympathy. By hiding this information, the daughters lost the opportunity to obtain social support. Because they were not emotionally open and did not express their feelings, their personal relationships often were not satisfying or meaningful. Social isolation and loneliness commonly resulted.

Alicia provides a good example. She transferred to a college that was closer to her home, so that she could care for her father on weekends. She felt as if she were "a lost soul." She felt needy and that her life was empty. Alicia does not consider herself lonely now (some twenty-five years later), but she does describe an ongoing difficulty with relationships. She fears losing friends because of being too needy. As she faces her elder daughter leaving the family for college, she experiences anxiety. Having experienced loss in her family of origin during this time, she describes this as "the end of family time." Trisha also returned to college after her mother's death, and found it difficult to make friends. College roommates encouraged her to talk, but then became overwhelmed when she did. Some students reacted by telling her, "Oh, you're so strong"—a comment Trisha did not know how to handle. She soon learned to hide the fact that her mother had died. Because Trisha has a twin sister, and they are very close, she may be less lonely than some other women in the study.

Veronica is another woman who returned to college after her mother's death. She reports on how sad and lonely she felt there. Veronica, like Trisha, didn't tell people that her mother had died, fearing they would think she was seeking sympathy. Veronica stated, "I think I was depressed for most of my college years. . . ." Holly, who became an orphan when her mother died, moved onto her college's campus after a short time. She did not share her history with other students. "It's an issue that makes people uncomfortable." Holly said she was in a different emotional "place" than other students at college. "There were some feelings of isolation."

Late adolescent women are experiencing a time of life in which they form intimate attachments; these relationships potentially provide a path out of loneliness. Alicia married shortly after her father and stepmother moved into a new home. She has a very protective husband, who took on an almost motherlike role. Ruth, whose marriage ended, feels that she may have picked her husband because "I needed somebody to talk to."

Many women selected a life partner based on characteristics of his family. Ruth speculated that she was attracted to her husband in part because of his very close family. "I felt a part of something." Janice is not sure if she is more attracted to her boyfriend or to his traditional family.

Long-Term Impact

Two themes were identified for late adolescents for the long term. These were chronic grief/depression and loss of mother's support.

Chronic Grief/Depression

This study did not measure levels of depression in the participants; however, it is clear that some, but not all, in the late-adolescent group exhibited high levels of sadness, and described themselves as "depressed." Many were still experiencing chronic grief. According to theories of the grieving process, one stage is a denial of the death, during which the bereaved seeks the deceased. Only when the bereaved person truly realizes that the deceased cannot be found does the grief resolve. Perhaps because many of the late adolescents in this study did not have an opportunity to grieve, they experience chronic grieving as adults. Veronica experiences a lot of sadness on the anniversary of her mother's death ("Everything is all gloom"). For Veronica, and many of the women who lived the "little women" experience, taking on the role as the "strong one" in the family during and after the crisis seemed to forestall a strong grieving response. One consequence may be a long-lasting depression. Janice finds that each anniversary of mother's death "hits [her] with a vengeance," suggesting unresolved grief. She asks, "How do you hold on to the person?" Linda (Appendix III) says her mother's death "took a lot of the fun out of [her] life. I'm no one's child. When your mother goes, you're alone, and that's it." Linda recently has gotten a little dog whose devotion gives her some comfort.

In summary, the late adolescent women whose mothers died from breast cancer were left with long-term sadness and often depression.

Loss of Mother's Support

Another theme for these women when their mothers died involves missing their mothers at critical times in their adult lives. Parents usually continue to provide emotional support to their adult children. The women in this group discussed how they missed having this help at stressful times, such as when having children or, more simply, when they needed emergency baby-sitting. They regretted that their children never had a chance to know their own grandmothers.

Veronica missed her mother's help with her wedding. Ruth (Appendix III) wished her mother was around for the "girl" things, and she continues to miss the opportunity to have a model for growing older. She also identifies everyday things, such as having her mother to fix her dinner when she is feeling overwhelmed. "It's the really simple things that I miss." Betty (Appendix III) also feels that her mother would have helped her with school, housing, and money as she moved into adulthood. Linda (Appendix III) missed the support a mother would have provided when she had young children and later, when her daughter needed help with a learning disability. Like many others, she misses having a mother to spoil and fuss over her children. (Linda feels this has affected her parenting. She gives her kids too much, to compensate for their not having grandparents.) Linda admits that she sometimes feels jealous of others who have more family support, a sentiment that was common in this group. Holly (Appendix III) also believes that the lack of extended family affects her parenting. She envies those who have access to the kind of support that grandparents provide.

The traditional developmental literature describes the young adult moving away from the family of origin as a method of achieving independence. In contrast, the women who lost mothers in late adolescence emphasize the difficulties they experienced by not having a mother to support them through the major transitions into adulthood. Theories of female life-course development suggest that ongoing ties with families (especially mothers) are important throughout the life cycle. Mothers continue to provide important support for their daughters, even as the daughters separate and move into adult roles and relationships. One reaction for women in this age category was to seek mother figures or mother-type relationships, after the mother's death.

SUMMARY

This chapter focused on the experience of daughters who were late adolescents when their mothers died from breast cancer. The cases of Janice, Trisha, Alicia, and Veronica were presented, and were supplemented by the cases of Linda, Ruth, Betty, Sally, and Nancy, which can be found in Appendix III. See Box 6.1 for a summary of the major themes experienced by late adolescent daughters.

During the illness period, these women often found themselves suddenly playing major roles in the home, often for the first time. During this period, many of these women's relationships with their mothers shift from a somewhat contentious mother-child relationship to a more adult relationship. After the mother's death, the late adoles-

---

**BOX 6.1. Themes Found in Daughters
Whose Mothers Died When They Were
Late Adolescents**

Phase I: Mother's Illness and Treatments

    1. Little women
    2. Moving toward an adult relationship with mother

Phase II: Following Mother's Death

    1. Oedipus again?
    2. Incomplete grieving
    3. Loneliness/isolation

Phase III: Long-Term Impact

    1. Chronic grief/depression
    2. Loss of mother's support

---

cent daughters often took on many of the mother's responsibilities, such as care of fathers and/or siblings. These young women often were isolated from others their age, or from others who had similar life experience or similar losses. They typically experienced a profound loneliness when they returned to college.

The long-term impact of their experiences suggests a chronic grieving. Although the women in the late adolescent group are theoretically *able* to grieve, the women in our study often did not. This may have been due to heavy family responsibilities. In addition, their bereavement was "out of synch" with most people in their age group; friends had little experience with death or bereavement. The lack of intense grieving after the mother's death may result in a long-term depression in the daughter.

As adults, these women focused on the loss of their mothers' support. This often was expressed in terms of loss of help with children, or children's lack of grandmothers. Equally important was the loss of general support in life, such as money, someone to help prepare a meal, or offer recipes.

The practice implications of these themes are discussed in Chapter 11.

Chapter 7

Experience of Young Adult Daughters When Mothers Die from Breast Cancer

This chapter explores the experience of daughters who lost their mothers to breast cancer when they were young adults. Four case studies are presented: Andrea was only a young teenager at her mother's diagnosis, but she was thirty-two when her mother died; Elizabeth and Sarah were both twenty-seven at mother's diagnosis and twenty-nine when she died, and Felicia was twenty-nine at mother's diagnosis and thirty-one at time of mother's death. Following the four case studies is a discussion of the common themes in the experience of these young women. As in the previous three chapters, the themes are organized into experiences during mother's illness, experience after mother's death, and long-term impact.

CASE STUDY #1: ANDREA

Age at Her Mother's Breast Cancer Diagnosis: 13; Age at Time of Her Mother's Death: 32

Background

Andrea was the younger of two sisters. Her mother's marriage to Andrea's father was her second. Her mother stayed at home when her children were young, and later had a number of jobs. She worked as a teacher, substitute teacher, and door-to-door salesperson. Andrea had a normal relationship with her mother.

> Probably like any adolescent daughter and her mother, we definitely fought a lot. I had periods when I just wanted to be left alone. I was a fairly normal teenager and I didn't want my mother going everywhere with me. It was a good relationship. We went shopping together and things like that.

She describes her mother as "a beautiful woman, very classy and sophisticated. She just loved her friends and her family. She was very popular. She had lots of friends. She was the most giving, generous woman that you would ever meet."

Experience of Her Mother's Illness

Andrea was thirteen when mother was diagnosed. Her doctor soon performed surgery. "Basically, she had a mastectomy, but she woke up not even knowing that she was going to be having a mastectomy. For her it was a shock to have her breast removed, and she had no idea." Andrea's mother had what was called a "one-step" procedure, in which biopsy and mastectomy are done in one operation. Andrea has little memory of that time.

> I remember her being in the hospital, and I remember my sister had her senior prom and she went to the hospital all dressed up so that my mom could see her. I don't remember it having a profound impact on my life at that time. It's strange to me now that I didn't do more or know more. Maybe it was just because of my age. I think I was so wrapped up in going to parties and going out with my friends that it really didn't have a major effect on me at that time.

Andrea now realizes that her mother protected her daughters from the potential seriousness of her illness. "My mother was so good at not worrying her children, and always protecting us and shielding us. I don't remember it being a big deal, and I don't know if it was because she covered it up." Andrea saw her mother's scar, and knew that she used a prosthesis.

> She never had any cosmetic surgery. She had something that she would just stick in her bra. I don't remember really ever asking her how she felt about her body, because I'm sure that it had to have bothered her. I didn't want to draw attention to that.

Andrea's father had little involvment with her mother's cancer. "My father was never all that supportive at the time when she was originally diagnosed." After the surgery, the family was certain the cancer was gone. "I think she thought that that was it. And we all thought it was gone." Mother returned to her active life. "You would never know looking at her that anything had happened. Unless you saw her naked. She was an avid tennis player. She won a lot of trophies. She was very active again, and working again."

When Andrea was eighteen, her parents divorced.

> I remember being told that they were going to be separating. That had a profound effect on me. It was shocking. There was no sign of it. At the time, the divorce kind of really overwhelmed me, and outweighed the importance of the cancer.

After the divorce, Andrea's mother started her own business. "She was extremely independent and very strong-willed. She really enjoyed her work. She loved what she did and she built a good company." Andrea went away to college, and then moved to another city, where she had a job in the publishing industry.

Twelve years after the original diagnosis, her mother's cancer recurred. Andrea was twenty-five.

> She had gone on a trip, and she cracked her rib. That's when they realized that the cancer wasn't in remission. It was the cancer that caused the bone to break in her rib. She started on the regular treatments. At that point, our relationship really changed. I was older and I could understand and relate to it more on an adult level.

Learning that the cancer had returned was a shock for Andrea.

> It was extremely scary. At that time, I was much more aware of what cancer was and how serious it was. I remember calling her oncologist from my office cubicle, asking him to explain to me what was going on and how serious it was. He said, "I wouldn't give her more than two years." He likened it to being on a roller coaster—that there were going to be these ups and downs. That was horrible. I remember being at my office and I was left just hysterical with the realization that her time was finite.

Over the next seven years, her mother's health gradually worsened.

> It certainly deteriorated her physically. She shrunk. She could joke about everything and she would say, "Thank God that I was so tall!" Because you know, she shrunk, like, five inches. She got hunched over. She had surgery on her neck. Honestly, she must have had at least eight surgeries, all for different parts of her body. Late in life, she was walking with a cane.

The therapy also caused hair loss. "It was difficult, but she just managed to overcome it. She got wigs. She got scarves. She went out." Andrea's mother remained upbeat.

> I never heard her complain about her illness. She always found the bright spot. She was full of life. Mother continued to run her business. She didn't want people to know and she didn't want to lose her accounts. She didn't want people feeling sorry for her. A lot of people were shocked [when they found out] that she even had cancer. And I was shocked, like, "How could you not notice?" She would say, "I had a car accident." That must be how she handled it because she never talked much about it. She just wanted to get on with life. It was there. It was a fact of life, but it wasn't something that we'd belabor. She had found a way to live with it and to live an extremely fulfilled and happy life.

Andrea's family followed her mother's philosophy at that point: "Taking one day at a time. Taking each step."

During the period between the recurrence and her mother's death, Andrea, her mother, and her sister became extremely close.

> We certainly could connect with each other on a different level at that point in our relationship, as opposed to [when I was] growing up. The three of us were extremely close. We really enjoyed doing things together. My mother would come up, and we'd go shopping and we'd go to the museums, and we just really had a lot of fun together. We talked a lot more candidly about life, and all of our experiences, and death. The history of our family. What Grandma was like, and Great-Grandma. We have that on videotape.

Andrea thinks that her mother's illness improved their relationship.

> I see some of the relationships that my friends have and they're not as open. I don't know that I would have been as forthcoming with personal details of my life, my dating life. I don't know. I was very open with her, and she was very open-minded and very understanding. It was just a good relationship.

During this period, Andrea and her mother also took some trips together.

> We went on an incredible cruise to Alaska. We went to New Orleans. I really don't think I would have gone on vacation with my mother if I didn't know she had cancer and was going to be no longer living in a couple of years. Yet these are some of the best memories that I have of my life.

Despite their open, very positive relationships, Andrea's mother continued to try to protect her daughters from her illness.

> She really shielded us. Initially, there were a lot of questions that my mother never asked. She just couldn't handle everything at once. I spoke to her oncologist a lot over the years, and went to see him myself. It wasn't until a month before she passed away that my sister, my mother, and I actually all three went to the oncologist together.

A pattern of mutual protection developed in the family. Andrea's mother tried to limit her daughters' involvement; at the same time, the daughters protected their mother from information they felt she would not want to know.

> I had several conversations with her oncologist that she never knew about. I think she thought she was protecting us, but really, we had turned into adult women and were taking charge of the situation. I would often just go behind her back and call him myself. I certainly did not share the information but certain things I really needed to know. Things that she didn't ask, and maybe she didn't want to know.

Because her sister was married and had two children, most of the caregiving responsibility fell to Andrea.

> She had surgery on her neck, and I came down for a couple of weeks. She just couldn't lift her head up. She couldn't get out of bed. That's sort of really when I learned to cook. I stayed with her and cooked every single meal for her. Brought it in to her, took care of her, bathed her. It was extremely difficult to be in that role. I was thirty-two years old and I still feel very young. It's not something that I wanted to be doing.

Eventually, Andrea moved in with her mother.

Six weeks before her mother's death, Andrea married an oncologist who was involved in her mother's care. "Ironically, my husband was one of my mother's doctors when she was treated. They were extremely close. He was very fond of her and she adored him. So that made it easy for me. He was very understanding." At the wedding, Andrea's mother was "not in great shape"—but she was there.

> She looked radiant. She really did. It was our celebration, but there she was, surrounded by all her friends, and friends from all over the country that she doesn't get to see. It was a great way to see everybody and almost say good-bye for the last time. It was a great farewell.

Because of her mother's illness, Andrea did not have a lengthy honeymoon. "I only went away for four days, and I was calling her every day. I was really anxious to get back." After she returned, she had a hard time juggling the demands of her mother's illness with her desire to adjust to her new marriage. "I had just gotten married. I was new to married life, but I wasn't really with my husband. I was sleeping there [mother's apartment]. I wanted to be with my husband. I wanted to be having fun." At this point, her mother had a feeding tube.

> She couldn't even eat anymore. And it never really worked. So we'd have to change the dressing on the tubing three times a day. This dressing change was horrific. It was disgusting. It was unbelievable. It wasn't something that I wanted to be doing and it wasn't something that I felt qualified to be doing. At the time she wasn't getting any home care. She was adamantly opposed to getting home care. I thought maybe it was time that we got a nurse or hospice care. In the end, I got angry at her because I had to do this. I just couldn't even take it anymore. Just the stench coming from it, and the sight of it and everything else is not something that I wanted to remember about her. So I told my sister she had to come down and help me. All along we both kept saying, "Mom, it's time that we get somebody in here. We can't be doing this anymore." That went on for several weeks where we had to keep doing that. She [mother] said, "I'll let you know when I need the help. I don't need somebody here now. I'm fine by myself." And she probably wasn't, but that was how she wanted it. She really didn't want somebody caring for her. It was very hard for her to take help. She wasn't good at asking for help and it was difficult for her to receive [it].

Finally, Andrea's mother agreed to hospice care.

> We were really fortunate because she always wanted to be [die] at home. She wanted to be in bed, surrounded by her family. And that's exactly how it was for her in the end. It was extremely peaceful, and because she was still mentally coherent, we were able to say everything. I'm very fortunate because I don't have any real regrets and there's nothing left unsaid. She had the people around her, really, that mattered the most. It was her brothers and her friend and my sister and I. She didn't linger. Once she was too weak to get out of bed, it was just a realization that nothing more could be done. I mean, she had no interest in going on that way. That was why she never wanted the home nurse. She didn't want to, I guess, admit that it had reached that point. She would hear my sister and I trying to make arrangements for the nurses, and she would say, "I don't want . . . I hope I'm not here. I don't want that. Don't waste your time getting the nurses. I really hope that I'm not here for it." I found that comforting, because that's what she wanted in the end.

Even until the very end of her life, Andrea's mother was active.

> She was always so good at remembering people's anniversaries and all her nieces' and nephews' birthdays. She was sitting at the kitchen table, writing cards to people. She had, you know, twenty-four hours to live, and she's writing cards. "Happy Birthday!" That's the kind of person she was.

When her mother had been bedridden for several days,

> we would sit on her bedside a lot and sort of talk to her, but we felt like she was sleeping. She was so out of it. And I felt like, *It's definitely going to be today.* I guess I felt like, she's sort of on this journey now, and maybe we shouldn't bother her. We should let her rest in peace. I'm really so thankful to this nurse that we had. She said, "It's good if you go in there and talk to her. She can still hear you. Tell her how much you love her. Just talk to her." We went in that evening and just said everything again. She was not responding, but I do think that she heard us. We said, "It's okay now, Mom. [You] can let go and we will be okay. We will take care of each other." And it was that night that she died.

Andrea's mother's personality affected the manner in which she died.

> For her, everything had to be in order, and she had to know that when she was going to be leaving, everything would be taken care of. I think it was wonderful for her to have seen me get married and know that I would be taken care of with my husband, and my sister would be taken care of with her family. . . . She took care of so many things. She left all of her finances and everything in such good order. She left explicit instructions for us. I remember sitting on her bed in the last week and dividing up some of her jewelry. Afterward, we had to pack up all of her things. She had left, like, yellow Post-it notes on her dishes and things: "These dishes go to Andrea." My sister and I were just amazed. When did she do this? It was unbelievable how well taken care of things were.

Experience Following Her Mother's Death

Our interview with Andrea was only six months after her mother's death. Andrea was having difficulty visiting her mother's grave.

> I would like to believe that she is somewhere having a wonderful time, that her spirit is living on, but I'm not really sure. I had a difficult time with it at the grave site. And I go back there often. I had a lot of dreams about that. I don't really like the idea of being underground. My hus-

band keeps telling me, "That's not your mother. It's a body. That's not her anymore." I don't know. I have a hard time with the cemetery. I still feel a need to go to the cemetery.

Andrea also finds herself driving by her mother's former apartment.

I tend to go there often and just sort of sit outside in my car and spend time there. It is extremely difficult for me. I lose it right when I get off of the exit. I find myself sitting in front of her apartment. I have to drive by there and I sit and stare at her apartment. I have all of these memories.

Andrea finds comfort in talking with her mother's brothers and best friend. "I see them and I feel more of a connection."

Andrea also has some guilt about the feelings she had while caring for her mother.

Now, I feel guilty about feeling that way [resentful about having to provide care when she was a newlywed]. How selfish of me to feel that way. Now I wish I could have more time to go up there. But I never let her [mother] know that. No. I pretty much held it all in and did the dressing changes and stayed with her. But she knew anyway that that's not where I wanted to be.

Andrea and her sister packed up all of their mother's things several weeks after her death.

We tried to get everything out of there as soon as we could. She was renting her apartment and my sister and I didn't want to have to incur the cost of another month's rent. We were in such a daze when we were doing it, really. We got rid of a lot of stuff, and we ended up getting two storage units downtown. It was too hard to go through it the first time. I'd like to keep it.

Andrea's husband is not always sympathetic to her grieving.

There's a lot of things that he doesn't understand. I'll still just start crying, and anything could trigger it. It could be something major like the unveiling [of the headstone], or it could be just something as small as driving past her exit [the freeway exit for mother's apartment]. I'll just start crying, and he won't understand. He'll say, "What happened? What started that? You were doing so well!" It's hard for him to understand, and I'm getting tired of explaining that it's still there. It's not gonna go away. It's not like, "It's over. Closure. We're moving on." I mean, life's moving on, but it's not the happiest days for me.

Andrea experiences a similar lack of understanding from other people.

> With a lot of friends, you know, nobody really asks how I'm doing anymore. People don't call as much anymore. You have a lot of attention right afterward, and then everybody's on with their own lives. They do expect you to be over it. A year later, it's "What's wrong with her? She's still upset?" I have a problem with that, because I think I'm always gonna be upset about it. I'm sure I'll find a way to live with it, like I'm doing now, but it's always gonna be a painful thing for me.

Ten months after Andrea's mother's death, Andrea's husband got a job that involved moving to another city.

> It's kind of strange. It's a great opportunity for him, and I'll be close to my sister. It will be nice, when I have children one day. She has two kids, and they can grow up together. We're very close. It's just strange how things happen. I know she [mother] would have wanted me to be closer to my sister. I'd like to think that maybe she had something to do with all that. It would have made her very happy to know my sister and I would be together.

Although she was happy to move closer to her sister, Andrea felt as if she had lost a home. Andrea and her sister had considered their mother's place "home." "My sister and I both feel like we have no place to come home to anymore. It's strange because I'll be leaving and I don't really know when I'll be back." Her mother hosted holidays and other family get-togethers. "She was the one that always had holiday dinners. That's where we always gathered. That's where I would always stay." She anticipates the feeling of being unable to visit her mother's apartment.

> That will be hard. It's comforting for me to have that. It was just a great place to go. My sister would come down with the kids. We don't have that now. It's just hard because we have no home base anymore. Her [mother's] brothers are here. Her friends are here. I run into her friends shopping at the supermarket and, for me, it's really nice. When I move away, I'll lose all that. My mother was just such the connection for everything. I miss the connection. On the other hand, maybe it will be better for me that I won't constantly be driving by her exit and feeling sad. I mean, it's difficult for me to drive around that area without having all of these memories. So maybe it's better for me to relocate and start anew.

Regarding her new home, Andrea says, "Once we get our new place, I can certainly put all of the pictures of my mother out. I'll have all of her things around me so that I'll still have her there."

Andrea does not have a close relationship with her father. "My father is remarried. We don't have much [of a] relationship with his wife. I don't even know how to get to his apartment, and it's not a home for me."

Long-Term Impact

Although Andrea's mother had died quite recently, Andrea could already identify some effects the death was having on her.

> I think there's nothing more important to me than family. I've always really felt like family was the most important thing, but I feel that way even more so now. Having close friends and people that really love you, and having a support group around you [are critical].

She also has thought differently of her job.

> I'm in a job right now that I don't entirely love. I'm not going to stay there anymore. I guess when you lose your mother, you realize that life is extremely short. It can be taken at any time. It's pointless to stay in positions that don't make you happy. I feel like her death maybe was the impetus for me to get on with my life and do things that would make me happier in my career.

Andrea also thinks the association she has made between breasts and cancer has affected her sexual expression.

> I wonder what my husband would do if one day I don't have my breasts. I think, "Is he still gonna want me and is he still gonna love me if I don't have them?" But sometimes, too, I don't even want him touching them. I don't want it to be part of a sexual act at all, because . . . I just don't know why.

Andrea believes having a family would be a way to keep her mother alive. "And I certainly want to have a big family. I want to have a lot of children. And I hope to God I can have a relationship with my children like I had with my mother." She says,

> I really want my mother—I want to bring her alive through all my children. Since my mother's death, I have felt much more strongly that I really would love a daughter. Daughters are more curious. More inter-

ested in Grandma's things, and what Grandma was like. It's important for me for my mother to be a big part of my children's life, even though she's not here. I want her to still be a big part of them.

Andrea now feels that her mother lives within her. "I just feel sort of empowered now. I feel like I have my mother inside of me. I feel like I'm going to always carry her with me. I pull on her strength a lot when I need it." Andrea intends to continue some of her mother's roles and hobbies, including hosting holiday dinners and taking up tennis. "I'm going to start playing tennis again, because she did that for so much of her life. Just things that she really enjoyed, I'm going to incorporate more into my lifestyle." Andrea says she does these things partly out of fear that her mother might be forgotten. "I don't want to ever forget her. I can't imagine that I ever could. But I want to keep her alive. It's important to me to keep her alive."

Andrea feels that these changes have made her different than some of her friends.

I felt myself gradually changing [during the caregiving period]. I feel more grown up, more mature than some of my friends. I feel stronger, and like I have a better perspective. Things don't upset me as much as they used to. Work is just not that important. I'm going to take advantage of everything that life has. I think it's such a simple philosophy to live every moment to the fullest. People all try to do that and very few people really achieve it. My mother was really, really able to do that.

Risk

Andrea recently has become more concerned about her health.

I exercise regularly and I watch what I eat. I've sort of always been that way. I'm certainly paranoid about getting breast cancer. It scares me and I constantly think I have a lump, even though I don't really feel anything, or I'm afraid to feel for anything. I just feel like something will happen. And I worry about my sister, because she doesn't exercise and she doesn't really eat well. I couldn't imagine having to go through this, for her or for me, again.

Andrea is uncomfortable doing breast self-exams.

I constantly think I feel something under my armpit before my period. I have some swelling, and I'm afraid to feel for it myself, so I don't really do anything about it. I feel lumpy things all the time. I just feel like I won't really be able to tell. I'm afraid that I'll actually find something. It's crazy because I know that the earlier you find something the better off you are. I read a lot about it, and I'm in a very high-risk category. I do try to take care of myself, but I kind of feel, in a way, if it's gonna happen, it's gonna happen. It's a genetic, "cell" thing anyway. I mean, my mother was extremely active, never smoked, watched what she ate. She was really the picture of health, so . . .

Andrea has started getting mammograms.

I got the first one when I was thirty, so I feel like that will cover me for a couple of years, if it will show up on there, which I don't believe. I don't really believe that mammograms are gonna show anything, but I convince myself that I'm covered.

Before her mother died, Andrea went to see her mother's oncologist.

He told me that I could just cut off both of my breasts, if I wanted to minimize my risk. So that I wouldn't have to worry about it. I thought that was extremely radical. I was not really ready to do that. Plus, I want to have children, so I really wouldn't want to do that now, but I don't know. It's something to think about after I have children, maybe. Just to be one hundred percent certain nothing like that would ever happen.

Andrea has not considered having genetic testing.

I don't know what it would entail, or how accurate it is. I don't know that I'd want to know, either. If you do have the gene, does that mean that you're definitely gonna get breast cancer? Can they do anything about it? I mean, it's kind of like, do you want to know the day that you're gonna die? I don't. I'd rather kind of let fate . . . I don't know if I'd want to know that.

Current Situation

At the end of the study, Andrea (thirty-two) and her husband were considering another move, as his job did not meet his expectations. Andrea decided to change careers, as she wants to have more meaningful work. She is considering becoming a writer. She also wants to do volunteer work for charitable organizations.

CASE STUDY #2: ELIZABETH

Age at Her Mother's Breast Cancer Diagnosis: 27; Age at Time of Her Mother's Death: 29

Background

Elizabeth, the second of four children, came from a small town. Her father was a dentist, and her mother a nurse. "I consider myself to be very lucky. I had a really good relationship with my mother. She was a very good friend, and there wasn't anything that I couldn't tell her." Elizabeth describes the family as "very traditional," in that although both parents worked, her mom was the one who took the children to after-school activities, participated in the PTA (Parent Teacher Association), and so on. "We always knew that we came first." Elizabeth's older brother went into the medical field and became an oncologist. After college, Elizabeth got a job in hotel administration and lived in another city.

Experience of Her Mother's Illness

Elizabeth's father called her at work with the news about her mother's illness. "I knew it was big because he never called me at work—ever, ever, ever." He told her that her mother was in the hospital; her breast and lymph nodes had been removed.

> I was just stunned. We were all very, very healthy and very active. So it was just very surprising. I mean, my mother smoked, so we were concerned that she would get lung cancer. Breast cancer was something that never, ever came to mind.

All of the children came home. "We were all home within twenty-four hours. All four of us. And she was feeling much better. My brothers had her laughing." Elizabeth found comfort in the strength of her family. "Even though it was scary, it was comforting to have us all there, just all rallying around Mom."

Her mother began chemotherapy and radiation.

> It's like Mom and Dad are these rocks of Gibraltar and they're always supposed to be there and help you and kiss you when you need it. For these roles to be reversed, all of a sudden, was a little discomforting.

Her mother refused to rent a hospital bed for the home, and was not interested in any programs for cancer patients. The family did their best to entertain her during her recovery. "For a while there was one of us home every weekend. Since I lived the closest, I was going home a lot." Despite the difficulty of the treatment, Elizabeth's mother maintained her sense of humor. "She never complained or bellyached or 'Woe is me' or 'Why me?' or any of that." Elizabeth felt bad for both of her parents. "It should have been her time with my dad. This should have been a time when they could travel and enjoy life. Do all the things that they worked so hard for."

About eight months later, the family rented a beach house for a week. "It was gorgeous. We all went, as a family. And it was really great." During this vacation, her mother mentioned that she did not feel well and thought she might have a stomach virus. "So we all just thought it was the flu, but my older brother said later that he knew immediately what it was." After the family returned from the beach, it became clear that the cancer had spread to her liver.

During the next months, Elizabeth's mother never talked to her about the diagnosis. Instead, she would say things such as, "I'm not feeling well today" or "I'm not having a good day." She would make light of her situation, commenting, "I have a room with a view, but the room service is not so hot," when she was in the hospital. She usually would redirect the conversation to focus on Elizabeth's life. Her mother didn't want to reveal her innermost thoughts and feelings to her children. "She would allow us to be supportive, but just so far. She still wanted to be 'Momma' and look out for us." The family looked into experimental or alternative treatments, but nothing looked promising. "She was getting worse. It was very anxiety producing. I talked to the rabbi, and went to the synagogue a lot. But the reality was that she wasn't going to get better." Elizabeth and her brothers and sister went home frequently and often talked about their mother's illness via telephone. She felt somewhat frustrated with her older brother (the physician), because he was "very clinical, Mr. Never-show-emotion, with the 'doctor facade.'" At the same time, Elizabeth was angry because her brother could not "fix" their mother.

Elizabeth's mother wanted to have a big New Year's party; all of the children came home.

It was like she was saving all of her strength for that day and the party. She looked pretty and she really was in her element. She just loved having all the activity around. We all stayed for a couple of days before we had to go back.

About a month later, Elizabeth's father called. Her mother was back in the hospital. When it became clear that she was dying, all of the children returned home. "There was always somebody in the room with her. The hospice nurses were absolutely wonderful. They're just an amazing breed. That night, I just kissed her on the forehead and I said, 'I love you, Mom.'" Her mother died early the next morning. Elizabeth awoke and knew immediately.

Experience Following Her Mother's Death

Her mother's funeral was the first Elizabeth had been to. "It was absolutely awful." Although Elizabeth did not find the service meaningful, she enjoyed having so many old friends around. "There were a lot of tears but a lot of laughter and joy as well." Elizabeth had a more difficult time after she returned home. "For the longest time, it's like I wanted to run away from myself, but couldn't. I always had to be in motion. I lost a lot of weight. Cried a lot." Elizabeth's sister entered to a bereavement program and shared her "homework" and readings with Elizabeth. "It was very good. I wish there would have been something like that here. I think it would have been extremely beneficial for me."

Elizabeth's father took on some of her mother's family roles.

Now, he's a friend. What I used to be like with my mom, now I am with my dad. He's much more mellow. Much more laid back. Things that used to send him through the roof just don't phase him now. He's much more verbal in saying things like, "I love you" and "I'm so proud." And he's much more willing to try things or to concede that he's wrong.

Elizabeth considers this new relationship with her father a final gift from her mother.

About four or five years after his wife's death, Elizabeth's father decided to remarry.

I was just angry, not so much that my father was getting remarried. We were happy if he was happy, and he has a lot to offer, but I guess I was just angry because this should have been the time he was enjoying with my mother. I was crying a lot, I wasn't eating. I wasn't even eating chocolate, so that is a sure sign that something is wrong.

Elizabeth began counseling. Elizabeth did not like her father's new wife; she felt that she was destroying her family.

> She wasn't sincere. She was manipulative. My mother was none of those things. She was just very different from my mother. She was very hurtful and very spiteful toward us. She would never let us have any private time with my dad.

Elizabeth's counselor told her that, "It was like I was championing my mother's cause. I was still standing up for her." At the suggestion of the counselor, Elizabeth asked her father to spend a weekend with her so they could talk things out.

> We just sort of duked it out. It was great. I really felt like I had unburdened. I didn't like [stepmother] any better, but I got my eyes opened a little bit from his perspective. He let me see that they [Elizabeth's parents] had a good marriage, but it wasn't perfect. I was lucky that he was willing to participate in doing this. It just made me feel better about the whole thing.

Despite this conversation, the situation between the children and their stepmother did not improve. Once, Elizabeth called her older brother to complain. "He was really good. He said, 'I will not let that woman destroy this family.' He called my dad. He really did some good. He and my dad were on the phone for about two hours." Soon after this incident, Elizabeth's father left his new wife. They were divorced after only seven months of marriage.

Long-Term Impact

Elizabeth has periodic crying spells that she calls "a big cry."

> Every couple of months, I just need to have a big cry. It's just stress and aggravation in my life. It's like my quarterly cry. The Jewish holidays are hard, and Mother's Day. We send my dad a Mother's Day plant. Thanksgiving is very hard, 'cause Thanksgiving was always my mother's holiday.

Elizabeth's sister writes their mother a letter on her birthday, and she calls Elizabeth to ask if she wants to include anything special. The anniversary of her mother's death also is a difficult time. "February is such a 'do nothing much' month. It's hard because the world still keeps going on." Elizabeth does not only miss her mother on holidays and special days. "Sometimes it's just a mom thing, and she's not here. I get angry still, that she isn't here when I still need help."

Elizabeth still keeps her mother in her life. She has numerous pictures of her in her apartment.

> I think about her every day, and I talk to her almost every day. Now, I just truly, truly appreciate all that she really did for us. Sometimes I can feel her presence, which is really cool. When I get really hyper or really anxious about something, every now and then I'll just all of a sudden be very peaceful, and I'll feel like someone's hugging me from behind. It's like I know she's around.

It is especially difficult for Elizabeth when other women are not appreciative of their mothers.

> I hear so many people who don't get along with their mothers, and it just makes me sad. I think, *Get that shit resolved now and appreciate what they have to offer.* You have to understand that they did the best they could with what they had. Since I don't have my mother, I just expect everybody else to love theirs dearly, and they don't.

Risk

Elizabeth is not worried about getting breast cancer.

> I think a lot of my mother's cancer and her sister's cancer also was a lot of anger toward their mother. A lot of it was repressed anger. I think that was a big contributing factor. So now I'm not worried about it at all.

Elizabeth tries to lead a healthy life by exercising and eating well. She limits her smoking and drinking. However, this is not because she fears breast cancer.

> I'm not worried because I'm very healthy, and then, part of me just knows that my mother wouldn't ever let anything bad happen to me. It is just more spiritual. I meditate a lot. I pray a lot, and I just really don't think about it.

Elizabeth gets annual mammograms, and "I try the breast exams, but I really can't tell in all honesty what's what."

Current Situation

At the time of the interviews, Elizabeth was thirty-seven and work-ing in the hospitality industry (she has a master's degree in this field). She has since taken a position in health care administration, which she loves. Elizabeth has been a volunteer for organizations dealing with factors related to her mother's death. She served as a hospice volunteer for several years. Recently, she served as the organizer of a breast cancer symposium for a local foundation. "It just makes me much more compassionate toward other people. My brother is now a hospice director. I think it's made him a much better doctor." She was planning to be married, but then broke off the engagement. She still hopes to get married and have children.

CASE STUDY #3: SARAH

Age at Her Mother's Breast Cancer Diagnosis: 27; Age at Time of Her Mother's Death: 29

Background

Sarah was the oldest in a Catholic family with four children. Sa-rah's parents remained married, despite many marital difficulties. Sarah's mother was the principal's secretary in a Catholic high school. Sarah was married in 1986, and had a child in 1988. She lived only four miles away from her parents' home, and she and her mother were very close. "We were best friends. We shared everything—thoughts, dreams. We talked on the phone almost daily." Of her fa-ther, she says, "He was never there. He was always a very distant father." One of Sarah's younger sisters was "always in trouble" grow-ing up. She moved out, then got pregnant and eloped. Sarah's youn-gest sister attended a local college on a part-time basis while living at home with her parents. Sarah worked for a data processing company in the insurance business.

Experience of Her Mother's Illness

Soon after Sarah's child was born, Sarah's mother found a lump the size of a small marble in her breast. She immediately called Sarah, and together they decided that she would see Sarah's new doctor. Within days, the biopsy and other tests were done. Sarah's mother was diagnosed with breast cancer. A mastectomy was recommended. Sarah was not worried at that time. "I figured, 'Okay. She just has her breast removed, and they'll do the chemo and she'll be fine.'" The week before the surgery, the family took their traditional beach vacation.

> We [Sarah and her mother] spent some time talking that week. She was scared, but my mom had strong faith. She believed that God was with her and that she would get through this. She was just beginning to make changes in her life. She had started working full time. She was really finding herself as a woman, separate, apart from the family.

Sarah prayed for her mother. "I said the rosary daily for her." The week of her mother's surgery was not an easy one for Sarah. Her husband had recently had major back surgery, and her sister and her child were staying with Sarah afer escaping an abusive family situation. Then, Sarah's uncle (her mother's younger brother) died unexpectedly of a cerebral aneurysm only a week before her mother's surgery. "So while we're all going through trying to help Mom on this, all this other stuff is going on too." To make matters worse, the evening before the surgery was to take place, Sarah's father started to have chest pains.

> So we called nine-one-one and they took him to the hospital for a possible heart attack. So I went with my mom to the hospital and we were sitting there and she said, "I knew he would do something to me like this. It's always about him. It can never be about me." She was right. My father has to take the spotlight off of her to focus on him. She was really upset about that. He was fine. He had an anxiety attack.

Sarah wanted to take time off work to be with her mother for the surgery, but her boss wouldn't let her. "She was just a workhorse. She was a matronly woman with no family, and she couldn't understand that I had family. She wouldn't give me the day off, so I left work sick. I needed to be there." When the surgery was completed, the doctors told Sarah's mother that the lymph nodes were clear. They recommended chemotherapy as a precaution. Sarah knew that breast cancer was serious, but "I guess I didn't realize how serious this was going to be."

Her mother started chemotherapy, and lost her hair.

> She was upset about the hair loss. She got a wig. We kind of handled some things with humor in our family, and my brother cracked a joke, and she went from tears to laughter. He had her laughing so hard. It helped.

Always a deeply religious person, Sarah's mother also used religion to help her through this period.

> She prayed daily. She had her set of saint cards, and she would pray every day. I brought her a rose or a bunch of flowers once a week. It's Saint Teresa's little flower. Mom believed strongly. She never knew when I was going to bring the flowers and it seemed like every time I brought them, it was just when she needed that extra boost.

Sarah's mother continued on chemotherapy for six months; when she was finished she quickly regained her strength. "One of her life-long dreams was to go to Hawaii. My father wouldn't go with her. She went anyway. She and her sister went to Hawaii in April."

Life returned to normal for Sarah. She was ecstatic when she found out that she was pregnant with her second child. Soon after, her mother took a weekend trip to a shopping outlet, where she tripped and broke a bone in her foot. The next week, she noticed a lump in her shoulder. After some blood tests, the family learned that the cancer was back. This time, her mother did not tell Sarah.

> My father came over. Mom didn't want to worry me because I was pregnant. He sat me down in a chair and said, "I have something to tell you. Your mother is dying of cancer. She's not going to . . ." I said, "You've given up all sense of hope! I don't even want to hear that!" I was, like, really angry at him for that. I said, "There's treatment out there! There's things we can do!" That was the first time ever in my life that I had yelled back at my father.

Sarah and her sister decided to take matters into their own hands.

> We didn't understand why we couldn't talk to Mom about this. He wasn't telling Mom. [Father said,] "The doctor and I decided not to tell your mother." My sister and I, we weren't putting up with this. I could not imagine that with my mother. Mom was very up front about wanting to know what was going on. So we got a hold of Mom's doctor. He explained to us that the cancer had metastasized, and the outlook for recovery was grim. And we were like, "Well, what can you do about it?" And there was nothing that we could do. But there were some experimental studies that he might be able to get her into. We were still in

flat-out denial. There had to be something that could be done. We were not willing to accept a death sentence, because to see my mother then, she was still full of life, vibrant. There was no sign of the disease. We couldn't understand.

The next doctor thought that with treatment, Sarah's mother might live six to twelve months. With her daughter's encouragement, Sarah's mother decided to undergo more radiation and chemotherapy. "And the hell that she went through! Radiation was *terrible*. Megadoses of chemotherapy. But nothing seemed to stop this cancer. Nothing." She goes on:

We were kind of working on two levels. We were working on this real hopeful level, that everything was going to work. But if we let ourselves think about it, we realized that three of the six months were gone already. That she was dying. That we were going to have to deal with this.

One of Sarah's strongest memories of this period was when she and her mother took a drive out to a park.

She started preparing us for her death. She told me that the last bone scan came back, and the cancer was still spreading. She was still going to try to fight it. But it might not work. She wanted me to understand that. So we started talking, in terms of, she wanted me to handle the funeral mass. And we cried. We talked and we cried. She said she was okay with dying. She goes, "I've done all that I've wanted to do. I've raised you four. You're healthy. You're established." Mom and I could talk real open and honest about that. She talked about what it was like after her mother died and she told me how I would be feeling. She said, "If you have to cry, then go ahead and do it. You will get through it."

Later, Sarah and her mother attended a support group together.

The family worked together to help her mother through her last weeks. Sarah went to her parents' home every morning before work to make breakfast. Her sister stopped in at lunch, and her brother visited in the afternoon. "Dad just wasn't handling it at all. He shut off emotionally." Sarah continued to provide her mother spiritual support.

I'd bring her communion. I'd pray with her. We'd talk about death, about her funeral. Which songs she wanted. We picked the readings together. We had some really beautiful conversations about death and sin and forgiveness and God. She wasn't afraid of death, but she was afraid of getting to death. We talked about the light at the end of the tunnel. We talked about God's forgiveness and what that meant.

Sarah arranged a prayer service at her parents' home. "We had one of the priests come down and talk to us about Mom's dying and death, with her there. We were all together." The family had their last Thanksgiving together. "She was able to sit at the table for a little while." In December, Sarah contacted a hospice. "[My youngest sister] was begging me to get a nurse to come in." Close to her due date, Sarah resigned from her job. As a result of her experience with her mother's illness Sarah decided that she wanted to be home to spend more time with her children, and that she wanted more meaningful work. She soon found a part-time job as a youth minister at her church. Her mother was in and out of the hospital in the final weeks. On one visit, Sarah's and her sister's children played on the floor while her mother sat up in a chair. "We kept it funny and light. Christmas Day was spent home with family. That night, Mom took a turn for the worse, and she was taken to the hospital." The day after Christmas, Sarah visited her mother in the hospital.

> Mom's spirits were up. She was sitting up in bed. We were talking. She was clear. She asked me if I could clean her fingernails. She was like, "I don't want to die and be in the funeral home with dirty fingernails." So they got me the stuff and I cleaned and I did her nails. I filed them down. We sat there [for] an hour or two. We talked a little bit. She was in real good spirits. When we were getting ready to leave, we kissed her and told her we loved her and we'd see her the next day. We got into the hallway and Dad said, "She's probably not going to make it through the night." So I went home and I called her sisters and brother and said, "Get down there and see Mom tonight."

Later that night, Sarah's brother called. He told her to come to the hospital. When she got there, her brother said, "She's gone." Later, the nurse told Sarah, "I just want to let you know that I happened to be in there when your mom died. Your mom just turned and looked at me and smiled. She just went very peacefully. I wanted you to know that."

Experience Following Her Mother's Death

The next day, Sarah told her son (almost three) that "Mom-Mom went to heaven with Jesus last night." Sarah went to the funeral home and the church to make arrangements. "I met with the organist and said, 'This is the music Mom picked out.' I took care of the flowers. There were rose crosses from each one of the kids." Sarah got to the funeral home for what she expected to be a special time with her immediate family, to find her father's extended family there.

> I was not in the mood to allow any of that to happen. I stood there and I said, "This is the way things are going to be. We are going to go in first with our children. When we're done, then the rest of you may come in. But we need the time alone with Mom." They didn't quite like that too much, but at that point, I didn't care.

Sarah got much satisfaction from the way the funeral progressed.

> It was really good. We had a really good wake service and at the funeral the next day, we handled that well. I had a lot of control, and Mom had given each of us our responsibilities. We each had our own little parts to take care of that day.

However, Sarah was upset that her father took off her mother's rings before the casket was closed. "I wanted her wedding ring to be buried with her. My father didn't. [He said], 'I want mother's ring. I bought it. I paid for it. And I want it.' Mom was Irish so it was a party after the funeral."

Two days after her mother's funeral, Sarah's father called her. He said, "If you want any of your mother's stuff, you've got two days to get it out of the house."

> When I got down there, he had already started throwing her things in bags. I made three trips. We were all mad. We were crying and we were like, "How could he do this? I don't understand." He just said, "I want it gone by the time I get home." And he just left. So we did. We cleared out her closet. We cleared out the attic. I got most of her clothing because I was her height. We just brought it all in and we stored it, because I couldn't deal with going through a lot of that stuff right then and there.

One week after her mother's death, Sarah gave birth to her second child. Sarah did a lot of crying during this period.

> There were afternoons I'd sit here and cry and just cry. When I'd start to feel a sadness, I would hold on to him [baby]. Mother's Day was tough, of course. Her birthday was tough. You go through that whole grief process.

Sarah took a course in death and dying. "It was a real good healing process to go through. It helped me understand a lot of what I was going through and it helped me see what my family was going through."

One area of frustration for Sarah was the effect of her mother's death on the family, and her inability to prevent change.

> For the first two years after Mom's death, I tried so hard to keep the family together, and I got into so many conflicts that I just decided, the hell with it. I couldn't do it anymore. I was trying to take her place, and I realized I couldn't do that.

Conflicts broke out between Sarah's youngest sister and her father. When the family got together for their traditional beach vacation, it was not the same as it had been in the past.

> It was nice for us to be down there but tension had already set in. With her gone, the family no longer . . . We tried to keep things together the first two to three years. The holiday celebrations. The birthday celebrations. We were nice to each other but there were some tensions that, if Mom had been around, would have been easily squelched. But without that mediator, and they were not allowing me to fulfill the mediator role, we had to learn how to deal with each other again as a family. Mom's death was the end of the family as we knew it, because she was the person that kept the family together.

Sarah regrets that no support programs targeted to the families of women who died from breast cancer were available. "We all kind of are just handling it on our own. There were no support systems to help us through that."

Following his wife's death, Sarah's father also experienced a major adjustment.

> For the first time in thirty-two years, he had to go grocery shopping, he had to cook the meals, he had to do his laundry, he had to clean the house. He had to learn how to operate an ATM machine [laughter]. He started dating not long after Mother died. He needed someone to fill that void very desperately. He dated a couple of different people, and then he got engaged. He remarried about three years after Mom died, moved in with his new wife, and they sold the family home. There was a whole lot of tension over the belongings in the house. Mom made Dad promise to take care of [youngest sister], and Dad wasn't living up to his promise.

Sarah's youngest sister lived with each of her siblings for a while.

> She has diabetes, and she lost her partner [mother] in managing her diabetes. Dad never bothered to learn about the care. She's had to learn to become self-sufficient in so many ways so quickly, whereas we didn't. She doesn't have a home anymore.

Although Sarah gets along well with her father's wife, it is clear that her stepmother has not replaced her natural mother.

> Dad just turned sixty. [Her stepmother is] forty-two. I'd rather have the children call her by her name. She didn't want to be called "Grandmother" or "Nana" 'cause she felt she's too young for that. And I said, "Well, that's fine with me because you're not the children's grandmother. You're my father's second wife." We try to talk these things out. But she's still somewhat uncomfortable when we talk about Mom.

Long-Term Impact

Sarah says, "I've learned how to function without her in my life." She is comforted by remembering that her mother told her to expect to have a really good cry every couple of months. Her mother also told her that her crying would gradually decrease to once a year; this is what Sarah now experiences. Sarah misses her mother's support.

> She used to send me little cards all the time. If I got a promotion at work, or if I changed jobs, it was always, "CONGRATULATIONS!" She was my number-one supporter. So with her being gone, that's been a real struggle.

As Sarah approaches menopause, she would like to know more about her mother's medical history. She knows that her mother had a hysterectomy, but doesn't know why.

Sarah feels that she has been able to achieve a balance in her life between work and family, and that this is due in part to her mother's death.

> I went back to focusing on what it was that I wanted to do with my life. I wanted a family and I wanted children. I wanted to be a part of my children's lives, just like my mom was a part of my life. That means not working a sixty-hour-week job. It means being home during the day, being the den mother, being their coach, doing the sports, running them around, and being an active part of their life. I want a career, but I had to realign my priorities. I made a lot of life changes with her illness and death.

Sarah became a breast cancer advocate.

> I wear my pink ribbon during the months of May and October. May because of my mother's birthday and Mother's Day, and October because it is [National] Breast Cancer Awareness Month. I don't hesitate now in groups of women that I'm with—if someone mentions

something, I say, "Make sure you do your BSE [breast self-exam]. My mother died of breast cancer and it's important." I've become very aware of this.

Sarah also read about breast cancer, and came to regret that her mother did not seek more aggressive treatment.

Reconstructive surgery was not even an option for my mom. It's like, when you have the money, different things happen. I really do believe the more money you have, the better off you are in health care. The average woman, they're not getting the treatment that they deserve.

Risk

Sarah had a baseline mammogram when she turned thirty, and does breast self-exams every month. She would like to have more mammograms, but her insurance company won't cover them until she reaches forty. "There are three daughters. The chances are one out of three for family members. The chances are that one of us could develop breast cancer." Sarah has had one scare. She found a small lump after she stopped breast-feeding.

It was a very small lump. I went into his [doctor's] office, he found it, he sent me for a sonogram, he sent me to a surgeon. This is all within, like, four hours. This guy looked at it and just said it was fibrocystic. I kept checking it, and the next month, it was gone.

Sarah is interested in developments in the field of genetics and breast cancer.

I'm real interested in the genetic research they're doing. I keep my ear open because I want to be tested. I ask my doctor each time, each year, "Is there any test in place yet?" He says, "It's all in research." I don't want to be a part of that type of research, when you don't know whether you're on the real drug or a placebo. I would just rather have a blood test to know am I genetically . . . and if I am, then I know I still need to exercise and eat right and take vitamins. Eat broccoli three times a day [laughing]. Knowing that it might be genetic, you'd give special attention to it. Maybe you won't forget to do that BSE each month. Maybe if you're genetically disposed, the insurance company will pay for a mammogram every two years.

Current Situation

Sarah was thirty-four at the time of the interviews. She had three children. The middle child has a serious chronic illness, and his care and prognosis are a major focus in Sarah's life. She remains frustrated that she has not been able to keep her family together. She is close to her youngest sister, but her relationship with her other sister remains strained. She maintains a cordial but somewhat distant relationship with her father and his second wife.

Sarah still cries easily five years after her mother's death. Sometimes, Sarah prays to her mother. She still feels her presence, and feels as if she can rely on her. Sarah looks for signs from her mother, and feels supported and uplifted when she finds them. For example, when she recently completed her credits to graduate from college, she learned that the graduation ceremony was scheduled for her mother's birthday.

> I just really felt her presence. I mean, to graduate on her birthday! It was the most special thing. It was like her gift, almost, to me. She encouraged me throughout. Now I feel she even supports it more.

She continues to work with young people in the Catholic Church, and considers this a source of satisfaction. Sarah graduated from college in 1996 and was working on a master's degree in theology.

CASE STUDY #4: FELICIA

Age at Her Mother's Breast Cancer Diagnosis: 29; Age at Time of Her Mother's Death: 31

Background

Felicia, the older of two sisters, was raised in a very close African-American family in a small, rural community. The girls did everything with their parents and their many relatives who lived nearby. Felicia and her sister never had a baby-sitter while they were children. The family had a strong sense of their history; Felicia remembers that her great-grandfather would tell family stories from past generations.

Although her parents were not highly educated, they encouraged the girls to attend college. After high school, Felicia started working on her bachelor's degree, with plans to go to law school. However, when she was twenty-one, her father died suddenly of a heart attack.

> I cried every day for two years and I kind of had a breakdown. I broke out in hives, and was confined to bed for about a month. I just felt like one of the most important people in my life had just been snatched from me. So I was just helpless, crazy.

About a month after her father's death, Felicia went back to school.

> I was so young and I felt lost without my father. "What am I going to do? Who's going to take care of the car? The house?" I felt totally vulnerable to society. I'd never had a full-time job. I was not ready for prime time. Not ready at all.

After graduating from college, Felicia got a government job in a large city about an hour and a half from her hometown. She lived at home and commuted. Her younger sister had a baby, but continued to live with their mother.

Experience of Her Mother's Illness

Around this time, Felicia's mother began to feel some tenderness in one of her breasts. Although she had had a mammogram only six months before, she decided to have another. A biopsy was followed by a mastectomy. "I had a very close-knit family, and we were very open. I was residing with my mother when she found out, so we talked about everything. There's nothing we didn't talk about." In fact, the entire family (mother's mother, sisters, and daughters) all went to the biopsy, and, within two days, they all returned to the hospital for the mastectomy. Felicia got in touch with the American Cancer Society and tried to find a support group for her mother, but her mother did not want to join one. "She was very strong-willed and religious. That was just her way. She would talk to us about it, but not to other people." When her mother started chemotherapy, Felicia took her to doctor's appointments for six months. She also read everything she could find on nutrition and combating nausea during chemotherapy, and coping with cancer in general. Although her mother hated getting chemotherapy ("It tasted like drinking oil slick"), she never lost her hair. Following the chemotherapy, Felicia's mother returned to normal life.

Two years later, she had a recurrence. Felicia was angry. "She's done everything you possibly can do! She's always had her regular checkups, always been very conscientious about what she ate and all those kind of things, and I'm thinking, 'How could this happen?'" Felicia's mother's lungs began to fill with fluid and she was hospitalized several times to drain them. Once she had to stay in the hospital for forty-five days. During this stay she was given another round of chemotherapy. This time, her hair did fall out.

> Within a week, all of her hair just fell right out. I mean, like, we visited her one night and the next day she called me at work and she said, "You have to buy me a wig *today!* My hair is falling out in clumps!" and I was like, "Ma, you're exaggerating." Well, no, she wasn't. It just came out by the handfuls. So I went out and bought her a wig, which she hated [laughing]. But you know she was fine with it. My mother was very, very strong. I was scared to death. I thought she wasn't gonna come home. But she recuperated. She came home, and she even went back to taking care of my nephew. She went to church. But she would get tired really easily. She never bounced back to one hundred percent.

Felicia helped pay her mother's bills (mortgage, car, health insurance), and she applied for Social Security Disability for her mother.

After six months, Felicia's mother needed to go on oxygen. Felicia and her sister adjusted their work schedules so that one of them was always home. Mother lost her appetite, and ate less and less. As mother became bloated, caring for her got more and more difficult. "Getting her dressed for a doctor's appointment would take almost an hour. Just to get her in the clothes, because she was just so worn out, so out of breath, so full of fluid."

> By this point, she was bloating. I mean, she couldn't even wear her shoes. She wore slippers all the time, and we were getting bigger and bigger slippers. She was just wearing sweat clothes, or nightclothes. She couldn't even tolerate getting dressed.

Felicia shares a funny story from that period.

> We had to take, like, two tanks of oxygen everywhere we went, because the doctor's was a forty-five-minute drive, and we had to have enough to get home. One time, I took an empty tank [laughing] by mistake. What happened was the guy didn't fill all the tanks, and it's not

like you can really tell. And then, too, I was an emotional wreck. Just seeing her dying was too much for me. So she says, "I think my oxygen is getting low!" And I realized that I had this empty tank for backup. And I'm thinking, *Oh, God!* Luckily, we were near the oxygen place, so I drove over and they gave me [a new] one. She [mother] just laughed. She was never angry or anything like that. She was always pleasant. Just very strong throughout.

Eventually, Felicia's mother became more and more uncomfortable.

She was on painkillers so she was sleeping quite a bit, but she was having a hard time breathing, and her heart was really weak too. The fluid in her chest was getting to be more and more each day. I mean, her legs were, like, big, like, blown up. She could hardly move, and when you helped her to move, it was a lot for you to lift her and stuff. But she never admitted being in pain until the day she died. Never.

Her mother returned to the hospital, where she could get more oxygen and where the staff could help with lifting her. Felicia and her sister practically lived at the hospital. "I slept in a chair for three weeks. I took care of her, read the Bible to her, and we just talked. She never cried. I did all the crying." Felicia's mother talked openly about dying, making such comments as, "Don't worry about me."

Felicia's mother was in the "respite" area of the hospital, and she was expected to go home to die.

So each day the social worker would come down and she wanted me to take her home. "Your insurance won't pay for you to stay at the hospital. You have to go home to die." But my mother didn't want to go home. One day, she'd look at me and she'd say, like, "I know you're tired. Mommy's tired too. God knows when we're all tired and he'll take care of it." The doctors told me she would live another six to eight weeks. At that point, she was in really bad, bad shape. When I brushed her teeth, her gums would come off on the toothbrush. She wasn't skin and bones—she had fluid—but her face was a lot thinner, and her skin was like a newborn baby's, but it was gray.

Felicia has very vivid memories of the day her mother died.

All that day, it snowed and snowed. And blackbirds kept coming to the window. I don't know if you've heard people say that when blackbirds come, somebody's gonna die. Well, there was a big pine tree outside of her hospital room, and the whole tree was full with blackbirds. I mean, the whole tree.

That night, Felicia's mother started gasping for breath. The nurse said, "Something is seriously wrong." After taking vital signs and offering Felicia's mother pain medication, she turned to Felicia and said, "If you want to call the family [do so now], because she isn't going to live much longer." Felicia recalls, "She just laid there and rested. The last thing she said was my name, and she smiled. She died with a smile on her face, about ten minutes later. I was a basket case." Felicia was angry. "My mother had become my best friend. It was hard. I was real upset. I just felt like, 'Why?'"

Experience Following Her Mother's Death

After her mother died, Felicia's small community pulled together in support of the family.

> They were very supportive. They would come up, bring us a dish, you know, just talk or just call and say, "If you need anything, we'll do it." My sister picked out what my mother was going to wear. The whole family went to the funeral home together. My father's brother, my mother's brother, all of my mother's siblings went. Even my little cousins went. So we all picked out the casket.

Felicia also was appreciative of her co-workers' support. "Most of them came down for her wake on Sunday night. I was really shocked. I mean, people came out of the woodwork. That was a long drive for them!" She describes the service, remembering that "it was so packed there was no place for people to sit." Speaking about the funeral, Felicia admits,

> By that time, I think I was really tired. I had lived at the hospital for three weeks, and I was exhausted. I was sad, but I was at peace too. You know, when I saw her suffer through all that. At that point, she was ready. When I look back at it I think, *God, she suffered more than she wanted us to know.* You know, it just hurt me to my heart.

Following their mother's death, Felicia's sister began to have difficulty sleeping. "My sister started sleeping on the floor outside of my mother's old bedroom." Her sister also kept herself very busy, to block the pain. "She kept very busy day and night. She and my nephew, they were always just ripping and running." Felicia took on some responsibility for her younger sister.

> My sister is very strong, but dependent. Quite dependent on me. Right now she's unemployed. Since my mother died, I think I've spent at least three years weaning my sister. And I guess weaning myself some too. I took the mother role, and I've babied her. At first, we could not convince her to go to college. Now she is going and she has thirty-eight credits.

Felicia stayed at her mother's house for several weeks, but then moved to a large city. "It was hard. I cried every night." Felicia has not had any counseling or been to any bereavement workshops, but she has prayed a lot. "I'm my own best counselor," she says.

Felicia also broke up with her boyfriend after her mother died.

> I changed my whole life. When she died, I broke up with my boyfriend, who I'd been dating for eleven years. It had been coming, but I was just too occupied with other things. It was just a bad relationship and I should have gotten out of it a long time ago.

Long-Term Impact

Felicia's philosophy on life changed after her mother's death.

> I decided I would never spend another day mulling over things that weren't important. Worrying about he said, she said. I would not entertain anything that was not benefiting me or someone else. It had to be something worthwhile. I just took on a whole new outlook on life. I think we're so materialistic and we take too many things for granted. I decided I was gonna concentrate on me for once.

Felicia put more emphasis on her spirituality, and also on nurturing herself. "I started doing things that made Felicia happy for the first time in my life."

Felicia still feels the loss of her mother, but has learned to take meaning from her death.

> Whenever I missed her or felt bad, I thought about how she suffered, and that kind of helped. It still hurts, but it's a different hurt. It's a hurt that you can cope with, and it doesn't bring you down or knock you off your feet. We learned a whole lot. How to love and what unconditional love is truly all about.

Felicia thinks that because of her experience she can better help others who are in pain.

Based on what she [mother] did for me, I've been able to help other friends and talk to people. I think that's a therapy in itself, if you can help someone else get through their experience. I do that very freely. My thing is, if you can help someone else to get through a bad situation or help their pain to be a little less, then I think you've done a great thing.

Risk

Felicia is aware that cancer is prominent in her family's history.

My mother's brother died of colon cancer, and my mother's aunt died of cancer—I think it was female, but I don't know. Older people don't tell you exactly what is what. My father's mother died of cancer. She had cancer of the uterus.

Felicia gets a yearly mammogram but does not do her BSE every month. "I do check, but I don't do them every month." Once, her sister found a lump that needed to be biopsied. "We were scared stiff. She had it removed, and they said it was just fatty tissue. So, she's fine."

Felicia watches her diet and exercises, but she is not interested in genetic testing.

I think diet is a big thing. Exercise, I have been lacking on, but I'm getting back on the track with that. You know, preventive medicine. I do mammograms and the self-exam. I don't think you really can do much more than that. I don't want to know if I have the gene or whatever. You can't get rid of it. I know that heredity has a big part to do with it. But I also believe that diet and those things can counteract heredity too. I'm going to continue to eat healthy and pray a lot. I won't even worry myself with all that. That's not even a concern with me.

Current Situation

At the time of the interview, Felicia was thirty-six and single and worked for the government. Five years after her mother's death, Felicia still returned home every weekend to be with her sister and other relatives. She talks on the phone with her sister, her aunt, and her cousin every day. "We spend a lot of money on the phone bill!"

Felicia is concerned about her sister:

My sister has been really sick lately. I mean, like really emotionally sick in that she has heart palpitations. She has phobias. She's claustrophobic and she doesn't like heights. She has fits about riding the elevator. The doctor says it is the stress of being independent and on her own. She was director of a day care center, and that was very stressful.

Although Felicia is very close to her family, she is also trying to achieve some independence. "Last November, I went to New York with my friend for Thanksgiving. They were very upset. They just won't hear of that. That's not allowed. You know, even with a lot of closeness, sometimes you do want some space." She and her sister frequently share memories of their mother. Her aunts have been telling her that, as she ages, she looks and acts more and more like her mother. This makes her happy.

Felicia has been engaged twice and at the time of the last interview had just broken up with her fiancé.

> He was really wonderful. I really thought he was the love of my life, but it didn't work out. He has kids, and he's not willing to do some of the things he needs to do. You know, when my mother died, I decided that I'm not going to waste time and energy on people who will not do what I think is right.

She hopes to marry and have children one day. "I hope I have triplets!"

DISCUSSION

In this section, common themes are developed for women who as young adults lost their mothers to breast cancer. In the period during mother's illness and treatment, three themes are discussed: taking charge, superwoman (balancing care of mother with adult-life roles), and adult mother-daughter relationship. During the period after mother's death, the themes are healthy grieving, walking in mother's footprints, and Cinderella grows up. The section on long-term impact identifies changing priorities and the big cry as major themes. In addition to the four case studies (Andrea, Elizabeth, Sarah, and Felicia), the cases of Cheryl and Lily, whose cases are described in Appendix III, are also included in the discussion.

Daughter's Experience of Her Mother's Illness

Taking Charge

Most daughters in this study, even those who were very young, provided some care for their mothers; however, the adult daughters carried much more responsibility and were able to offer much more help than were adolescents or young children. Adult daughters helped by communicating directly with the mother's physician, locating and arranging medical and social services, and providing financial assistance. In Andrea's words, "We had turned into adult women and were really taking charge of the situation." Andrea spoke directly with her mother's physician so as not to upset her mother, who did not want to talk about her illness. Eventually, Andrea moved back home to help her mother by providing comprehensive care, including changing dressings and operating a feeding tube, a very difficult task. Sarah was involved from the time her mother discovered a lump, and helped her mother locate a suitable doctor. Later, when mother's cancer recurred, Sarah and her sister went directly to the doctor for information, and to identify alternative treatments. Because of Sarah's background in the church, she took on the role of spiritual advisor and counselor for her mother. Felicia provides another example. After her mother was diagnosed, Felicia identified services (support groups) for her mother, and read "everything she could find" on cancer. She took on many caregiving tasks, such as taking her mother to appointments and, later, managing her oxygen supplies. Cheryl (Appendix III) became an advocate for her mother at the hospital, "making sure [she's] cared for, and that the physician sees [her] as a person." When her mother could no longer work, Cheryl took over her house payments and set up a trust to ensure ongoing ownership of the home. She also cared for her mother's many pets. In fact, it was Cheryl who paid for her mother's funeral expenses. Lily (Appendix III) also talked to her mother's physician directly.

In summary, young adult daughters provided more comprehensive care than did younger daughters, including direct contact with physicians, arranging services for the mother, providing financial help, and, in one case, serving as a spiritual counselor. This case went beyond the supportive care offered by daughters who were younger by including "taking care" of the care.

Superwoman

One common issue for the young adult daughters was the strain they experienced in balancing the need to care for their mothers with other demands of young adult life. This was most obvious in the women who were married, had children, and worked. For example, Sarah carried multiple responsibilities at the time of her mother's illness. In addition to caring for her mother, she dealt with a pregnancy, her husband's back injury, her young child, her father's problems, her sister's crisis, her uncle's death, and a demanding job. As her mother's health deteriorated, Sarah went to her home almost daily, visited her mother in the hospital, and helped manage her dying process.

Other women who were married but did not have children took on caring for their mothers in addition to maintaining their marital relationships, managing a household, and working. Andrea, for example, moved back home after her mother's breast cancer recurred, and got married only six weeks before her mother's death. Although her husband was an oncologist and very understanding of her situation, Andrea was caught between wanting to be with her new husband and caring for her mother. Her honeymoon was cut short, and she spent much of it on the phone. Cheryl (Appendix III) and her husband also moved to be closer to her mother, and she later changed jobs to have the flexibility she needed to be a caregiver.

Young adult women who were not married exhibited less role conflict, but they too show strain between work and lifestyle issues and the demands of caring for their mothers. Elizabeth was working on establishing a career and a lifestyle away from her family. She was not the main caregiver, so the conflict was not as great as with other cases, but she did go home on weekends. Felicia was living at home at the time of her mother's diagnosis, but she worked in a city an hour and a half away. When her mother's illness progressed, Felicia and her sister had to adjust their work schedules so that one of them was home at all times. Felicia basically lived at the hospital (hospice) until her mother died.

Women in the later twentieth century have tried to "have it all." In the past, most women had to choose between being either housewives and mothers or working. The modern woman, in contrast, has children but continues to work. Many women today feel that they are able to do an adequate job with any one of these roles (mother, wife, worker), but they have difficulty managing to do all three. Add to this the burden of caring for a mother when she is ill, and that the strain can be enormous.

Most literature about the difficulty of balancing family demands and caregiving for parents comes from studies of midlife women caring for elderly parents. This literature has generated the concept of the "sandwich generation" (Brody, 1985; Dautzenberg, 2000; Horowitz, 1985). Similar to midlife women, young adult daughters whose mothers have breast cancer find themselves sandwiched between the demands of young adult life and the mother's need for care.

Unfortunately, little literature is available on the young adult stage of life (Rossi and Rossi, 1990). The major roles of the "young adulthood" phase of life are thought to be those of worker, spouse, and parent. "Young adults are learning to engage in intense and meaningful relationships in marriage, with intimate partners, with friends and with co-workers" (Newman and Newman, 1995, p. 522). Emphasis is on the difficulties of early married life, and the need for the young adult to learn to communicate, deal with conflict, develop a satisfactory sexual relationship, and manage dual careers (Newman and Newman, 1995). Rolland (1994) suggests families of young adults can be seen as in a centrifugal phase, during which young adults focus on their own families, and do not regain closeness with families of origin until later, when parents become elderly. When a parent of a young adult becomes seriously ill, it is considered "out of synch" or nonnormative (Rossi and Rossi, 1990). Dealing with life events that are considered "untimely" is often more stressful because these incidents are unexpected and can be difficult to explain to others (Nolen-Hoeksema and Larson, 1999).

> When a disabling or life-threatening disorder occurs earlier [than expected], it is out of phase in both chronological and social time. When such events are untimely, spouse and family lack the psychosocial preparation and rehearsal that occur later, when peers are experiencing similar losses. The ill member and the family are likely to feel robbed of their expectation of a normal life span. (Rolland, 1994, p. 186)

The young adult daughters interviewed were stressed by the caregiving demands caused by the mother's breast cancer. Those who had competing responsibilities, such as children, husbands, and work, were especially overwhelmed. However, even those without children (e.g., Andrea) or without husbands (e.g., Elizabeth) were dealing with added and unanticipated responsibilities at a time of life when these were not normative. They would have preferred to be with husbands, building relationships; at work, building careers; or with their children. If they did not have these relationships, they would have likely preferred to participate in other age-appropriate activities.

Adult Mother-Daughter Relationship

The young adult daughters in this study became closer to their mothers as a result of the breast cancer. Andrea's case illustrates this shift in the mother-daughter relationship brought about by her mother's illness. "At that point [mother's recurrence] our relationship really changed. I was older and I could understand and relate to it more on an adult level." Because of her mother's illness, she and her mother took trips together—something they would not have done under normal circumstances. After her mother died, Andrea especially cherished her memories of these trips. Cheryl (Appendix III) describes how her relationship with her mother improved. Before, she had taken her mother for granted, but after her mother became ill, the two became "closer than ever." Sharon (Chapter 8), whose mother survived, contrasts her postillness relationship with her earlier relationship. "Once you get older . . . you start to see your parents as not your parents, but as human beings."

Some young adults did not experience a dramatic shift in the mother-daughter relationship. Elizabeth comments, "It's like she wouldn't allow that part of herself to be revealed. She would allow us to be supportive, but just so far." This role seems to be more of a "mutual mothering" relationship, in which the mother withheld parts of herself in the interest of protecting the adult child. Felicia's relationship does not shift dramatically, in part because she never had a period of adolescent conflict with her mother. One factor may be that Felicia comes from a rural, extended family and close community. In this type of social structure, commitment to family and community is often valued over individual development. Felicia's case also is different because her father died when she was in college; this may have put her on more adult-adult terms with her mother earlier than other women.

In normal life-course development, the mother-daughter relationship is the most intimate of all the parent-child relationships (Rossi and Rossi, 1990), especially after the daughter reaches the age of twenty, and the rough adolescent period has passed. "Whatever stain mothers and daughters experience during adolescence is lost once the daughter reaches maturity" (Rossi and Rossi, 1990, p. 314). Generally, mothers and daughters have frequent contact, with about half of daughters in America living within thirty minutes of their mothers, and two-thirds speaking on the phone at least weekly (Rossi and Rossi, 1990). Normally, despite this ongoing interaction, the mother-daughter relationship is highly ambivalent (Troll, 1987; Bassoff, 1987), with daughters needing to stay connected to their mothers, and at the same time needing to let go. Although this pattern is characteristic of the struggle for independence for all adolescents, in mother-daughter relationship, the ambivalence continues into adulthood. Women may achieve a physical separation but remain emotionally dependent throughout their lives. Many mother-daughter relationships are not rated positively, but they remain strong. When the mother is seriously ill, it seems that the more conflictual aspect of the relationship is diminished or overlooked.

For daughters who have children, the mother's potentially terminal illness increases the importance of her role as grandmother. Sarah felt it was important for her child to spend time with her mother before her death. She was sorry her mother did not get to meet her second child, but enjoyed showing her mother the sonogram picture before his birth. Women who had not yet had children when their mothers died sometimes expressed regret that they had not "given Mother a grandchild," and also that when their mothers died, their future children also had lost a grandmother. The relationship between children and grandparents is highly valued in our society, by both children and the grandparents themselves.

Another aspect of the more adult relationship between mother and daughter is increased openness in communication. In contrast to the experience of younger daughters, the level of openness was high, and communication was shared on the most difficult topics, including mother's death. Sarah talked openly with her mother about her mother's death, and even picked out the music and readings for the funeral. Similar to Sarah, Felicia came from a highly religious family, and this topic formed the basis for discussions about mother's death. Felicia was involved with her mother's illness from the very beginning of the ordeal. Cheryl (Appendix III) and her mother discussed where her mother wanted to die, and had many intense conversations "on a level that's not superficial. . . . Everything from death to religion to relationships."

In other cases, the discussion of death was more guarded, and patterns of "mutual protection" developed. In Andrea's case, "We talked a lot more candidly about life, and all of our experiences and death," but her mother didn't want her daughters to attend visits to the oncologist. One month before their mother's death, the two daughters went to the oncologist with her. A pattern of mutual protection existed in the family, as daughters saw the oncologist independently, and did not share with their mother the information they obtained. Andrea speculates that her mother simply did not want to know, and avoided asking her physician direct questions. Although they ultimately achieved very open communication, earlier in the illness it seemed as if the mother and daughters colluded to "keep up appearances" and keep her illness a secret. The mother refused to let the daughters provide a home nurse, and insisted that they perform difficult nursing tasks themselves. It is not clear if this was a case of denial or whether she wanted to keep the knowledge of her condition within the family. Elizabeth's case provides a similar example. Her mother did not openly discuss her illness or death, in spite of using a hospice, and knowing that her death was inevitable. She used euphemisms such as "I'm not feeling well," and used humor to cope.

Lily (Appendix III) also said her mother protected her and her sister by staying positive. In her last conversation with her mother, on the phone, Lily "was trying to carry on like—not like she wasn't sick or she wasn't in the hospital, but to let her know that life's going on around her." This suggests an avoidant pattern in which family and friends try to "cheer up" the dying, or provide "positive thinking." This pattern is more common in earlier phases of the illness, when a "fighting spirit" is encouraged. It was usually not until very close to the death that a very open pattern developed. If the death occurs very rapidly, as in Lily's case, where mother went into a coma unexpectedly, mothers and their young adult daughters may not reach this level. Open communication about death also is more acceptable in some cultural and religious groups than in others.

Experience Following Her Mother's Death

Three themes were identified for the young adult daughters in the period following mother's death: healthy grieving, trying to walk in mother's footprints, and Cinderella grows up.

Healthy Grieving

Women whose mothers died when they were young adults grieved heavily following the death. In their grief, they made use of many conventional rituals and practices they found particularly comforting. Sarah is an example of a young adult who shaped the traditional rituals of death. She arranged for the music, readings, and flowers at her mother's funeral, and found satisfaction in that everything was as she wanted it to be. Later, Sarah took a course on death and dying, which she found very helpful. Elizabeth found support from the gathering of friends and relatives, and from "following along" when her sister took a course in grieving. Elizabeth said that at her mother's funeral, "there were a lot of tears, but a lot of laughter and joy as well." Andrea grieved by parking in front of her mother's apartment, crying and remembering good times. Felicia was exhausted at her mother's funeral, but felt supported by her family, community, and co-workers.

One important part of the "grief work" for many of the adult women in the study was the ability to keep their memories of their mothers alive. Many surrounded themselves with pictures, videotapes, or audiotapes of their mothers. Others shared stories and memories with family members. Elizabeth thinks about her mother every day, often in a casual way. "Mother would have loved that!" Cheryl (Appendix III) also engaged in a variety of grief-related activities, such as sending flowers to the church on the anniversary of her mother's death, listening to a tape her mother made for her, and setting up a scholarship fund in her mother's memory. Cheryl had grief counseling, joined a support group for motherless daughters, and sought comfort from friends.

This range shows that people need support to grieve, and that the young adults in this study had the resources to seek the kind of support they needed. On potentially sad occasions such as Mother's Day, Lily (Appendix III) spends time with her grandparents and aunts, focusing on what she has instead of what she has lost.

Some young adult daughters described sensing the presence of their deceased mothers. Elizabeth says she often feels her mother is with her. She describes feeling as if her mother is hugging her, "when I get really hyper or really anxious." Sarah too felt her mother "arranged" for her graduation ceremony to be on her mother's birthday. Andrea talks of her mother being in favor of her husband's last-minute job choice near Andrea's sister's home. She says she has a sense of her mother living inside her. Andrea's goal is to "keep her alive."

Another way young adult daughters were able to "keep mother alive" after death was to become like their mothers. Felicia, for example, enjoys hearing her aunt say that she looks and acts very similar to her mother. By having children, and actively passing on their mothers' legacy to them, adult daughters aim to include their mothers' legacy in their lives. Andrea, for example, wants to have a daughter so that she can re-create the kind of relationship she had with her mother, and make her mother an important part of her daughter's life.

One factor that affected whether a daughter could engage in meaningful grief activities was her living situation. Daughters who lived close to their families of origin and had ongoing contact with them had many opportunities to remember and share stories. However, when they move to another town (as in Andrea's case), these opportunities become more limited. (This is what happened to many late adolescent daughters who returned to college after the mother's death.)

Another factor is the extent to which their families and friends allowed them to continue to grieve and share their memories. Some families are not comfortable discussing those who have died, and may not allow the daughter to do so. Andrea's husband was uncomfortable with her ongoing grief. Some daughters lost touch with maternal relatives, married after the mother died (so the spouse did not know the mother), or have stepmothers who were not comfortable when the family shared happy memories of the deceased (as was the case with many of the younger daughters). However, in contrast to the younger daughters in our study, the young adults were usually able to create the opportunities they needed. They had the power to set the tone they wanted in their own families, and to shape customs and traditions in their extended families. They did not lose touch with the mother's family, as did younger women, because as adults, they usually could make these connections if they wanted to.

Trying to Walk in the Mother's Footprints

Young adult women in this study tended to move into the mother's family roles concerning their siblings and the mother's parents (especially if they were oldest daughters). These attempts to take over the mother's roles were not always successful, and when they were not, frustration for the daughters resulted. Young adult women who were older sisters often tried to "mother" their younger siblings. For example, Felicia took on some responsibility for her younger sister, who had a very difficult time after their mother's death. Although she has moved away from her mother's hometown, Felicia returns home every weekend to be with her sister, and to be part of her small, rural community. Lily (Appendix III) had always "looked out for" her younger sister, and continued to do so after their mother's death. (She uses the term "substitute mom.")

Sarah also tried to take on her mother's roles, but experienced frustration. "I tried so hard to keep the family together, and I got into so many conflicts that I just decided the hell with it! I couldn't do it anymore. I was trying to take her place, and I realized I couldn't do that." Cheryl (Appendix III) took on caregiving responsibilities for her grandparents after her mother's death. She helped them maintain their home. She also helped them financially. "Sometimes I feel I took Mom's place as their daughter." Lily also has stepped into her mother's role, in this case, as the communicator in the family. "I kind of feel like I stepped in my mother's shoes in a lot of places."

It is interesting to note that none of the young adult women in the study tried to take on their mothers' roles with their fathers, as many of the younger women in the study did. Sarah, for example, relates how much difficulty her father had after her mother's death, but she did not try to take on these tasks for him.

Cinderella Grows Up

The Cinderella pattern that was so difficult for the younger women in this study also resonated with the young adult women, but they were much less devastated. Fathers were likely to remarry; this may have been disappointing or upsetting to the young adult women, but they had many more resources available to help them to handle the situation. Sarah, for example, was angry at her father, but not just about his remarriage. He was never a supportive husband or father. She gets along with her father's new wife, but does not want this woman to be considered her children's grandmother.

Elizabeth's relationship with her father improved enormously after her mother died. At first, her father actually took on many of her mother's roles by keeping the family together and acting as consoler to and advocate for Elizabeth. However, when he remarried, Elizabeth reacted with much of the same fury as did younger women, but the outcome was quite different. In therapy, Elizabeth came to see that she was "championing mother's cause," feeling that being supportive of or liking her stepmother was being disloyal to her mother. As an adult, however, Elizabeth was capable of recognizing her father as a person, and (similar to Sarah) was able to let go of her more childlike view of her parents' marriage. She said, "Now that I'm old enough to understand . . . I got my eyes opened a little bit from his perspective." She was able to use therapy to negotiate a different relationship with her father. As adults, Elizabeth and her siblings also had resources and skills, which they used to wage war on their father's new wife. Eventually, they succeeded; their father divorced this woman.

As with the younger daughters in this study, those who lose their mothers as young adults may experience the loss of their childhood homes, and mourn the loss. However, they have already moved on from those homes, so the loss does not carry the same weight that it does for younger girls. None of the young adult women needed to find a new home when the father remarried or when the mother died. They often were able to salvage many of the mother's belongings from the home, and to incorporate these into their lives. Although Sarah's father quickly disposed of all of her mother's items, Sarah was able to take many of them to her home. Andrea also got most of her mother's things and planned to use them in her new home.

Long-Term Impact

The two themes that emerged related to long-term impact for the young adult daughters were changing priorities and the big cry.

Changing Priorities

Those who were young adults at the time of the mother's death often were able to reframe the experience in a positive way. Most took important lessons about how to live life successfully from the experience. In this sense, they often are ahead of their peers. Sarah changed to a more meaningful job and decreased her work hours, to spend more time with her family. Felicia makes a point of reaching out to others who are experiencing losses in life. Elizabeth is intolerant of other women who don't appreciate their mothers. Cheryl (Appendix III) always expresses her feelings for those she loves. She also does not invest in superficial relationships, and no longer feels she has to say yes to everything. "It certainly helped me focus my priorities on who's important to me, and that life is an adventure." Lily (Appendix III) also used her experience to change her priorities. She decided that "life's too short" and she learned "not to take people for granted, because they may not always be there." She also feels that she has gained strength from going through her mother's death. Comparing her current problems with that ordeal makes them seem insignificant. "If I can get through losing my mother, I can get through this."

Many of the young adults whose mothers died from breast cancer become politically or socially active in breast cancer advocacy. For example, Sarah encourages women to do breast self-exams and wears her pink ribbon to show support. She also participates in an advocacy group. Felicia contributes financially to cancer causes. Elizabeth is active in breast cancer causes, taking leadership in breast cancer organizations, and volunteered in a hospice. Cheryl (Appendix III) set up a scholarship fund in her mother's name and participated in the Race for the Cure in memory of her mother. These activities can serve several purposes at once. They help with grief resolution, channeling energy into constructive causes. At the same time, they provide social support and combat isolation, by placing the bereaved daughter in contact with others with similar experience. They also provide an opportunity for the bereaved daughters to reach out and help others. This enhances self-esteem and provides "helper therapy."

The Big Cry

The long-term grieving of some young adult women involved periodic "big cries." In our culture, this outlet is available to women (and not to men), even though long-term grieving is often frowned upon. Sarah speaks of having a "really good cry" every couple of months. Elizabeth also has periodic crying spells. "Every couple of months, I need to have a big cry."

Lily (Appendix III) says that, although she is not depressed, "You have a long-term feeling of sadness and loss." Lily stores up her sadness, not expressing it inappropriately but has a "good cry" periodically. "I'll cry for a couple of hours . . . a good cry . . . heaving sobs . . . disabling . . . a 'cry-yourself-to-sleep' kind of thing." These women describe a controlled venting of accumulated sadness. Elizabeth notes that her cries are not necessarily triggered by memories of her mother, but by the accumulation of life stresses. It is not until the end of the crying spell that she realizes that everything goes back to "not having Mom there when I need a mom."

Sarah notices the loss of her mother's support in the little, everyday situations—the times when life is stressful, and she needs someone to talk to, share with, laugh with. When this is lacking, stresses accumulate, and crying provides a welcome relief. The need to cry periodically, even many years after the loss, suggests how profound the loss of a mother is for a young woman, and how much ongoing grieving needs to be done. What is important here is the comparison with women who lost mothers when they were younger. The young adult women were able to grieve actively (painfully) at the time of the death, and to gain relief later from crying when tensions built up and they missed their mothers.

SUMMARY

This chapter has used case studies of young adult daughters to illustrate themes common to women whose mothers die from breast cancer (see Box 7.1). During the illness period, the women took an active role in the mother's illness, including direct communication with the physician. They also experienced role conflict as they tried to balance the demands of the mother's care with the needs of their own families and the demands of careers. They also developed adult relationships with their mothers, which often included open communication about death. Following the mother's death, they grieved heavily, able to benefit from rituals and support from friends and therapists. Many took on their mothers' roles, trying to mother their younger siblings and, in some cases, care for grandparents. They were not always successful, and some felt frustrated when unable to keep the family together.

Another theme in this period parallels that of many of the younger women: Cinderella. Fathers tended to remarry, and daughters did not accept their stepmothers. As did younger daughters, they lost their homes. However, this was not nearly as devastating for them, because

---

BOX 7.1. Themes Found in Daughters Whose Mothers Died When They Were Young Adults

Phase I: Mother's Illness and Treatments

1. Taking charge
2. Superwoman
3. Adult mother-daughter relationship

Phase II: Following Mother's Death

1. Healthy grieving
2. Trying to walk in mother's footprints
3. Cinderella grows up

Phase III: Long-Term Impact

1. Changing priorities
2. The big cry

---

they had their own homes at this point in life. They also had the power to decide how they wanted to relate to the new family situation, if at all. They could change relationships if they wanted to. In the long term, these young adult women found that their mothers' deaths led them to change their priorities, and often became advocates for breast cancer prevention. Some also tended to have a periodic "big cry" to deal with stress. During the mother's illness, and following her death, young adult daughters are propelled into adult roles, relationships, and activities. They take on active roles to support their families, to grieve, and to structure their lives in meaningful ways.

Implications of these findings are discussed in Chapter 11.

Chapter 8

Experience of Daughters Whose Mothers Survive Breast Cancer

Although the previous four chapters have focused on the experience of daughters of women who died, in fact the large majority (about two-thirds) of women survive breast cancer. Therefore, the majority of women whose mothers have had breast cancer have a surviving mother. This chapter presents stories of six daughters of various ages whose mothers survived breast cancer. A discussion of broad themes regarding the impact of the mother's cancer on the daughter follows. This chapter is organized somewhat differently from the previous chapters. When mothers die, "phases" are fairly clear-cut, with definable beginnings and ends; however, the key phases of the experience are different for women whose mothers survive. The periods up to the time of the mother's death (phases 1 and 2) are essentially the same, but no period similar to the period after mother's death exists. Instead, the period after the acute phase of the illness merges with the long-term impact phase. The phases for the case studies in this chapter are background, experience of the mother's illness, and experience following the mother's illness.

Because the experience of daughters in the early phases of the disease has already been covered in Chapters 4 through 7, this chapter focuses on the period after the initial illness and treatment are over. This chapter begins by introducing the following cases: Ramona (age eight at mother's diagnosis), Lisa (age ten) and Jane (age eleven), Mandy (age fourteen), Jamie (age seventeen), and Sharon (age twenty-one).

CASE STUDY #1: RAMONA

Age at Her Mother's Breast Cancer Diagnosis: 8

Background

Ramona was raised in a Protestant family in a small town in the Midwest. She had a brother who was two years older than her, and her parents were professionals. Both sets of grandparents lived about two hundred miles away and Ramona saw them mostly on holidays. She also spoke of a housekeeper who "was like having a third grandmother."

Experience of Her Mother's Illness

Ramona was in the third grade when her mother was diagnosed with breast cancer. On the day of her biopsy, her mother was "very confident and convinced that nothing was wrong. She was very in control." Ramona stayed with a neighbor while her mother had "something checked out." Soon after that, she says,

> I saw my father sitting on the floor talking on the phone. I'd never seen him sit down before; he's a really hyperactive person. And I saw him crying and that was . . . the first time I really knew this was really, really, really serious.

Ramona's mother had a radical mastectomy and remained in the hospital for more than a week. Ramona had a test at school on the day of her mother's surgery ("My mother wanted to preserve my normal day") and she was embarrassed because "I don't think I got any of the answers right." Her grandmother came to stay with the children. Ramona visited her mother once in the hospital. She said "she seemed kind of far away."

After Ramona's mother returned home, Ramona got sick and developed a high fever. When the doctor recommended a particular type of treatment (wrapping her in frozen sheets), Ramona begged her mother not to fo this. For the first time, Ramona's mother gave in to her demands, and Ramona attributed this reprieve to the illness.

Ramona never thought her mother would die.

> She [mother] told me that in a small town sometimes there are rumors that people are sicker than they know. She said that if anybody said anything to me about her dying of cancer or anything, that it wasn't true. She told me she was gonna be fine and that it would take a little while just to get better because she had a big incision and, you know, that I shouldn't worry.

Ramona's mother explained the medical aspects of the disease, showed Ramona the scars, and explained the function of lymph nodes, but Ramona knew not to ask questions about her mother's feelings. "I think the precedent had been laid down where we couldn't talk about emotional things." Her family never used the word *cancer,* especially around her father. "He just didn't want to be reminded minute to minute."

Experience Following Her Mother's Illness

Ramona felt that her mother rushed her to grow up, because she was worried that, if she died, her husband would not know how to raise a girl. For example, Ramona's mother began very early to give her information about menstruation, puberty, and sex. Ramona believes this "sort of robbed me of my childhood. . . . I never was a very playful child. I never really was encouraged to just pretend and be silly. I was very serious."

Ramona's mother battled cancer off and on for the rest of her life. She had two recurrences in her middle and later years and passed away shortly before Ramona's interview. During the recurrences of her mother's disease, Ramona became more involved in her mother's care and treatment. When her father was having a difficult time, she took care of her mother so he could get some rest. Her brother was never very serious or helpful. Once he told her, "It's not a guy thing; it's kind of a girl thing." However, after Ramona confronted him, he started to visit his mother more regularly and became more supportive.

Risk

At puberty, Ramona became very anxious. "When I started getting breasts, I told her [mother] I thought I had lumps." Ramona was mortified when her mother couldn't tell and asked her father to check the breast tissue. "I became kind of phobic about it." Ramona feels that her anxiety about doing breast exams extends back to this time. She has difficulty distinguishing between real lumps and normal tissue. Ramona started getting mammograms at age thirty-five, choosing not to start in her twenties out of fear that any extra radiation would increase her risk for breast cancer. Ramona attributes her mother's breast cancer to radiation exposure in her laboratory work.

Ramona planned for her pregnancy and breast-feeding to be completed by the time she was thirty-three (the age at which her mother was diagnosed) in an effort to reduce her risk. She got married at age thirty and had her daughter at thirty-two. She chose not to have any more children. "I was sure that when I was thirty-three I would also have breast cancer and if I was breast-feeding, I wouldn't be able to find a lump and it would go [undiagnosed] too long."

Ramona does not believe genetic testing is appropriate for her because she lacks a strong family history of breast cancer. She pays attention to breast cancer issues and stated, "I read everything I can." She once lost a significant amount of weight after learning that weight was a risk factor. She does not drink alcohol for the same reason, but says this is not a great sacrifice because she does not particularly enjoy it anyway.

Current Situation

At the time of the interview, Ramona was forty-seven. Her mother had passed away from a complication of breast cancer treatment about a year before. Ramona was married and lived with her husband and her teenaged daughter. She was working on a PhD in epidemiology. Ramona now has a good relationship with her brother although they live far from each other. Ramona's father remarried and her relationship with him is now strained because of this new marriage. For example, when her new stepmother said that she would always be welcome to visit, Ramona thought, *You're telling me that I'm welcome in my own house?* When her father and stepmother redecorated the house, they informed Ramona that she could retrieve her belongings if she wanted them. She was upset when she found her precious things (very old letters and family mementos) set out on the back porch.

Ramona tries to raise her daughter in a more carefree fashion than she was raised. She is particularly grateful that her daughter has not had to experience the issues of puberty in the same way. "This is so nice, you know, that she hasn't had to deal with this." After participating in the study, Ramona decided to participate in the Race for the Cure, in honor of her mother.

CASE STUDY #2: LISA

Age at Her Mother's Breast Cancer Diagnosis: 10

Background

Lisa was born into a Jewish family, the oldest of two daughters, and lived most of her life in Texas. Lisa's parents' relationship involved much conflict. "My father had a problem holding down jobs, and he also had many affairs. He drank. They fought all the time."

As a child, Lisa was devoted to ballet.

> I remember my mom always . . . she really wanted me to be a ballerina. That was her dream life. So I was in ballet forever, which I loved to death. But, like, six days out of the week, from five to ten every night. She was always taking us, and bringing us back, and getting us new shoes, and finding those pointe shoes. Ballet was a huge thing. My mom was a huge supporter of all that. All the money my parents forked out, going through millions of pairs of pointe shoes, tons of heartache with eating, not eating, not being flexible enough. My mom was great about it. She really was great about it.

When Lisa was eight, she started seeing a therapist.

> They thought I had an eating disorder. It wasn't because I was dancing. It was more along the lines of me being a perfectionist. I just have to have everything perfect. I wanted a perfect body. I actually don't remember the anorexia part so much. It was more with my grades, and having things organized. If they weren't perfect, I would flip out. I also had this huge thing that I thought I was gonna choke if I ate anything except baby food. So, Mom used to buy me all these candy bars to con me into eating.

Lisa's relationship with her mother has always been close. She remembers her mother baking (her mother owned a cheesecake company), and gardening, and "just being a caring mom." Lisa had a grandmother and several maternal aunts, but no other relatives lived in the Texas area.

Experience of Her Mother's Illness

Lisa has no memory of being told about her mother's cancer.

What I remember about it is just, I think what any ten-year-old child would remember. Seeing their mom lying in bed. I just didn't know what to think. I remember seeing her once in the hospital. It was right after surgery. I walked in there, and she looked really pale. She was to the point where she was almost blue. I remember her showing us her scars; because of the wound, it was purple. She seemed actually really alive at the time. Like she made it through. Like, "Wow, it was great!" I guess to me at the time, I was just like, "Oh, it was just an operation." But then, when I found out she had to have chemotherapy, I was like, "Oh, my God. What's chemotherapy? Is my mom gonna die? What's going on?" Chemotherapy just hit me the most [emotional]. I remember her coming home after chemotherapy and just getting straight into bed. And I wanted so much from her. She was always telling me what to expect, like, "I'm going into chemotherapy in two days, and after that, I'm not going to be able to provide for you." And then she'd come home and she'd lay in bed and throw up, and do all that stuff, and the door would always be closed. I didn't know if she was going to make it. I didn't know what was going to happen. [She was] just always asleep, sick. So I would just sit there and watch her and wait for her to be like Mom again, you know [emotional]? So I went through that. I went with her to chemotherapy once. She warned me what it was gonna be like. But when I walked in there and saw all these cancer survivors, with their hair gone and everyone so sick, I was just like, "Why is my mom here?" I mean it was really, really scary. I knew that cancer killed people, and the fact that she was totally out, just laying there as if she was dead. It was just like, "How can she possibly be okay if this is how she is reacting?" I think the hardest thing was that my mom can't get up and go to the grocery store, my mom can't cook dinner, my mom can't, like I said, be a mom. If the cancer's gone, then she should be fine.

Lisa recalls her thoughts on the possibility of losing her mother:

The fear that she might die was just reinforced by the fact that I had to . . . I don't think they ever said, "Okay, you're going to have to be a big girl now and take Mom's place," but I felt as though I was. I was looking after my little sister when my dad was at work, and cooking dinner and cleaning and doing laundry and doing the dishes. Things I thought I shouldn't have to do as a daughter. And I saw a lot of my mom's friends coming in and helping out, which was also kind of weird. I just didn't like it. I was just like, "Why can't people leave us alone? Let my mom get better!" Having people bring over dinner, or taking my sister and I out just to let my mom rest, to me that was so abnormal. I didn't like that. I liked normal routine, and this was breaking it. It was the thing you do when something is not right. So that kind of reinforced that something was not right. My mom was sick. And that scared me.

Lisa was grateful that her parents didn't hide the illness from her. "I really thank my father for, like, opening the door, letting me look and be involved and know that she was okay and that she was still there. He didn't close me out at all."

After her mother recovered from the treatment, life for Lisa went back to normal. She continued with her ballet studies.

Then, in the seventh grade [Lisa was twelve], she [mother] was driving me to ballet one afternoon, and she's like, "I have to tell you something." And I asked her [emotional], "Okay, What's going on?" And she's like, "They found another cancerous lump." And this is right as she's dropping me off for three hours of ballet. I was totally upset. I was so furious with her! I was like, "How can you do this to me? How can those doctors screw up? This is so terrible!" So I just got out of the car, slammed the door, and went to ballet. I don't even remember what happened after that. I can't believe I thought this now, this is so terrible of me, but I was just like, "Oh, great. So now my mom's gonna be bald in front of all my friends! How can she do this?" I was just freaking out about that.

However, her mother recovered from this recurrence, and life again returned to normal for Lisa.

When Lisa was fifteen, her father took a job on the East Coast and moved away from the family. Around this time, Lisa decided not to continue her ballet studies. "It was so serious. When I was fifteen, I just realized this is not how I want my life to be anymore." She became interested in social problems, such as poverty, drug abuse, and homelessness, and decided to become a social worker.

Her parents divorced when she was seventeen.

When I found out that my father was having an affair when I was fifteen, I talked to my mom. I said something about, "So, I guess you and Dad don't have sex anymore." And she said, "Lisa, he hasn't touched me since I lost my breast." And of course, I just lost it. I was so irate I was bawling my eyes out. I think he views my mom like a cripple.

Lisa admired her mother for the way she dealt with these problems.

I really respect my mom. She really got herself together, dealing with her health, dealing with my father leaving, her having to find work and raising two kids. Really, my respect is so enormous for her. That's when we started becoming close. I had my first boyfriend when I was fourteen, so that's when I started talking about boys, and that's when I realized I could trust her and discuss things. It's just been great ever since. I mean it just gets better and better each day. We talk about everything. Absolutely everything.

In college, Lisa made friends with a girl whose mother also had had breast cancer. Lisa said they could share each other's pain and fears. "So we would just cry together."

Experience Following Her Mother's Illness

Lisa has had many relationships with men, but they tend not to last.

They are, like, five minutes! I cannot hold down a relationship for the life of me. My mother and I have talked about this so many times. I think it is for two reasons. One: I really have not had a good male figure to look up to, obviously. I'm quite apprehensive about men and trust and all that. And the other thing she [mother] says is, when a boy comes into the picture, I become very mean. I just become short with everyone because they're causing me such a headache. So I'd rather not have them than take it out on my sister and my mom. I hate myself when I'm like that. So she [mother] says, "I think that you don't want to date people because you don't want to share yourself between me and someone else." I can agree with that. To me, it's a lot more comforting at nine o'clock at night when I come home from work to pick up the phone and call my mom than to pick up a boy and have to deal with this and have to deal with that. Too much of a headache.

Lisa also feels that her perfectionism plays a role in this aspect of her life.

I want someone perfect in my eyes. But that's almost a safeguard. I know there's no one perfect, so I'm gonna keep searching for someone perfect, knowing that I won't ever have to be with anybody. I mean, yeah, I do want to get married someday. A lot of my friends are getting married now, and it sounds like a lot of fun. But I have a long way to go.

Lisa is now living far from her mother, but they still have a very strong connection. She says,

I know I'm really scared of losing her now [emotional]. The biggest effect was that now we're like the best of friends. I mean, I speak to her every day. This weekend, I was visiting my dad and his girlfriend, and I was very depressed. And I realized that I'm just depressed because I'm not near her. Since I hit college, I go through a lot of roller coasters, like going through depression of not being with her, and I just mainly cry the whole time. I mean, I can't even [tearful] explain my fear about losing her. I can't even imagine not having her around; I really, really can't. I mean, I tell her *everything*. Absolutely everything. I want her to live right next door to me, but she thinks I'm a little insane. [She thinks] I'll never find a husband that wants to live right next door to his mother-in-law. That's my biggest thing right now. I'm just like, "I wish she would just move in with me." I really want to go overseas, and my mom has no problem: "Go!" But whenever I get the opportunity, I don't go because I'm scared that I'll like it over there and stay there a long time. And I know that she's not moving [there]. So, I cut my experience short because I want to be close to my mother. So, my moving here has been a baby step. Another baby step will be going to New York. Maybe I'll be able to go overseas at some point and feel like, "Okay, everything's gonna be okay with my mom." Probably not, though. I really need her by my side.

Risk

Lisa was afraid when her breasts started to develop.

When I just started having my period, and for about two years after that, I would go through these phases when I would think . . . I would check my breasts every month. I would always run to my mom's room and have her check my breasts for me because I was so paranoid. I still have a huge paranoia. Like last week, I woke up in the middle of the night thinking something was going on. And I called my mom, and she said, "If it feels like a bruise, then I don't think you have anything to worry about." I definitely have a huge fear of it.

Lisa hopes to prevent breast cancer through maintaining a healthy lifestyle.

I'm very, very cautious [about] what I put in my body. I really believe that my mom got cancer from, besides the fact that she and my dad had a terrible relationship, she owned a cheesecake company, and spent years, instead of eating healthy foods, just licking up the cheesecake batter, which is full of carcinogens. I really believe that was a huge trigger. I eat no dairy and I eat no meats. I eat almost completely macrobiotic. I exercise a lot.

Lisa does not expect to get breast cancer at the same age her mother did.

No, no, not at all. I haven't even thought about that. I really haven't thought that I'm gonna get cancer. I'm just, like, I really want to prevent it. I'm more like, I have it within me to prevent it. So I'm gonna do what I can do.

Lisa also is aware of the genetic factor. "I know it's genetic too, 'cause it does run in my family. I think this can trigger it." Lisa is more fearful for her sister than for herself.

She started developing and got her period at a very young age, like my mother. Like my mother's aunt, who is the last person to get it [breast cancer]. And she's not overweight, but she is short, and she could definitely stand to lose thirty pounds. So those things are weighing toward her having it. She doesn't watch what she eats. She exercises, but she's just half [hearted] about it. I wish that I could scare her a little bit more so that she would start watching it herself. I need her to start taking care of herself. It's like you're playing with fire. I tell her, and she's like, "I know, I know." You know, I just can't stop every chocolate chip cookie going into her mouth.

Current Situation

When we interviewed her, Lisa was twenty-three and living on the East Coast, where she hopes to enter social work school. Her mother lives in the Midwest and owns a successful business. Lisa sees a therapist and continues to deal with her anxiety by talking with her mom.

CASE STUDY #3: JANE

Age at Her Mother's Breast Cancer Diagnosis: 11

Background

At four years old, Jane saw her father have a fatal heart attack. Her mother was pregnant with Jane's brother at the time. This event had a tremendous impact on Jane and her family; several months later her mother was hospitalized for depression. Two years after her father's death, her mother married a man who had teenage children.

Experience of Her Mother's Illness

When Jane was eleven, her mother was diagnosed with breast cancer. At that time, she and her mother, stepfather, and brother were living abroad. The family came home for Christmas that year and Jane did not want to return to Europe. "I was eleven and I didn't appreciate that kind of stuff then." She remembers thinking, "Please let something happen so we don't have to go back." Jane felt very guilty at the time of her mother's diagnosis, believing that she may have caused the illness. She later confided this to her mother, who was very understanding and reassured Jane that it was not her fault.

Jane heard about her mother's illness by telephone. She was at her grandmother's home when her mother called from the hospital. Her mother waited to tell her until after the biopsy because, "She wanted to be sure that it was cancer before she told us and got us all upset." Jane's mother did not want to tell her son about the illness, but Jane didn't feel that was fair.

> So I put him on the phone and she talked to him. And I remember going in the other room and my grandmother was talking to my aunt in Italian. I was trying to figure out how you say *breast* in Italian.

Jane's mother had a radical mastectomy that included the removal of lymph nodes. She also had chemotherapy. It was difficult for Jane to see her mother so ill.

> All her hair fell out and she was just very sick and kind of irritable. She couldn't do much. I guess for me, seeing her like that was hard because she was so at the mercy of those chemicals. Just as she started looking better and feeling better she'd have to go back again [for more chemotherapy].

Jane remembers "sitting on my bed, looking out the window and saying, 'Please, please, don't let her die.'" It was around this time that Jane's aunt told her that her mother had tried to commit suicide after her [Jane's] father's death. "It was such a shocking thing for me to think about losing my mother along with having lost my father."

Jane began experiencing headaches and insomnia. "The reason I couldn't sleep was because I'd get in bed and my mind would start going off in all these different directions." Jane also remembered becoming withdrawn during this time. "I'm very much an extrovert and very outgoing, but I had just sort of turned into myself and was very self-absorbed. I was dealing with so much that I think I just had to be that way." Despite being close to her mother, Jane did not feel she could share her feelings with her. "I didn't want to burden her with what I was going through, because I knew she was going through so much."

Jane had a different reaction to her mother's illness than her brother.

> He'd yell, scream, cry . . . do all this really external stuff. I never did that. Everything was kept inside. And I don't think I ever really talked to anybody about how I felt or what I was going through. I just remember feeling scared and hurt.

Jane's stepfather sometimes unleashed his anger on Jane.

> I remember him blowing up over stupid things, like leaving my backpack in the living room instead of taking it upstairs. I really tried not to make waves. He was supportive in some ways, but not in others.

For a while, Jane's mother became too ill to participate in family life. This was a particularly difficult time. "My mom really held the whole thing together. When she was incapacitated, we all just sort of went off in different directions and didn't know what we were doing . . . including Dad."

Experience Following Her Mother's Illness

Jane describes her relationship with her mother as

> very, very close. Always have been. I think that is a result of my dad dying. Because in the space of time between when my dad died and my brother was born, we were just inseparable. She would go to the bathroom and I would go with her. As an adult, it's been hard to set a boundary, but I think we're doing better with that. We're getting to the point where we can be friends.

Jane also has experienced depression. "I suffered with bouts of depression throughout college." She describes herself as an "angry" person.

> I'm still angry. My mom says I'm mean to her. I've really tried to change that. I'll pick on her gently, not anything bad. I think I was angry because my dad died. I was angry with her for getting sick. For having the audacity to presume to leave.

Jane believes her mother's breast cancer had a great effect on her own body image.

> I think my weight problem has to do with my mom having cancer. That was my form of rebellion when I was a teenager. I ate and I gained weight. "I can do whatever I want." It makes me less desirable and that, I think, has always been a fear of mine. I have a really hard time with men paying attention to me. I don't like that at all.

Risk

Jane regularly performs breast self-exams and also plans to start getting mammograms by the age of thirty-five. Although concerned about breast cancer, she is more concerned about getting heart disease.

> I have risks on the other side of my family for heart disease. I look much more like my father than I do like my mother. So I would think that that would be more pressing for me. Breast cancer is a much more treatable thing, I think, than heart disease. With heart disease you can prevent it, but once you've got it, you're stuck with it.

Jane doesn't feel genetic counseling would be helpful.

> I worry about my own risk, but I'm not obsessed about it. There's really nothing I can do. I think that if I did it [genetic counseling], it would make me feel doom and gloom. If I don't have the gene it doesn't mean that I'm not going to have cancer. It just means that I don't have the gene. So I don't see the point in putting myself through it.

Jane does not follow a specific diet or exercise regimen. She does take medication for high cholesterol. She lost weight at one point, but her cholesterol went up. She notes that much conflicting advice about prevention exists. "One day they'll come out with this, and next day it's something else. You never really know what is good and what is bad."

Current Situation

Jane, twenty-two at the time of the interview, describes herself as "family-oriented . . . maybe more so than someone my age." She also would like to have children someday.

> I don't have anybody to marry right now, but I've decided that if I'm not in a committed relationship by the time I'm thirty-five, I'm going to have a child on my own. I have no intentions of foregoing children.

CASE STUDY #4: MANDY

Age at Her Mother's Breast Cancer Diagnosis: 14

Background

Mandy, the youngest in her family, had an older sister and brother. She described her relationship with her mother and siblings as "really close." When she was seven years old, her parents divorced, and Mandy and her siblings remained with their mother. Later, Mandy was depressed and in therapy because of relationship difficulties with her father and difficulties transitioning to high school. Her mother began dating a man who is now Mandy's stepfather.

Experience of Her Mother's Illness

Mandy was fourteen and in the ninth grade when her mother was diagnosed with breast cancer. Her brother and sister had already left for college, although her sister often returned home on the weekends. Mandy's mother told her daughters about the cancer, including the fact that it had already metastasized. "I didn't know what that meant. She said that breast cancer was becoming more treatable now and she tried to make it seem as if it was not serious."

At first, Mandy accepted her mother's explanation. At that time, she had a job at Baskin-Robbins, where she was learning cake decorating. When her mother was diagnosed, Mandy and her sister made a cake that said SORRY ABOUT YOUR BOOB on top, planning to give it to their mother when she got home from the hospital. "My sister and I felt horrible, because we [had] thought it was no big deal. We thought it was just a cyst." After they realized how serious their mother's diagnosis was, "my sister and I went upstairs, bawled, and ate the entire top layer off the cake, just so she wouldn't see it."

Mandy's mother had a mastectomy and eleven lymph nodes removed. She also underwent chemotherapy, radiation, and reconstructive surgery. Mandy became the primary caregiver for her mother, providing hands-on care and taking care of the house. Meanwhile, her sister commuted from college in a nearby city on the weekends to run errands. Mandy's aunt (mother's sister) also provided some support for a time. Her brother lived in a different part of the country and was not able to come home often.

Because of her depression, "it was hard for me to take care of myself and take care of Mom. So instead I just opted to take care of my mom because that's really all I had the energy for." Mandy describes feeling anxious about her mother's illness, and being scared about what would happen to her if she died. At one point, she slept with her mother at night. "It made me feel better that I could see her get up in the morning and listen to her sleep at night."

Throughout her illness and treatment, Mandy's mother remained supportive. For example, her mother called the school and told Mandy's teachers and coach about her illness and encouraged them to provide extra support to Mandy. At one point, her mother asked her [mother's] boyfriend to leave for a period of time because he was not coping well with the illness and was taking out his anger on Mandy. Sometimes, she used humor to help Mandy feel at ease with the disease. For example, during chemotherapy, her mother would have Mandy vacuum the hair off her head.

Mandy found support from adults, but had a more difficult time relating to her peers. "My friends sort of took off when my mom got cancer. It made them feel really awkward. I think it was that they didn't want to say the wrong thing so, instead, they just didn't say anything." She also was going through puberty and developing breasts at this time.

> It wasn't one of my main concerns at the time, but I was sort of angry. I thought, *I'm just starting to get these now and they're gonna have to go soon*. . . . It scared me to think that now that I'm getting breasts, I can get cancer.

Experience Following Her Mother's Illness

Mandy and her mother remained close throughout her mother's illness, but they faced some adjustments after recovery. "We had open communication during and before the breast cancer. But then after the breast cancer, I was often afraid to bring things up, in trying to protect Mom." Overall, she feels that her relationship with her mother grew closer as they supported each other. "I feel fortunate that I was here and that we have this special bond . . . that it's something that we did together and that I know I was here the whole time."

Risk

Mandy tries to keep a realistic outlook on her risk of breast cancer. She does not feel particularly anxious about it, recognizing that genetics is only one cause of breast cancer. "It just happens. The two major risk factors for breast cancer are being female and being a certain age." Nor does she feel that her situation requires genetics testing or a prophylactic mastectomy. Instead, she feels that genetic testing could harm women by giving them a false sense of security because they may only hear what they want to hear. However, she does believe in the importance of regular mammograms and self-examinations.

Current Situation

Mandy was twenty-one at the time of the interview. She and her family are very active in local breast cancer support groups and her mother is the editor of a newsletter for breast cancer patients and survivors. The family also participates in breast cancer awareness events, including the Race for the Cure benefit. Mandy refers to her family as "the breast cancer family." "Every time there's a new article, everyone gets it, everyone reads it. The more active we are, the better we feel about it."

Mandy's current boyfriend is a source of support; he understands her need to participate in support group and awareness activities. He also supports her attempts to lead a healthy lifestyle, including eating healthy foods and exercising. Most important of all, he is emotionally supportive. "It's so nice to have someone to take care of you and to understand."

Mandy plans a career in nursing. She became very interested in a medical career as a result of her experiences with depression as a teen and with her mother's illness.

> I really watched the nurses and how they took care of her. . . . They gave her a little pillow for her arm that one of them had made. . . . They do this for all the women who have breast cancer. . . . I want to be in that role.

CASE STUDY #5: JAMIE

Age at Her Mother's Breast Cancer Diagnosis: 17

Background

Jamie comes from an African-American family with a single mother and an older brother. She describes her family as fun-loving and very close.

> When I was little, my mother was very top-heavy. She was large. Short but heavyset. She was, like, a double H. I used to sleep on my stomach on my chest and say, like, "Ya'll are not gonna grow." 'Cause I didn't ever want to be that big.

Experience of Her Mother's Illness

When Jamie was in the twelfth grade, her mother told her that she had a lump and was going in for a biopsy. "She would go regularly for mammograms and regular checkups. And I guess it was like you never would think it would develop into anything. Nobody else in my family had ever been diagnosed with breast cancer." Soon after that, Jamie returned home from school and received upsetting news.

> I was walking down my alley and I saw all these cars parked. I walked in the house and my aunt said, "Have you talked to your mother yet?" and I was like, "No." And she said, "Well, I think you should go upstairs and talk to her." And I went up there and she was still in the bed, and she said, "Okay. I went to the doctor today." And before she could get the whole sentence out, she said, "It's cancer! I'm gonna have this surgery." She just burst into tears and I just hugged her and it was like a whole lot of thoughts flashed through my head. It was like, "Oh, my God!" It was so overwhelming and I thought, *My mother is a single parent and it's always been her to take care of me. That person that I could always count on.*

Jamie continues:

> First, she was treated with chemotherapy. That's a really strong drug and my mother had been wearing her hair short for years and the thing that you most notice about taking chemo is that your hair comes out. She tried to prepare herself as much as she could so she got her hair in a scrunchy, laid-down style. She thought it would kind of sit up there a little bit longer. And that did not work. Her hair was coming out. She

crept in the bathroom with her bag, and she just pulled it out clump by clump, and she just put it in her bag. There was this tension through the whole house. You could feel it. That hair experience, that was one of the hardest parts. 'Cause you have a lot going on inside, but that is the part that you see. That brings to you the reality of what's actually going on.

After her chemotherapy, Jamie's mother had a mastectomy and major reconstruction [tissue was moved from her abdomen to form a new breast, and a reduction was done on the other breast]. Jamie was quite fearful before her mother's surgery.

A lot of things don't scare me, but I needed to brace myself. The closer it got to that time, the more scared I got. It was like, "Oh, my God. This is major surgery." My mother is that kind of person that sees the upside, and she pranced around all the time, "I'm getting a new body! I haven't had on a bathing suit for so long!" Her stomach was going to be flat. She just thought that was the greatest thing.

Coping with the stress of her mother's illness was not always easy for Jamie, but she tried to keep her feelings from her mother.

I would do the praying thing. I would talk to friends if it came to a point when you have to let it out. I could pick up on her up and down days. I remember one time it was really, really hitting her. I walked into the kitchen and she was sitting there with the light out. She had the radio playing. It was a Sunday, and the song [went] "The Battle Is Not Yours. It's the Lord's." I guess if you're a person that's recovering, it helps that much to have somebody around you to bring you up. So I would just put on a happy face, even if I didn't feel like it. Even if I was extremely tired.

Jamie took on some of her mother's roles.

It was right before Christmas, and like I said, I have a big family and every year my family comes over to my house for Christmas and brunch. The whole week before Christmas, it's major chaos around my house. I was coming home from college. I thought, *I've got to clean up the house, make sure everything is presentable.* It wasn't just the tension there, but nothing like this had ever happened in my family. I think they were very nervous too. Everybody just got it out in their own way. My aunt is a "doer." She was at my house every day, doing stuff. That was her way of getting it out.

Jamie's new role in the family continued after her mother's surgery.

> I remember when she [mother] first came home from the hospital. I was at home, in bed, on a Sunday morning. I heard my aunt downstairs just yelling and fussing. She was like, "You sitting around this house and you didn't get up and cook my sister's breakfast!" And it bothered me a lot. I was like, *Oh my God, she's right. I didn't fix breakfast, and my mother can't just get up and fix breakfast for herself.* I was really offended because I am very close to my mother. Don't think that I didn't fix breakfast because I don't love my mother. It just didn't occur to me because I had never been in this role. But now I was, and that clicked: *I've really got to take care of her.* So for months, it was as if it were my house that I was running. I got up, I cooked, I cleaned. You have to make sure she's not there by herself, because she might need or want something. You have to make sure she's eating enough, and that it's something well balanced. Make sure she's waking up to take her medicine. Make sure she doesn't get bored to death or lonely to death sitting up there in her room.

Jamie had help from her brother, her aunts, and a friend from church.

> People are very, very kind. People from church, people at my mother's job would bring her food if they had luncheons at work. They would bring her check. They would send flowers. People constantly called. They constantly came by. They sent money and everything. It was like everybody really came through.

Jamie was also involved in her mother's medical care.

> Usually, things don't gross me out. So when she had all these cuts and things, she said, "Well, I don't want to make you puke, but I kinda need some help changing my bandages." I told her it was no problem.

Jamie got real satisfaction from her caregiving role.

> There's one song that always comes to mind, "Count on Me." I like that song a lot because cancer and healing are something that you go through together. 'Cause I do say my mother is like my best friend. It comes down to a lot of support. In the relationship between us, I depended on her all my life, but then it was my turn to help her, and she had to depend on me.

Experience Following Her Mother's Illness

As her mother's health improved, Jamie was able to spend less time at home and more time in her dorm and on campus. At first, she didn't tell her roommates that her mother had breast cancer, but when they teased her about going home every weekend, she finally told them. Jamie's grades suffered due to her efforts to juggle the two roles of student and caregiver. "My first semester of school, I got all C's because I couldn't concentrate or focus as much." Jamie's grades went up the following semester.

Jamie's brother had a friend whose mother died from breast cancer.

> I remember one time my brother said to me, "I was just kinda think-ing—Mommy could have died." All the time I just felt like I was really re-ally blessed. 'Cause I would look at my brother's friend, and I was like, *He doesn't even have a mother anymore.* But it could have been the other way for me as well.

Jamie learned some important lessons from her experience.

> It was a long experience and it opens your eyes to a lot of things. I've always been very close to my mother but, dealing with cancer, I learned that these kinds of struggles and pains make you stronger. And they pull you even closer together. But this experience was some-thing that, if you're close to somebody, you go through with them, and in your own way, just as much as they do. I do have to say that life has its ups and downs. And this was a down, but it had a pretty good out-come. Not that things don't happen to me, but just that, I deal with them.

Another thing Jamie learned from her mother's illness was how important it is to have family and friends.

> It's a hard thing to go through. It's probably even harder if you don't have anybody and have to go through that by yourself. That's one of the things that my mother counted on was family and friends to just be there.

Risk

Jamie suspects that her mother's smoking contributed to her breast cancer. "I know my mother used to smoke at one point in time, a long time ago. I was little. I don't know if that had any impact on her or what."

Thinking about her own risk, Jamie says,

> My boyfriend asked "Is this going to happen to you?" And I was like, "It could." But it would be easier because it would be familiar to me. I would know what to expect. I try to think of it in terms of not being prepared, not to look forward to it, but, to just be on the lookout.

Jamie continues:

> I've made some personal health choices, but not because of her experience or anything. They do tell you that people who have mothers who have breast cancer are more likely to have breast cancer. So I know it's not to play with and I need to check ever so often for myself. But other than that, just be thankful for the health that you have.

Current Situation

Jamie was nineteen and a college student at the time of the interviews. Two and a half years after her diagnosis, Jamie's mother was doing very well.

> It's given her a refreshment. My mother was like a kid at heart, a fun-type person anyway. She calls it her second chance at life. She went back to work. She's out there. She's really active and everything. She's joined a dance class. She's joined a support group.

Jamie is pleased to see her mother so happy.

CASE STUDY #6: SHARON

Age at Her Mother's Breast Cancer Diagnosis: 21

Background

Sharon was the older of two children in a two-parent Catholic household. She had a brother three years younger than herself. Her father was in the military, and the family frequently moved around when Sharon was growing up. When she was a teenager, her parents' strictness caused strain in her relationships with them.

Experience of Her Mother's Illness

Sharon was a sophomore in college when her mom was diagnosed with breast cancer. Her father called and told her that her mother was in the hospital and that "it would be really nice if you could come and visit." Sharon's parents did not share a lot about her mother's condition and tried not to make "a big deal out of it." Only after visiting her mother in the hospital and reading brochures about breast cancer did Sharon realize "just how serious of a situation it was." Her concern was increased when she found out that her maternal grandmother had also had breast cancer.

> It wasn't until after my mom got better that she told me that my grandmother had also had cancer and she had to have a whole breast removed. And my grandmother had never even mentioned it to me. . . . Apparently my mom had flown out for the operation and they just kept it really quiet. . . . And I think that's when I got really upset . . . because I wanted to know these things.

After spending three to four days in the hospital, Sharon's mother began follow-up treatment. "That was during the time when they still didn't really tell me that much about what the follow-up was and what was going on. It wasn't really discussed that much. It was just that 'Mom is better.'" Sharon would call home from college and talk to her brother about her mother's condition in order to find out what was really happening.

During the summer following her mother's hospitalization, Sharon took classes

> so that I could block it out. I think it was an excuse not to have to go home and deal with what was going on. . . . And I think that summer, that's when it really hit me . . . that something really bad could happen to her.

Sharon stated that she really had no friends to talk to about her mother's disease. Sharon sought out therapy on campus and became active at the college's women's center.

> You have friends, but it's kind of hard to talk to your friend about your mother having breast cancer. So that's why I would go to the women's center and talk to someone there and they seemed to be understanding and really into these kind of issues.

Experience Following Her Mother's Illness

Many aspects of Sharon's life changed following her mother's illness. For example, Sharon's involvement in the women's center made her reconsider her career goals. She switched her major from accounting to political science and became interested in nonprofit organizations. "Working in a nonprofit setting, I would feel better about what I'm doing versus working in an office all day just pushing paper for money." She met her husband in a women's studies class. "I think I chose somebody who was very open about his feelings and not closed up like a lot of men are."

Sharon's relationships with family members also improved over time. She became particularly close to her mother after she recovered from breast cancer. Sharon said that she and her mother now speak very openly with each other, and that she demands that she be told about what's occurring in her parents' lives. Sharon has been the catalyst in her family for opening up communication. Whereas her family once had a closed communication style, she now feels they talk much more openly because, "I have a big mouth." Once, her father was out of town on business and her mother was not answering the phone.

> I got worried because I kept thinking, *What if something happened to her at home?* I got so worried because I called her at work and they said that she was sick. She hadn't been in to work for a couple of days. . . . I remember leaving work here and driving all the way out to her home [in another state] and noticing that the trash had been taken out. The house was really clean. I remember even feeling her toothbrush to see if she had been there that morning and being really upset that I didn't know where she was. . . . And it just turned out she had gone away for a couple of days.

Sharon and her husband visit fairly often with her parents either at their home or at her parents' home in a nearby state. Sharon says that if her father should die before her mother, she would like her mother to move closer to her so that she could care for her. This is in part why she is also not interested in having children. "I think, when you have to think about the fact you might have to take care of your parents someday and juggle kids at the same time, it's a scary proposition."

Risk

Sometimes, Sharon is deeply concerned about her own health: "If my grandmother had cancer and my mom had cancer, that means there's a big likelihood that I'm going to have to go through this." She focuses on trying to maintain her health so that she can be a survivor as are her mother and grandmother. "I'm not really obsessed about dying of cancer. I'm more along the line of, 'If this is going to happen to me, and there's a chance it's going to, I'm gonna survive. I'm not going to die from it.'" Sharon tries to stay health focused, despite having recently gained weight.

Sharon finds it difficult to go in for her yearly gynecology appointments.

> I get scared to death going to my gynecology checkups every year. I really worry about that, because I think about . . . getting closer and closer to that age when I'm going to really have to start worrying about the possibility of that happening. . . . I worry about if I do find something . . . how am I going to handle that?

Sharon will start getting mammograms soon because, although she is only in her late twenties, she thinks her family history warrants extra caution.

Sharon opposes genetic testing; she is concerned that it will lead to discrimination by health insurance companies and possibly employers. "If that kind of information is put in the computer, who can get access to it? Not to sound paranoid, but you have to be careful in the computer age." Sharon also has made an effort to have adequate health and life insurance.

> I make sure that I always have good [health] insurance in case I get something like breast cancer. And I have life-insurance coverage, so in case something happens to me, my husband can pay off the house and take care of the bills.

Current Situation

Sharon was twenty-seven at the time of the interviews. She and her husband live about two hours from her parents' home. Sharon works for a nonprofit human service agency and describes herself as a feminist. She and her husband are renovating a historic home.

DISCUSSION

The following section begins with a discussion of how the variable of the daughter's age differs for cases in which the mother survives. Then it briefly considers the impact of the family background and the experience of mother's illness and treatment on the women whose mothers survived. (See Chapters 4 through 7 for more extensive discussion of daughters' experience during the mother's illness.) This is followed by a discussion of the daughter's experience after the active phase of the mother's illness. The themes discussed in this section are worries about mother, close to mother, difficulty with intimate relationships, and change in priorities. In addition to the six cases just presented, the discussion includes cases of women whose mothers survived that can be found in Appendix III. These are: Chloe, age six at mother's diagnoses, Tina, age fourteen, Jody, age seventeen, Betty, age eighteen, Tomasina, age twenty-one, Laura, age twenty-four, and Dora, age twenty-six.

Impact of Daughter's Age When Mother Survives

Daughter's age was an extremely important factor in the cases of women whose mothers died from breast cancer, and as such, it provided the primary organizing framework for Chapters 4 through 7. However, the impact of a daughter's age and her psychological development in women whose mothers survived is quite different. Unlike the situation in which a mother dies, in this case the mother-daughter relationship evolves as it goes through various developmental stages and a variety of life experiences. Ramona, the youngest at time of diagnosis in the case studies in this chapter, provides a good example. Ramona experienced many of the themes that were discussed in Chapter 4, in the phase "experience of mother's illness and treatment," such as limited communication and a push to independence. However, this wasn't the end of the story. Because her mother survived, they were able to renegotiate their relationship. When Ramona had questions about her mother's illness, she could discuss what happened again and again as she developed increased cognitive and emotional abilities. This is in sharp contrast to the women whose mothers died, who were left with many unanswered questions and unresolved issues. Sharon's case illustrates how daughters of survivors can create changes in how the illness is handled. As a young woman, Sharon was protected from information about her mother's condition. However, she was unhappy with this, and as an adult actively and effectively worked to change the pattern of secrecy in her family. Daughters whose mothers survive have many opportunities to resolve problems that may have developed at the time of the mother's illness. This may not happen for many years, but because both mothers and daughters change during these years, old issues can be settled at any time. For this reason, the age of the daughter at her mother's diagnosis was less of a defining factor for women whose mothers survived than it was for those whose mothers died.

When the mother survives, breast cancer becomes one in a series of events that shape the family story. As time goes on, it recedes in significance and other events take its place. For example, Lisa's father left the family years after her mother was diagnosed. Jane's father died of a heart attack when she was only four. Mary's (Appendix III) mother died of a heart attack several years after her breast cancer. In other cases, if life is without other major crises, the breast cancer can be a major event, even when the mother survives. At the other extreme, when life has been a series of major crises, the breast cancer may be considered just one more hurdle (Laura, Appendix III).

Impact of "Family Background" When Mother Survives

The family structure prior to the breast cancer, family communication style, and the level of other family problems are important factors for daughters whose mothers survived (as they were for women whose mothers died). For example, in some families (Mandy, Dora), the parents were divorced. Jane's father died when Jane was a very young child. Lisa and Mandy both had problems (anorexia and depression, respectively) prior to their mothers' breast cancer. These issues impacted how the families experienced breast cancer, because the daughters had a different type of relationship with their mothers before the diagnosis. Jane, for example, describes how she and her mother became extremely interdependent after her father's death; this may have contributed to Jane becoming her mother's caregiver and confidante.

Experience During Mother's Illness and Treatment When Mother Survives

The experience of the daughter during the early phases of the illness and treatment does not differ from that of women whose mothers eventually die. The age-related themes identified in the previous chapters apply to the cases in this chapter. Ramona, for example, illustrates the themes of "loss of independence" and "lack of communication" discussed in Chapter 4. Lisa and Jane, early adolescents, illustrate the focus on body integrity of many adolescents (Chapter 5), and Jamie illustrates how older adolescents take on household responsibilities (Chapter 6).

Again, as for daughters whose mothers die, the experience of daughters whose mothers survive is affected by which treatments the mother has initially, and whether the cancer recurs. If the mother's cancer is detected very early, treatment is minimal (lumpectomy), and no recurrence develops, the impact on the daughter may be minimal. The other extreme would be a case in which the mother experienced more aggressive treatments (mastectomy, chemotherapy), needing more help from the daughter. These treatments also are more physically represented and more likely to interfere with the daughter's denial of the seriousness of her mother's illness. If the mother has one or more recurrences, the effect on the daughter will be magnified as more chemotherapy is required and the mother's prognosis worsens.

Experience Following Mother's Illness and Treatment

The fact that a mother has had breast cancer can impact the mother-daughter relationship; this can affect other aspects of the daughter's life. An understanding of this impact begins with consideration of how mothers and daughters interact under normal circumstances. The relationship between a woman and her daughters is probably the most complex of all family relationships. Little solid research on this topic exists. The titles of many self-help books—*Don't Blame Mother: Mending the Mother-Daughter Relationship* (Caplan, 1989); *When You and Your Mother Can't Be Friends* (Secunda, 1991); *Mending the Broken Bough* (Zax and Poulter, 1998)—suggest that this is a problematic relationship for women. Popular fiction and films such as *White Oleander* (Fitch, 1999) and *Divine Secrets of the Ya-Ya Sis-*

terhood (Wells, 1997) also commonly portray problematic mother-daughter relationships.

Although breast cancer researchers consistently have found that women with breast cancer are extremely concerned about their daughters (Oktay and Walter, 1991; Wellisch, as cited in Tarkan, 1999), the daughters' perspective on this has not been studied. Nor has much research occurred on how the mother-daughter relationship is affected when the mother (or daughter) experiences a major illness.

For women whose mothers survived, four themes were identified in the period after illness and treatment: worries about mother, close to mother, difficulty with intimate relationships, and change in priorities.

Worries About Mother

Daughters of women who survive breast cancer often express worry about their mothers, a feeling that would not normally be common at their stage of the life course. Lisa says, "I know I'm really scared of losing her now." Sharon got so worried that when she couldn't reach her mother, she drove all the way to her house in another state. Tina (Appendix III) says, "I worry that she'll have stuff go wrong and be afraid to go to the doctor." Jody (Appendix III) is afraid to think that her mother might die because she might bring her mother bad luck. Although many daughters of survivors did not say they worried about their mothers directly, 92 percent of them checked this category on the final questionnaire.

To understand the dynamic that takes place between mothers with breast cancer and their daughters, it is helpful to look at the situation from the mother's perspective. Protection of the vulnerable child is central to the nature of motherhood, and although it is strongest when children are very young, it continues throughout the life course. Women are held responsible for their children's health and safety, even when they do not have control of the factors that affect it (Lerner, 1993). When a mother gets diagnosised with breast cancer, her sense of control may be shattered. She realizes that if she dies, her children will lose her and her protection at the same time. Thus the tension between responsibility and control is exacerbated.

Kathy Weingarten (1994), a family therapist who was diagnosed with breast cancer, writes eloquently about this dilemma in her book, *The Mother's Voice: Strengthening Intimacy in Families:*

> I cannot promise them the one thing I believe they need more than anything else from me, the one thing I need. I cannot tell them that I will live, that I—their MOTHER—will always be there for them. I cannot assure them that I will be ultimately responsible always. I cannot tell them—because I do not believe it—that they will be all right without me, that my death will not damage them. From my breast, from which has come the milk that has sustained, comes a poison to kill, not just me, but them too. (p. 47)

Weingarten (1994) discusses how difficult it was when she was diagnosed to express her own vulnerability to her children.

When a mother is diagnosed with breast cancer, her health and life are threatened. At the same time, the disease threatens her children. Some mothers tried to protect their children from the realities of the illness, by keeping it secret (Sharon, Tomasina) or by controlling the information about the illness (Ramona, Mandy). Ramona's and Mandy's mothers both continued to try to protect their daughters. Ramona's mother taught her how to deal with insensitive comments by people in her small town, while Mandy's mother contacted her teachers and made them partners in her quest to help Mandy adapt to the illness.

Daughters often later repeat the same behaviors. When the mother is vulnerable, daughters protect their mothers in the same way that they were protected. Some daughters become experts at hiding their true feelings and maintaining a cheerful demeanor. For example, Jamie describes how she learned to "put on a happy face," so as to keep up her mother's spirits. Jane keeps her fear and hurt feelings hidden from her mother, not wanting to burden her. Mandy, too, mentions that after the acute phase of the illness, she tried to protect her mother from her own negative feelings. These daughters don't share aspects of their lives that might be painful to the mother. This "mutual mothering" leaves both mother and daughter feeling good about being able to protect each other (Fischer, 1986).

The pattern of daughters worrying about their mothers may result from the mutual protection between mothers and daughters. Mothers protect their daughters from threatening information and from scary or negative emotions during the illness. Later, daughters continue to worry about their mothers' health, but they protect their mothers from knowing that they worry, feeling that this might upset the mother. The failure to communicate, the mutual protection, leads to increased worry among the daughters.

Daughters in single-parent families (Lisa and Mandy) or those in which the father does not take on a caregiving role may be especially likely to take on a protective role. At a time when daughters would normally be developing more independence, they are relied on to provide care. If the daughter is an adolescent, she may postpone or forgo rebellion, and may not achieve the kind of separation needed to become an independent adult. These daughters may continue to feel a need to protect their mothers long after the breast cancer has passed.

Close to Mother

Most women whose mothers survived breast cancer feel very close to their mothers. Fifty-eight percent of these women indicated on the final questionnaire that the breast cancer made them feel closer to their mothers. This may come from their recognition of mothers' vulnerability. Lisa, for example, states that although she and her mother always had been close, their closeness was strengthened as she saw her mother endure the illness and a divorce. "My respect is so enormous for her. That's when we started becoming close." Now, Lisa talks with her mother every day, and she even prefers talking with her mother to dating. "It's a lot more comforting at nine o'clock . . . to pick up the phone and call my mom than to pick up a boy and have to deal with this and that." When Lisa is not near her mother, she becomes depressed. Jane also describes her relationship with her mother as "very, very close," going back to the time of her father's death, long before her mother's diagnosis. Now, Jane says, "It's been hard to set a boundary." Similar to Lisa, she describes herself and her mother as "friends." At the same time, she admits that she is "mean" to her mother, taking out her anger on her. Mandy, too, describes her relationship with her mother as "close." She feels that by being there to care for her mom during the illness, "we have this special bond." Jamie says she has always been close to her mom. She comments, "These kinds of things [illness], they pull you even closer together."

Sharon also describes her relationship with her mother as close, although they were not especially so at the time of the illness itself. Now, Sharon enjoys her mother's visits and hopes that her mother will move to live near her if her father should pass away.

In normal life-course development, as children reach maturity, they move away from their parents, and toward independence. This process begins in childhood, as a child's world expands beyond the home, but it accelerates in adolescence. According to Erikson (1968) two major tasks of adolescence are autonomy and intimacy. In order to achieve independence from the family of origin, a certain amount of separation must take place. This separation allows the adolescent to form an independent identity, and to eventually establish a separate family of his/her own.

While the applicability of Erikson's model to women has been questioned (Chodorow, 1999; Jordan et al., 1991), many girls also go through a rebellious phase, when they outwardly reject the mother and all she stands for. Adolescence is usually perceived as a low point in mother-daughter relationships. This distance is related to the daughter's sexual development; girls may need some distance from parents to develop a sexual self. This idea is embodied in the Greek myth of Persephone, who must leave her mother to establish a sexual relationship and become a wife, much to the mother's chagrin. Research shows mother-daughter relationships tend to be most distant in adolescence. After adolescence, the relationship grows gradually stronger (especially after the daughter has a child) (Rossi and Rossi, 1990). The closeness is based on the mother and daughter helping each other, which continues through much of the life cycle.

When the mother is seen as strong by the daughter, the daughter may rebel against her, often using the conflict as a way to define herself as "other than mother." Pipher (1994), a therapist who specializes in adolescent girls, describes cases of adolescent daughters who "hate" their mothers, but who spend all of their time in therapy talking of nothing *but* their mothers. A mother's very strength allows the daughter to attack her, to move away and find a separate identity (including defining a sexual self), without fear of losing her, or even of seriously hurting her.

However, what happens when a mother is ill? Daughters of mothers who are ill, or who are weak in other ways, become fierce defenders of their mothers. Instead of attacking them, they quickly move into a "mothering" relationship in which they become the mother's protector. Fischer's (1986) stages of mother-daughter relationships are also relevant here. (See discussion in Chapter 7.) The cases of daughters whose mothers survived reflects such a pattern. Instead of attacking a strong mother, and moving away, the daughter forms a repressed recognition of the mother's weakness. The daughter fears losing her, stays close, and protects her.

Difficulty with Intimate Relationships

Some women whose mothers survive do not form adult attachments to partners and commitments to children. Lisa, for example, indicates that her relationships with men are short and superficial, and she prefers to be close to her mother. Sharon, who is married, is reluctant to have children. She fears that her mother will need her if she becomes ill again, and thinks having children might prevent her from helping her mother. Jane is overweight and recognizes that this may be a way of avoiding sexual relationships. In these cases, the failure to separate from the mother, due to her perceived vulnerability, may mean that the daughters get "stuck" and do not move forward in their life-course development. This theme is closely related to the discussion in the previous section. Literature on women's life-course development suggests that women need to separate from mothers to develop sexual relationships (Bassoff, 1987). The very closeness described may make adult attachments more problematic. This category was checked by one-quarter of the survivors, suggesting that it does not happen for all daughters. However, it remains a potential problem.

Change in Priorities

As with the women in the previous chapters whose mothers died, some of the women whose mothers survived also changed their priorities or their direction as a result of their mothers' illness. For example, Mandy became a breast cancer advocate and is studying to be a nurse. Sharon also changed her career direction, not to health care, but to something more meaningful to her than the business career she was pursuing. Jamie learned how important the family is in times of crisis, and now puts more emphasis on this area of her life.

The women who were younger reorganized different types of priorities. Ramona emphasized how she was trying to give her daughter a more carefree, fun childhood than she had. Jane focused on the impact of her mother's illness on her body image and weight problems. These topics reflect some of the themes identified in the daughters whose mothers died, as discussed in Chapters 4 and 5.

SUMMARY

This chapter has presented six case studies of women whose mothers survived breast cancer and discussed several themes related to the post–breast cancer mother-daughter relationship (see Box 8.1). Four themes were identified: worries about mother, close to mother, difficulty with intimate relationships, and change in priorities. The first three themes may be part of a pattern; it is possible that the daughters' worry results in an unusual level of protectiveness and closeness that precludes the daughters' ability to move away and form intimate partnerships with others. This pattern may be affected by factors such as the extent to which another adult (e.g., father) takes on the parenting roles in the family, the level of communication in the family, the birth order of the daughter, the mother's way of coping with the illness, and the extent to which she maintains a protective role in spite of the illness. In addition, the stage at which the breast cancer was diagnosed, the treatments received, and whether or not the illness recurs influence the extent of this pattern. The effect on the daughter may be minimal if the family has had no prior problems; open communication exists; the daughter has an older sister; the cancer was caught early; or the mother had limited treatment and no recurrence. (See Dora, Appendix III.)

The impact of the illness on the progression of the mother-daughter relationship has very important implications for the quality of life

---

BOX 8.1. Themes Found in Daughters
Whose Mothers Survived

1. Worries about mother
2. Close to mother
3. Difficulty with intimate relationships
4. Change in priorities

of both mothers and daughters. Because most women survive the disease, large numbers are affected. Unfortunately, little research on this topic has been done. This study suggests breast cancer can improve relationships, moving mothers and daughters toward greater closeness and a more mature relationship. However, in some cases, a pattern can emerge in the mother-daughter relationship which may interfere with healthy development in the daughter. Because the relationship is constantly evolving, mothers and/or daughters can address these issues and change negative patterns.

Implications of these findings are discussed in Chapter 11.

Chapter 9

Daughters and the Risk
of Breast Cancer

When a mother has breast cancer, a disease that can be genetic, the daughter does not only experience having an ill mother and, in some cases, losing a mother—she also lives with the knowledge that she may get the disease herself in her lifetime. This chapter provides some background about the two breast cancer genes we now know influence the risk of breast and ovarian cancer. In addition, the ways that the daughters in this study think about their risk, how they try to prevent the disease, and how they deal with their fears are discussed. This chapter uses cases presented throughout the book and includes daughters in all age groups. Women whose mothers died and those whose mothers survived are compared.

The following discussion presents the major themes based on analysis of what the daughters in this study said about their own risk. It is important to note that although the study originated from an interest in how "high-risk" women (due to their mother's cancer) thought and felt about their situation, we found that when given an opportunity to tell their stories, the women focused much more on their experience when the mother was ill and/or after her death. Some didn't even mention their own risk, and those that did, did so as an afterthought. Risk was not the central focus of any of these women, even among those whose mothers survived. Nevertheless, their thoughts and actions about their own risk are important.

The material on risk is divided into five categories: fear, assessing risk, actions to help prevent breast cancer, actions to help in early breast-cancer detection, and coping.

FEAR

Daughters of women who had breast cancer fear getting breast cancer themselves, and this fear is a major component of their lives. Some examples of how this fear is expressed include the following quotes from the case studies:

TRISHA: I get nervous getting close to people, being that it runs in my family. My grandmother had cancer and my mother had cancer.

JANICE: I thought about it a lot when my mother died. A lot. "I'm gonna die. We're all gonna die of it."

ALICIA: I worry tremendously about my own health. All the time. I've worried about breast cancer since the time she died.

KARA: I was so afraid. I thought to myself, *I'm going to die! Because this happened to my mother, this is going to happen to me.*

RITA: I was born with a [genetic] defect. My mother was obviously born with one too. . . . I do not honestly believe that I have any control over this anymore.

CAROL: So cancer is definitely a theme in my family. It was just another block to add to the fear column. Something that is going to happen to me someday.

NORA: I worry about it more than I think I will [get it]. . . . Am I fearful? Absolutely!

ANDREA: I'm certainly paranoid about getting breast cancer. It scares me and I constantly think I have a lump. . . . I just feel like something will happen.

SARAH: There are three daughters. The chances are that one of us could develop breast cancer.

RAMONA: I definitely have a huge fear of it.

SHARON: If my grandmother had cancer and my mom had cancer, that means there's a big likelihood that I'm going to have to go through this.

The fear of breast cancer may be constant, at certain times it becomes especially intense. Finding a lump and going through the process of having it assessed is frightening for all women, but it is especially stressful for these daughters. In addition to the time when lumps are found, fears are especially strong shortly after the mother's illness (or death), and when the daughter approaches the age at which her mother was diagnosed (or died):

ALICIA: Every birthday that comes, I get more and more depressed, because it's getting closer to fifty-three, and fifty-three is the big number.

BETTINA: I detected it [lump] myself. It was terrifying, because I was forty, a year younger than my mother.

When daughters survive past the age of the mother's death, the fear may dissipate. Bettina, for example, says, "As I approached and then passed the age at which Mother's cancer was diagnosed, I became a little more nonchalant about it. And at this point, I'm barely able to remember to do any breast self-examination." This suggests that the overestimation of risk prior to the age of the mother's cancer or death may be replaced by an underestimation once the daughter is past that dreaded age.

Another particularly stressful time is when adolescents begin to develop breasts. Several women in the cases mistook breast tissue for lumps and were terrified. (See Chapter 5.) Daughters also worry when their daughters reach the age they were when their mother was diagnosed (or died).

A high level of fear in daughters appeared in a number of studies. For example, Facione (2002) found that women with a female relative with breast cancer overestimate their own risk, and Trask and colleagues (2001) discovered that two-thirds of attendees at a high-risk breast cancer clinic worried about breast cancer so much that it interfered with their functioning. Interestingly, attempts to reduce worry through genetic counseling and education do not result in more accurate estimates of risk for those who are most anxious (Rothemund, Paepke, and Flor, 2001). This high level of fear has implications for breast-surveillance behaviors, and also affects quality of life for daughters and their families.

Our questionnaire results suggest that women whose mothers died were more likely to fear breast cancer than were those whose mothers survived. Forty-five percent of daughters whose mothers survived indicated that they feared getting breast cancer themselves, while 79 percent of those whose mothers died indicated that they fear the disease. Those whose mothers died from the disease also were more likely to expect to get breast cancer at the same age as their mother (45 percent) than were women whose mothers survived the disease (23 percent). This finding is consistent with other research, which also found that the level of fear is highest in women whose mothers died (Erblich, Bovbjerg, and Valdimarsdottir, 2000; Zakowski et al., 1997). In fact, the outcome of the mother's disease is not predictive of whether the daughter will be diagnosed. However, if the mother survived the daughter's fear may be lessened. In daughters of survivors, breast cancer may be seen as an illness that can be overcome, rather than a death sentence. In some cases, mothers who survive may encourage their daughters to feel that they are not at risk; perhaps the possibility that they may have passed on a genetic propensity to breast cancer to their daughters is too threatening or upsetting to them.

ASSESSING RISK

Daughters in this study assess and reassess their risk, based on a combination of factors. This assessment often is based on a woman's "explanatory model" (Kleinman, 1980), or what she thinks of as the cause of her mother's breast cancer. This may be a cognitive process that parallels the more emotional (and sometimes irrational) fear. Some relevant illustrations follow.

Alicia assessed her risk by comparing herself to her mother: "She smoked. I've never smoked. She was heavy, didn't exercise. I exercise a lot. I eat a healthier diet. . . . Emotionally, I'm a lot healthier. I'm happy. I don't think she was happy." Gloria attributed her mother's illness to her marital problems. "He [father] was abusive to my mother and, looking at it now, they say that blows and things can cause reactions within your bloodstream and cause you to have cancer. I mean, even stress." Rita saw similarities between personalities. "I think that I have the personality of somebody that gets cancer. My personality is similar to my mother's. And we both had really bad childhoods. That's more likely to give me cancer than anything else." Ramona attributed her mother's cancer to exposure to radiation at her job in a laboratory. Lisa focused on her mother's diet in combination with marital stress.

I really believe that my mom got cancer from, besides the fact that she and my dad had a terrible relationship, she owned a cheesecake company, and spent years, instead of eating healthy foods, just licking up the cheesecake batter, which is full of carcinogens.

Elizabeth also compared herself to her mother, and concluded that she was not as vulnerable to cancer.

I think a lot of my mother's cancer and her sister's cancer also was a lot of anger toward their mother. A lot of it was repressed anger. I think that was a big contributing factor. So now I'm not worried about it at all.

By developing an "explanatory model" for their mother's breast cancer, and then comparing themselves to the factors in their model, the daughters assessed their own risk. Although these models did not necessarily fit the risk factors accepted by the American Cancer Society (ACS) (2002) (age, family history, age of menarche, age at first pregnancy, breast-feeding, obesity, alcohol use, and hormone therapies), these recognized factors are based on statistical correlates and are not accurate predictors of individual risk. In fact, about 80 percent of women diagnosed do not have any of the risk factors (American Cancer Society, 2002). However, only daughters who were closely involved in the medical professions (Gloria, Veronica, Mandy) based their levels of risk on known factors. Women seemed to develop explanations for their mothers' breast cancer and then compared themselves to their mothers in these areas. When the daughters found differences, these explanatory models provided them comfort. When the daughters focused on similarities to their mothers, breast cancer was perceived as a virtual certainty.

ACTIONS TO HELP PREVENT BREAST CANCER

The women in this study were well aware of the recommendations of medical professionals regarding prevention and tried to incorporate them into their lives. Exercise was often mentioned (Janice, Alicia, Linda, Cathy, Carol, Andrea, Elizabeth) as was diet (Janice, Alicia, Cathy, Kara, Lisa, Elizabeth). Respondents commonly indicated that they tried to lead healthy lifestyles but were not always successful. One problem was that they knew there was no guarantee that these activities would prevent breast cancer; they often presented evidence of others who exercised and ate a healthy diet but still got cancer. For example, Kara told us that she just lost fifty pounds, and then added, "I have an uncle who got colon cancer. He was telling me how my aunt made him eat broccoli because it had cancer-fighting nutrients. He was so angry when he got cancer anyway."

Smoking also was mentioned frequently as a possible cause, and the daughters avoid this habit. However, although smoking is known to cause lung cancer and heart disease, it has not been found to increase a woman's risk of getting breast cancer.

Most risk factors on the ACS list are not controllable. One factor that can be controlled is age at first pregnancy. Kara took a "risk test" on the Internet: "I didn't realize that not having had children by thirty was another risk factor. I realized that I needed to have a baby, not at thirty, but I needed to push one out before then." Ramona also planned her life to be sure that her pregnancy and breast-feeding was completed by the time she was thirty-three, the age at which her mother was diagnosed. A danger here is that these risk factors are based on statistical correlations on large groups of women. No evidence supports that having a child at thirty instead of at twenty-nine protects a woman from breast cancer.

Other preventive behaviors mentioned by the women in our sample include avoiding hormones such as birth control pills (Janice) and hormone replacement therapy (Alicia). The drug tamoxifen was found to lower breast-cancer risk while the study was in progress, and one woman mentioned this but concluded, "More and more I thought about the side effects, and the possibility of me not getting it [without the tamoxifen], and I thought, this is really going to the extreme." The same type of assessment was made about prophylactic mastectomy. Several respondents mentioned it, but rejected it as too extreme. Andrea's mother's oncologist told her about it. "He told me that I could just cut off both of my breasts, if I wanted to minimize my risk. . . . I thought that was extremely radical. I was not really ready to do that."

According to questionnaire responses, women whose mothers died were more likely to take action to prevent the disease (95 percent) than were women whose mothers survived (69 percent). This may be a result of their higher levels of fear discussed earlier.

ACTIONS TO HELP IN EARLY
BREAST CANCER DETECTION

Clinical Exams, Breast Self-Exams, and Mammography

Although it is well known that breast cancer is more easily treatable if discovered when the cancer is still small and has not spread, the existing tests are far from perfect in detecting when a cancer forms or spreads. Three methods of early detection are recommended: clinical breast examination, breast self-examination, and mammography.

Of these, clinical breast exam was valued highly and used by all women in our study. Some women were able to arrange for clinical exams more than once a year. Because insurance does not pay for these extra exams, they often used their own funds.

Mammography was also generally accepted, but it was not available to the women who were in their twenties, and many in their thirties. Unfortunately, mammography has not been shown to reduce breast cancer mortality in women under forty. Even those in their forties often do not benefit, and screening for these women is controversial. This is very frustrating for daughters, especially those whose mothers were diagnosed in their thirties or forties. These daughters understandably want to have mammograms, and are frustrated that they are not recommended. For example, Rita's mother died at thirty-two. Rita was told she could not have a mammogram until age thirty (after the age at which her mother was diagnosed). Veronica started getting mammograms at age thirty-two although her insurance company would not pay for one until she was thirty-five. Without her doctor's input, Nora decided to have a mammogram at a young age. She paid for it out of pocket. Bettina got a mammogram at age twenty-five, on her own, and when she found a lump at age twenty-seven, she was glad she had. Sarah's insurance company would not pay for a mammogram until she was forty, which frustrated her. The other side of the mammogram issue is raised by Ramona and Rita, who worried about the possible cancer-causing effects from the radiation exposure of too many mammograms.

Breast self-exam (BSE) was a much more difficult issue for daughters than clinical exams or mammograms. Most women found BSE extremely anxiety provoking and, as a result, impossible to do.

JANICE: I just can't [do BSE]. I've never done it.

ALICIA: I have a hard time doing breast self-exams myself. I don't do them.

CATHY: I do them, but you would think that I would do it every month, but there must be some psychological reason why I'm not. But I just can't.

NORA: It's [BSE] no big deal most of the time, but every now and then I get this little panic thing. . . . That's very scary.

A second consideration concerning BSE for many women was their lack of confidence in their ability to identify a lump. Cathy said, "I get discouraged 'cause I feel like I don't know if, when I feel a lump, if it's a cyst or not, and the process makes me a little bit nervous." Elizabeth said, "I try the breast exams but I really can't tell in all honesty what's what." Andrea said, "I'm afraid to feel it myself, so I don't really do anything about it."

Clearly, the two issues of anxiety and lack of confidence are not unrelated. Many women are unsure of their ability to identify a lump, but the fact that these daughters fear breast cancer makes this much more stressful for them (Lindberg and Wellisch, 2001). Some literature suggests that in some cases, anxiety about breast cancer leads to the other extreme, "excessive self-examination" (Epstein et al., 1997). Only two women in our study indicated that they were possibly overdoing BSE. Gloria, who is a mammogram technician, does breast cancer detection for a living, and says she is constantly examining her breasts. Ramona also was examining her breasts so carefully, and finding so many lumps, that her physician told her to do the exams with a special sheet over the breast, so that she wouldn't identify every little "lump."

A major problem with breast self-examination as an early detection technique is that lumps are common in breast tissue, and so the likelihood of finding a lump is high. Women cannot determine when a lump is cancer, and so finding a lump usually means having a biopsy. This process is very stressful for most women (Padgett et al., 2001), but it is much more so for the daughters in our study. To experience this level of stress every month was more than even the most dedicated daughters could manage.

Questionnaire responses also provided evidence that the mother's illness outcome affected the daughter's performance of BSE. Women whose mothers died were much less likely to perform breast self-exams (39 percent) than were women whose mothers survived (54 percent). Perhaps this was due to their greater fear.

Genetic Testing

Background on Breast Cancer Genetics

In the latter part of the twentieth century, important discoveries in genetics, including the discovery of the double-helix structure of the human genome, made it possible for scientists to begin to uncover the genetic bases of many diseases. The National Institutes of Health took on the task of "mapping" the human genome, creating the Human Genome Project. By studying the genetic tissue of members of families with high rates of an illness (e.g., breast cancer), and comparing the genes of those who were affected by the disease and those who were not ("linkage analysis"), scientists identified specific parts of suspect genes that were different. In this way, in 1994 a gene associated with breast cancer named BRCA1 was identified on chromosome 17 at the q21 location (Easton et al., 1995; Miki et al., 1994; Wooster et al., 1995). Mutations in this gene were found in families with high rates of breast cancer. Further work identified a second gene also associated with breast cancer: BRCA2, located on chromosome 13 at q12. Once these genes were discovered, scientists studied the families with a history of breast cancer to determine the biological role of these genes, the pattern of inheritance, and the implication of a specific mutation in the gene for an individual who had not been diagnosed.

Much research is currently underway, and new discoveries refine our understanding and knowledge frequently; however, a basic outline of what is now believed about these genetic mutations is summarized here. Approximately 1 in between 800 to 2,500 persons in the United States are thought to have a mutation in one of the two genes associated with breast cancer. Certain subpopulations have been found to have higher rates. For example, in Jews of Eastern European origin (Ashkenazi), about 2 percent of the population has a mutation in one of these genes (Strewing et al., 1997). The BRCA1 and BRCA2 genes are understood to act as cancer-suppressor genes, so that a mutation that leads to a malfunction in the gene makes cancer more likely. However, exactly how the gene functions normally or how it malfunctions when a mutation is present is not yet well understood.

The genetic basis for breast cancer is complicated in several ways. The two genes now known to be associated with breast cancer are large genes. This means that testing for possible mutations is not a simple matter, because hundreds of mutations in the gene are possible. For this reason, scientists prefer to look at the gene in someone in the family who has had breast cancer. If they find a mutation, they then compare it to the gene of a woman at risk, to see whether she has the same mutation. If this tissue is not available (as often it is not, especially if the mother died long ago), the test is both much more expensive and much less accurate.

The breast cancer genes BRCA1 and BRCA2 are inherited in an autosomal dominant pattern (Claus, Risch, and Thompson, 1994). The genes are not located on the sex chromosome. This means that the mutations can be inherited from either the mother or the father. Because breast cancer occurs more frequently in women than in men, it is common to think of this as only a woman's disease, and not to think of the father as a possible source. The disease has a dominant inheritance pattern, so a woman needs only to inherit the genetic mutation from one parent. For genes with a recessive inheritance pattern, both sides of the family must carry the defective gene. Fifty percent of children in a family that carries a mutation in BRCA1 or BRCA2 will inherit the defective gene.

Scientists are trying to determine the likelihood of getting breast cancer in women who carry a mutation in these genes. Estimates of the chance of getting breast cancer range between 55 and 85 percent in someone who had a BRCA1 or BRCA2 mutation. That is, 55 to 85 percent of women with a mutation would get breast cancer by age eighty, depending on the specific mutation and lifestyle factors.

Another complicating discovery was that the BRCA genes are associated with several types of cancer, and not just breast cancer. Those with mutations in these genes also are at higher-than-average risk for ovarian cancer and colon cancer. In men with the mutation, the risk for prostate cancer is higher, especially in those with a BRCA2 mutation.

In addition, although genetic mutations are necessary to get some diseases (e.g., Huntington's disease), they are associated with only a small percent of breast (and ovarian) cancer cases (5 to 10 percent). Most women who have breast cancer (90 to 95 percent) have no genetic mutation, and have not passed an increased risk on to their daughters. This makes the interpretation of negative genetic test results difficult, because when someone tests negative for a genetic mutation, it does not mean that breast cancer is not possible, only that one's chance of getting it is no higher than that of the general population.

The value of genetic testing for breast (and ovarian) cancer is somewhat limited by the lack of a guaranteed way to prevent the disease if a woman tests positive for a genetic mutation. The ways now known to reduce the incidence of breast cancer involve drastic surgery—removal of the breasts and/or ovaries (prophylactic mastectomy and oophorectomy). Recent research suggests that taking tamoxifen also is effective in reducing the incidence of the disease in those with genetic mutations (Narod et al., 2000). Because of the risks of these preventative measures, many women with genetic mutations decide against surgery or drugs and instead increase attention to surveillance and early detection. Genetic testing for breast and ovarian cancers is also problematic because of potential discrimination by insurance companies and employers (Hudson et al., 1995; Oktay, 1998).

The increased availability of tests for BRCA1 and BRCA2 mutations (based in part on marketing by private companies) is creating both new opportunities and new problems for women. Women most interested in having genetic testing include those who have had breast cancer and want to know if their cancer was caused by a genetic mutation, those who have one or more first-degree relatives who have had breast cancer (such as the daughters in this study), those who want to know if they carry a genetic mutation, and those who are not high risk but who are worried about their breast cancer risk. Many questions have been raised about the risks and benefits of genetic testing for cancer.

None of the women in the study had undergone genetic testing, but several had thought about it, and a few had gone to educational sessions or to genetic counseling. Alicia, for example, considered the effects of getting the test results.

> At first, I thought that if it came back positive I would go in and have mastectomies with implants. Then I decided that would be too radical for who I really am. I would just want to know genetically if I'm predis-

posed to it, for the estrogen purpose, and for my daughter. For my peace of mind. If it turned out yes, then I would just monitor myself even closer. If it was not, I wouldn't decrease what I was doing, but I might live my life a little freer. . . . To find out I'm not would be the greatest liberation for me, but I don't know if I can handle finding out that I could be.

Other women also focused on the potential negative effect of learning that they had the gene. Jane said, "I think that if I did it, it would make me feel doom and gloom." Andrea also said,

I don't know that I'd want to know, either. . . . I mean, it's kind of like, do you want to know the day that you're gonna die? I don't. I'd rather kind of let fate . . . I don't know if I'd want to know that.

Felicia emphasized the fact that nothing could be done to prevent the disease if the genetic mutation was found.

I don't want to know if I have the gene or whatever. You can't get rid of it. I know that heredity has a big part to do with it. But I also believe that diet and those things can counteract heredity too.

Another problem was articulated by Cathy, who went in for genetic counseling. "She [genetic counselor] made me aware of the fact that there was a great deal of information that I just don't have. . . . Then, there's the issue of locating my mother's tissue." Felicia also recognized that she did not have adequate knowledge of her family history. "My mother's brother died of colon cancer, and my mother's aunt died of cancer—I think it was female, but I don't know. Older people don't tell you exactly what is what." The genetic counseling process does involve putting together a family history, and often, accurate testing requires the tissue of an affected relative to be compared to that of the person being tested. Women who have lost mothers, especially whose mothers died when they were young, often do not have full knowledge of the family history, especially the mother's side. Also, tissue is not available unless the daughter can locate a frozen blood sample. Without this knowledge, or the tissue, the genetic testing often is not accurate.

Finally, the women with the most knowledge of genetic testing were the most concerned about the possibility that the test results would become known to an insurance company, and used against them. Sharon, for example, said, "If that kind of information is put in the computer, who can get access to it? Not to sound paranoid, but you have to be careful in the computer age." Alicia also said, "I'm so afraid of medical confidentiality. If I did it [genetic testing], I would pay cash, and use somebody else's social security number."

Because breast (and ovarian) cancer can be an especially frightening diagnosis, which may involve the possibility of disfiguring surgery, very unpleasant treatments (radiation, chemotherapy), and a potentially terminal outcome, many women have intense emotions regarding genetic counseling. If they have a family history, they bring to genetic counseling these emotions (perhaps long buried) surrounding cancer and possibly death. A textbook on genetic counseling states this effectively:

> Counselees may have specific fears concerning their own possible illness, disfigurement or death as well as the possibility of further illness and loss for their children and families. They may be experiencing anger, isolation, loss of control, grief over past and possible future deaths within the family, and guilt due to a sense of having failed to do enough for family members with cancer. Intense concern about their children's chance of developing cancer is also common. (Weil, 2000, p. 169)

Since the discovery of the BRCA1 and BRCA2 mutations, a substantial amount of research has been done on the psychosocial aspects of genetic counseling and testing (Lerman et al., 2002). Some researchers have explored the psychological impact on women who have had genetic testing (Croyle et al., 1997; Lerman et al., 1996; Lynch et al., 1997). Studies have shown that participants experience relief from learning of negative results (Schwartz et al., 2002; Lynch et al., 1997), but impact has varied for those who receive positive results. Lynch et al. (1997) found that over one-third of those who tested positive experienced sadness, anger, or guilt. One study found that most participants do not realize the distress that may be caused by a positive result (Dorval et al., 2000). This was not the case for the women in this study, who were very aware of the possible negative impact of learning that they had the genetic mutation (Alicia, Jane, Andrea). Alicia's concern about her daughter was consistent with research that suggests concern for risk to children is a common reason for testing (Lynch et al., 1997).

COPING

Breast cancer is the most feared illness among American women (Tracy, 2004), even though it is not the most deadly cancer (lung cancer is), or the largest cause of death (heart disease kills many more). As discussed earlier, the daughters in our sample were highly fearful of breast cancer. How do daughters cope with these fears? The major coping strategies found in this sample were fatalism, spirituality, "do the right thing," and hope.

Fatalism

Many women in the sample took a rather fatalistic position. Rita, for example, said, "I do not honestly believe that I have any control over this anymore. I think that whatever is going to happen is a done deal at this point." Andrea said, "I do try to take care of myself, but I kind of feel in a way, if it's gonna happen, it's gonna happen."

Spirituality

Some women used spirituality to help them cope. Felicia, for example, included prayer in her list of activities to prevent breast cancer.

> I do mammograms and the self-exam. I don't think you really can do much more than that. . . . I'm going to continue to eat healthy and pray a lot. I won't even worry myself with all that. That's not even a concern with me.

Elizabeth also took a spiritual approach, and also relied on the protection she believed her mother's spirit provided.

> I'm not worried because I'm very healthy, and then, part of me just knows that my mother wouldn't ever let anything bad happen to me. It is just more spiritual. I meditate a lot. I pray a lot, and I just really don't think about it.

"Do the Right Thing"

Although some had a sense of fatalism, daughters also actively did what they could to prevent the disease and to detect it early. They struggled to overcome their fears by doing breast self-exams, getting mammograms, and reading about breast cancer. At times this was very difficult for them. Nora, for example, said,

> There's very little you can do about it. I wouldn't say it's inevitable, but certainly my risks are high. So I've kind of told myself, "Don't freak out. Do the right things. You'll catch it as early as you can and you'll live with it."

Gloria said,

> At this point, nobody can really tell you where it's coming from. I thank God there's treatments. There's early detection. I have a slight fear, but I think the attitude of how you would handle it [is more important]. Seeing so many other women survive it.

Jamie also expressed confidence in her ability to cope with the disease if she needed to. "[If I do get breast cancer], it would be a lot more familiar to me now. I would know what to expect. [I] make sure—not to be prepared or to look forward to it, but be on the lookout." Jamie also emphasized positive thinking. "Just be thankful for the health that you have." Sharon mentioned a different kind of preparation: health insurance.

> I make sure that I always have good [health] insurance in case I get something like breast cancer. And I have life insurance coverage, so in case something happens to me, my husband can pay off the house and take care of the bills.

Hope

Finally, there was hope. Janice, for example, hopes for a cure before she is affected. "I hope in the next fifteen years, they find a cure for breast cancer."

Although these women focused on different coping strategies, most use all of these at different times. Despite an underlying sense that the disease is "inevitable," the women are still "doing the right things," and trying to be optimistic and hopeful. At the emotional level the fear is enormous, but at the more rational, cognitive level, the daughters can take appropriate action to protect themselves by knowing how to detect the disease early and staying informed. It is important to recognize the high anxiety levels of these women, and how difficult this makes it for them to act rationally.

HEALTH BELIEF MODEL

The model of risk assessment and preventative activity just discussed relates fairly well to the "health belief model," a cognitive model widely used to predict health prevention in many fields (Becker, 1974). This model has five components, and four of them are relevant to this situation: perceived susceptibility, perceived seriousness, cost of preventative action, and benefit of preventative action.

The process of risk assessment can be perceived as a method by which susceptibility is judged. In the cases of these daughters, this involved a process of developing an explanatory model of the mother's breast cancer, and then comparing themselves to this model. The assessment of susceptibility was an ongoing activity for these women, and it was affected by factors such as the daughter's age (heightening when the daughter is near mother's age at diagnosis or death), news items on breast cancer, hearing stories from friends and relatives, and breast cancer exams and scares. Consistent with the literature from the new field of genetic testing, the women in our sample seem to overestimate their risk. Many feel that getting breast cancer is inevitable, although even in families with very high rates of breast and ovarian cancer, individual risk is usually calculated to be fairly low when linkage or genetic testing is done. If the normal risk for someone without a genetic mutation is about 13 percent (one in eight), doubling this risk would be 26 percent. This is a lifetime risk, including the possibility of getting the disease after age sixty. Many of these women speak as if the risk is 100 percent.

Breast cancer is a serious illness; no evidence emerged to suggest any of the women avoided activities designed to prevent or detect breast cancer early because they did not think the disease was serious. On the other hand, evidence indicates that some daughters exaggerate the risk of dying from the disease. In fact, the prognosis of surviving breast cancer is fairly high if the disease is detected early (96 percent for localized disease), and even when it is not, the chances of surviving are lowered to 77 percent for regional disease and 21 percent for distant (metastasized) disease. Some women in this sample talk as if a diagnosis is a "death sentence."

It appears from our data that women whose mothers survived the disease are more likely to envision themselves surviving the disease than do those whose mothers died. This does not have a factual basis, but it is a completely understandable belief, given the mother's experience.

The health belief model predicts the likelihood of a specific health prevention behavior by considering how the individual rates the costs and benefits of the behavior. The main cost of early detection activities for daughters is anxiety. Some women get extremely anxious when they have a mammogram (Alicia) or when they do a breast self-exam. Women who feel that the disease is inevitably fatal may feel little benefit exists in knowing that they have it. This would suggest that the cost of the procedure would outweigh the potential benefit for these women. Many women in this study believe the cost of doing BSE outweighs the benefit. They feel that they will not be able to detect a lump, and that if they do, the resulting anxiety is not worth wondering if they have breast cancer. Most women prefer clinical breast examinations, which are done by health professionals. This takes the burden off the woman in deciding whether the lump is cause for concern.

Thinking about genetic testing in these terms (cost/benefit ratio) may help us to understand behavior in this new area. For those who were aware of the genetic test and decided against it, the cost may have outweighed the benefit. For the more educated women, the costs often were described in terms of possible discrimination in insurance or employment. Also, the potential psychological burden of learning that they have a genetic propensity toward the disease outweighed the potential psychological benefit of learning that they did not.

Although it is possible to apply the health belief model to genetic testing and prevention/early detection of breast cancer, the model suggests a more rational weighing of alternatives than was used by most women in this study. This very logical model does not recognize the high level of fear in the daughters, or the ways that they cope with it. Sometimes the fear is so overwhelming it makes the rational weighing of alternatives nearly impossible.

SUMMARY

This chapter focused on how the daughters of women who had breast cancer think about their risk, and how they handle it. Basic themes identified were fear, assessment of risk, actions to help prevent breast cancer, actions to help in early breast cancer detection, genetic testing, and coping (see Box 9.1). Many of the daughters have an intense fear of breast cancer, and many themes discussed in this book can be considered attempts to deal with this fear. Not surprisingly, the fear is highest in women whose mothers died. Anxiety was fairly pervasive, but was intensified by events such as finding a lump or approaching the age at which the mother was diagnosed or died. For adolescents, fears of lumps also were very high during breast development. The daughters in our sample were involved in an ongoing process of assessing their risks. When risk was exaggerated, it may have been affected by the "explanatory model" the daughter developed for understanding why her mother got breast cancer.

Daughters commonly used diet and exercise to prevent the disease. In addition, many used stress reduction or tried to generally reduce stress in their lives. Activities to detect breast cancer early were anxiety provoking. This was especially true for breast self-examination (BSE), which many daughters could not do. They were more accepting of mammography and clinical breast exam. When insurers did not cover mammography at the age of the mother's diagnosis, the daughters were especially frustrated.

The daughters in this study were not interested in genetic testing. Some were not aware of the possibility, and others explored it and found that either they could not get the information needed for a thorough family history or tissue samples, or that they did not want to face the possibility of a positive test result. Some also feared insurance

---

**BOX 9.1. Model on Risk for Daughters
of Women with Breast Cancer**

1. Fear
2. Assessing risk for breast cancer
3. Actions to help prevent breast cancer
4. Actions to help in early breast cancer detection
5. Genetic testing
6. Coping
   a. Fatalism
   b. Spirituality
   c. "Do the right thing"
   d. Hope

discrimination. The benefits of genetic testing were not believed to be worth the risks.

To cope with the fear of breast cancer, women used a variety of psychological mechanisms such as fatalism, spirituality, and hope. In addition, they tried to "do the right thing," and not let their fear or fatalism prevent them from monitoring their breasts and achieving healthy living.

Implications for practice based on the findings of this chapter are found in Chapter 11.

Chapter 10

Key Phases and Broad Themes in the Experience of Breast Cancer Daughters

In earlier chapters, themes for women whose mothers died were identified separately for each age group (Chapters 4 through 7). This analysis allowed the development of an in-depth picture of each of the age categories—especially for cases in which the mother died. However, the focus on the different age groups made comparisons between the age categories difficult. In this chapter, the findings are organized based on the phase of the experience. This makes it possible to identify broad overarching themes in each of the critical phases, and to see more clearly the impact of the daughter's age on the major themes. Grouping themes by phase also facilitates making recommendations for practice, since most practitioners work with women and families in distinct phases of the experience. (Practice recommendations are presented in Chapter 11.)

FAMILY BACKGROUND BEFORE DIAGNOSIS

Family Configuration

Family configuration connotes the basic structure of the family. Of particular importance to the daughter's experience was whether she was the oldest child or, especially, the oldest daughter. This was especially instrumental in determining the daughter's role if the mother was not able to function due to the illness. Older daughters carried the most responsibility for taking on the mother's roles. The presence or lack of a father in the family also contributed to the daughter's role and to her experience after her mother's death if her mother did not

survive. (Technically, age of daughter could be considered a component of family composition. However, it was of such critical importance that it was used to organize the findings in all of the sections,
and so it has been discussed elsewhere.)

Family Communication Style

Family communication style was also a critical factor in shaping
the daughter's experience. This factor determined the level of communication about the mother's illness. Many families had a pattern of
dealing with unpleasant information by using secrecy. In these families, information about the mother's illness and treatment often was
not communicated openly. In these cases, daughters often had exaggerated fears, and were deprived of the information they needed to
help them understand what was happening to the mother, and to prepare for the future. When mothers in these families died, daughters
were cut off from important information not only about the illness,
but also about the history of the family. In families in which the mothers survived, secrecy may have long-term effects on the daughters'
ability to trust and relationship with their mothers.

Prior Family Problems

Whether the family had prior problems was another important factor in the daughter's experience of the mother's illness. Families with
issues such as drug or alcohol use, chaotic lifestyle, or a history of
child abuse were less able to help a daughter cope with her mother's
illness. If the family did not have an active father due to marital
cirucmstances, the threat of losing the mother to breast cancer was
magnified. If the father was already deceased, the daughter was likely
to be especially fearful of losing her mother as well, and painful
memories of her father's death may have been reactivated.

These three factors—family configuration, family communicaiton
style, and prior family problems—interacted with one another, so that
the daughters who had the most difficult experience were those who
were oldest daughters in families that lacked an open communication
style and had prior problems. The daughters least likely to experience
difficulty were those who were younger daughters (especially if the
older sister(s) were capable of taking on some of the parenting roles),
and had families with an open communication style and no prior

problems. Even in the best of situations, serious illness and death of a mother creates a life crisis of major proportion. Nevertheless, these three family background factors can be used to identify those daughters who may be the most vulnerable, and which families may especially benefit from intervention. (See Chapter 3 for further discussion of this phase.)

THEMES DURING THE PERIOD OF ILLNESS

Communication

Communication during the mother's illness and treatment was an important theme for all daughters (see Table 10.1). For the youngest daughters, communication was very limited, as the mother and other adults tried to "protect" children from information about the diagnosis. Families had greater tendency to share factual information with young adolescents, but often, the emotional aspects were denied, ignored, or minimized. Young adolescents may have felt more comfortable communicating with peers than with parents, but if they did not have peers with similar experience, they often chose not to share in-

TABLE 10.1. Experiences during mother's illness and treatment.

Age group	Communication	Increased responsibilities	More mature relationship with mother
Children	Little or no communication	Daughter nurtures mother	Increased independence
Young adolescents	Limited communication (May focus on facts and not on emotions)	Daughter takes on increased household responsibilities	Daughter foregoes rebellion. Relationship with mother becomes less contentious
Late adolescents	Increased communication	Daughter takes on major household responsibilities	Shift to more adult-adult relationship
Young adults	Open communication (Daughter may protect mother from negative information)	Daughter juggles adult roles to aid in care of mother and family	Adult-adult relationship may shift to role reversal

formation about the mother's illness with anyone. For late adolescent daughters, the communication was likely to be more open, while with the oldest group (ages twenty-three and up) a reversal of the direction of protective communication sometimes occurred, in which daughters communicated directly with physicians and then filtered the information when communicating with mothers. In some young adult cases, mothers wanted daughters to collude in keeping information about their disease from ex-spouses, in-laws, younger children, or neighbors and friends. Although communication in the family was an important issue for all families regardless of the daughter's age, communication became more open as the daughter's age increased.

Increased Responsibilities

A second common theme during the mother's illness, regardless of age, is that of increased responsibilities. Role shifts in families have long been identified by health professionals as part of the impact of illness on the family (Mailick, 1979; Rolland, 1994; Oktay and Walter, 1991). When the ill person is a mother, depending on her role in the family, and on the specific treatments she undergoes, daughters may need to take on some of her responsibilities. In our study, the age of the daughter was important in determining what type of tasks she took on. The youngest daughters assumed the role of "nurturer of the sick," such as by stroking the mother's face, reading to her, and getting things for her. Adolescent daughters took on responsibilities such as housework, care of younger siblings, and care of the father in addition to care of the mother. Young adult daughters found themselves juggling adult responsibilities in marriages, at work, and with their own children with the added responsibilities brought on by the mother's illness. The broader pattern that emerges here is that increased responsibilities were taken on by all daughters, but older daughters had more significant responsibilities.

More Mature Relationship with Mother

A third theme during illness and treatment was that of the daughter beginning a more mature relationship with her mother. In the youngest daughters, this took the form of a change in their mothers' behavior and expectations toward them; many mothers suddenly treated them as if they were older and more independent. Young adolescent daughters reported that they shifted to a more compatible relationship with their mothers, often foregoing rebellion. For late adolescent and young adult daughters, a more adult relationship was possible. This included a sharing of confidences that often does not occur in the mother-daughter relationship until much later in life. In cases of the oldest daughters, this shift sometimes resulted in role reversal, in which the daughter became a "mother" to her own mother. Regardless of their ages, all daughters shifted to a relationship with their mothers that was characteristic of a later developmental stage.

Each of these overarching themes—communication, increased responsibilities, and more mature relationship with the mother—was affected by background factors. Whether the family traditionally handled difficulties with secrecy influenced how the mother's breast cancer was communicated in the family. Family structure influenced the extent to which daughters experienced problems in the period of their mothers' illness. Daughters who were oldest children or the oldest daughters were more likely to be given information, and were more likely to take on family responsibilities. (Of course, this was mitigated by other factors, such as family situation. In some families, a younger daughter took on the heaviest responsibilities because the older daughter no longer lived at home.)

Prior family problems also were closely related to family communication patterns, as secrecy often is used to conceal problems. Earlier problems also may have impacted the willingness of a daughter to take on some of her mother's responsibilities. For example, if the father had previously left the family, daughters and mothers may have already undergone some of the changes described in this section.

The broad patterns also are affected by the nature of the mother's treatment, which is in turn affected by the nature of her disease and the stage at which it was diagnosed. Recent advances in detection and treatment of breast cancer have changed how daughters experience their mothers' illness. For the youngest daughters in this study, the most disturbing experience was separation from the mother. This was generally experienced when the mother was hospitalized for a mastectomy. In the past, radical mastectomies required lengthy hospitalizations, while today, less invasive surgical procedures such as modified radical mastectomies and lumpectomies are common. Cost cutting also has shortened hospital stays. Today mastectomies are sometimes done as outpatient surgery. However, some women who choose extensive reconstructive surgeries may be hospitalized for considerably longer.

The side effects of chemotherapy, such as hair loss, were especially upsetting for young adolescent daughters. Today, chemotherapies are much more common and often are used, even in breast cancers that are diagnosed very early. Thus today's daughters are more likely to experience the side effects of chemotherapy than were daughters in the past.

For late adolescent and young adult daughters, increased responsibilities were most disruptive. Also, for these older daughters, the fact that their mothers had cancer was in itself very threatening. The loss of the mother's functioning (most difficult for the oldest daughters) is now associated only with the very late stages of the disease, after the cancer has metastasized.

The three broad themes (communication, increased responsibilities, and more mature relationships with mother) should be assessed in the context of the family background and the characteristics of the mother's illness and treatments, as well as the daughter's age. This will allow health practitioners, counselors, and families to anticipate and prepare for change of special importance to daughters.

THEMES DURING THE PERIOD
AFTER MOTHER'S DEATH

The period after the mother's death was an especially traumatic time for daughters. Mother's death meant the loss of the central adult in the daughter's life, the primary attachment figure and role model, at a time far earlier than expected, even for the oldest daughters in the study. Because the study included only daughters whose mothers were diagnosed before age fifty, and women's life expectancy is well over seventy, this is not a normative loss. The daughter's age was critical in determining not only what was experienced in this period, but what resources the daughters had to cope with these changes.

Looking across the four age groups, two overarching themes emerge in the period following mother's death: family changes and survival (see Table 10.2).

TABLE 10.2. Experiences after mother's death.

Age group	Family changes	Survival
Children	Cinderella pattern	Survive by being tough
Young adolescents	Difficult relationships with fathers Lack of parenting	Survive by being like everyone else (peer group)
Late adolescents	Oedipal issues reemerge with fathers Daughters take on household responsibilities	Survival through survival of the family
Young adults	Family changes less traumatic	Survival through healthy grieving (resolution)

Family Changes

Family changes were problematic for most daughters, but they were most catastrophic for the youngest daughters. Because women are traditionally the "heart" of the family, when a mother dies, the whole family is inalterably changed. Mothers' roles are central, especially if young children are involved, and arrangements should be made for their needs.

A mother's death sets in motion what is called the "cascade of events." At the emotional level, the adults or older siblings who might ordinarily have provided comfort and care for the children were emotionally devastated themselves. Many fathers seemed to cope with their loss by using escape, denial, or withdrawal, all of which made them unavailable to their daughters. Other women in the family, such as aunts and grandmothers, may have been more capable of helping the young daughters at the emotional level than were fathers, but they often were not easily accessible, especially if the father remarried. The result was that the youngest daughters (ten and under) experienced major family changes at a time when they had very little support. For these daughters, a "Cinderella" pattern was common. Some actively resisted the new family situation, some sought to escape, while others tried to "go along and get along." The Cinderella pattern was tied to the family configuration. It usually happened when fathers remarried. Daughters in families with no father are likely to be taken in by maternal relatives.

The situation for young adolescent daughters was different because, at least in this sample, their fathers were less likely to quickly remarry. This may be just a coincidence, or it may be that men with teenage daughters are less attractive as potential marriage partners. Perhaps when children are older and can do more for themselves, fathers feel less pressured to find a "replacement" mother for them. After the mothers' deaths, fathers and adolescent daughters had more interaction, as daughters took over some of the mother's roles, and this may have frightened fathers. Daughters in the young adolescent group described a disintegration of the family after their mothers' deaths, and felt a lack of parenting existed.

Late adolescent daughters often were away at college when their mothers died, and the mothers' deaths often led to the daughters returning home, under very different circumstances. These daughters may have already taken on heavy household responsibilities during the mother's illness (see previous section). The older daughters in this study often described their mothers as "the glue that kept the family together." After the mother's death, they often tried to fulfill this role, cooking for their fathers, cleaning the house, caring for siblings and, sometimes, grandparents. Often, they were resentful, angry, and hurt when their fathers began dating.

Young adult daughters also experienced family changes after their mothers died. Because most had already achieved independence from the family at this point in their lives, they were much less affected by the issues that were so traumatic for younger daughters. When fathers remarried, they may have been upset, but they could choose to distance themselves, or to try to effect change. When their homes were lost, they were saddened, but if they had their own homes at this point, it was not traumatic. They also had partners who could support them as they coped with these changes.

In summary, the overall pattern in "family changes" showed decreasing levels of traumatic change for older daughters. That is, the youngest daughters had to adapt to the most drastic changes with the least support, while the oldest daughters experienced less traumatic changes, and had many more resources to help them cope (see Table 10.2).

Survival

Survival was a very important issue for daughters whose mothers died. Mothers are heavily invested in protecting their children and ensuring their survival. When a mother dies, children are vulnerable. (In animal populations, they usually do not survive.) The type of protection mothers provide changes as children grow older, but usually continues well into adulthood. It is not surprising, then, that survival emerged as an important theme. When a mother dies prematurely, daughters feel that their own survival (and perhaps that of their own children) is threatened.

As with earlier themes, survival also varied with the daughters's ages. It was most profound for the youngest daughters, who developed a tough protective layer and hid their feelings of loss from themselves and from others. Young adolescents were more in touch with their feelings, but because they wanted to be like their peers, they too hid their loss. Late adolescents tended to seek survival for the family unit, and put the needs of siblings and fathers ahead of their own. In contrast, the young adult daughters experienced healthy grieving, cried heavily, and used culturally appropriate rituals to work through their loss and achieve resolution. This process contributed to their survival, as it allowed them to move on in their lives, and devote themselves to the creation of new families (see Table 10.2).

For both themes identified in the period after the mother's death (family changes and survival), a consistent pattern emerged: The younger the daughter, the greater the level of problems experienced and the lower the level of resources available to deal with them.

It is important to recognize that a relationship exists between the themes identified in the periods before and during the mother's illness and treatment and those identified in the period after the mother's death. For example, family background factors such as family configuration and prior family problems impact the type of family changes a daughter experiences after her mother dies. In families with no father, or if the father was unable to function (e.g., alcoholics), the family may completely disintegrate. Also, a family that is unable to communicate with a daughter during her mother's illness will be more likely to leave her unprepared for the drastic family changes she will experience after the mother's death. Because communication was most strained in families with young children, these children were the most vulnerable to traumatic changes in the family if the mother died. The same can be said for both "increased responsibilities" and "more mature relationships with the mother," as both of these occurred less often, and to a lesser extent, in children, and both could be helpful to adjustment after the death of the mother.

THEMES CONCERNING LONG-TERM IMPACT (AFTER DEATH)

Mental Health

Looking at long-term impact across the four age categories (see Table 10.3), a major theme seems to be mental health. For the youngest group, problems commonly mentioned included insomnia, anxiety, depression, and low self-esteem. Young adolescents may be at risk for post-traumatic stress disorder (PTSD). For late adolescents, depression was commonly mentioned. In contrast, daughters who were young adults at the time of their mothers' deaths had no clear mental health impact. However, many of these women reported having a "big cry" periodically to deal with life's stresses. In addition to different problems in varying age groups, the level of long-term mental health impact was greater in the youngest daughters, and gradually decreased with the oldest daughter.

TABLE 10.3. Long-term impact (if mother dies).

Age group	Mental health	Relationships
Children	Insomnia, anxiety, depression, low self-esteem	Strong independent personality
Young adolescents	PTSD	Problems in intimate relationships
Late adolescents	Depression	Feelings of being alone
Young adults	No mental health impact "Big cry"	Relationships gain high priority
		Stresses family as well as cancer-related activities and careers

Relationships

A second long-term impact on daughters whose mothers die relates to relationships. Daughters who were children at the time of their mothers' deaths indicated that their strong, independent tendencies made it difficult for them to accept the dependency inherent in intimate relationships. These women talked about how their insistence on handling issues independently created marital problems. Women who were young adolescents at the time of the mother's death mentioned fears of forming close attachments, knowing that the relationships might not last. Daughters who were late adolescents said that they always felt lonely, even when surrounded by friends or family. The oldest group of daughters in this study also reported an impact on relationships, but it tended to be a positive one. These women were more likely to value their relationships after their mothers died. They often restructured their lives, giving more time and attention to the close relationships in their lives.

For both themes, mental health and relationships, the broad pattern that emerges is again one in which the youngest daughters seem to experience the most profound difficulties. These long-term issues are most likely related to the patterns that developed in the earlier phases. For example, daughters who needed to develop a tough protective personality in order to survive the chaos in the family after the mother's death might have particular difficulty with developing intimate relationships based on mutual trust. The same could be true for those whose families used secrecy to hide the truth about the mother's illness from them. Mental health and relationships are closely interrelated, as good mental health is dependent on supportive relationships, and at the same time, those with better mental health are more able to provide support to others.

SUMMARY

This chapter has provided a broad view of patterns in each phase, based on a comparison of the experiences of daughters of different ages. In the period prior to the mother's illness, family configuration, communication style, and the existence of prior family problems are factors that shape the daughters' experience in important ways. During the period of mother's illness, three common themes emerged: "communication," "increased responsibilities," and "more mature relationship with mother." The youngest daughters experienced the least communication, while older daughters were most affected by increased responsibilities. All daughters shifted to a more mature relationship with their mothers. However, while younger daughters may have been unhappy with the mothers pushing them toward greater independence, older daughters appreciated a more adult relationship. Following the mother's death, two overarching themes were identified: "family changes" and "survival." For both, it was the youngest daughters who experienced the most profound changes, and who felt their survival most threatened. In the long term, mothers' death most commonly impacted daughters' "mental health" and "relationships." Although the impacts were different, the general pattern suggested that younger daughters experienced more negative long-term impact. The themes identified in the four main phases (Figure 10.1) are interrelated, and the experience of earlier phases impacts the daughters' experience in the later phases.

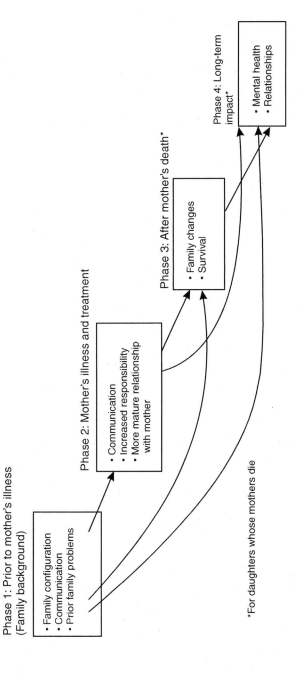

Phase 1: Prior to mother's illness
(Family background)

• Family configuration
• Communication
• Prior family problems

Phase 2: Mother's illness and treatment

• Communication
• Increased responsibility
• More mature relationship
  with mother

Phase 3: After mother's death*

• Family changes
• Survival

Phase 4: Long-term
impact*

• Mental health
• Relationships

*For daughters whose mothers die

FIGURE 10.1. Themes for daughters of all ages by phase.

Chapter 11

Conclusions

Although much attention has been paid to women diagnosed with breast cancer (commonly called "breast cancer survivors"), daughters of these women also are breast cancer survivors—psychologically and socially, if not in a physical sense. These other breast cancer survivors—daughters—have been almost invisible, and little is known about their experience and their needs. This book has provided an opportunity to hear the voices of these daughters and has identified key factors and themes from their stories. The results of this study have the potential to help all women and the health providers who serve them. Practitioners can use them to create more effective services for mothers, daughters, and whole families. Most important, daughters themselves can benefit from hearing the similar stories of others. Hopefully these stories will make them feel less alone. This final chapter summarizes the study and the major themes that were identified. The results are then discussed in the context of other research, and implications for future research are discussed. Finally, recommendations for practice are presented.

Daughters are now an especially important population now because the discovery of genes associated with breast cancer has made genetic testing for the disease possible (see discussion in Chapter 9). As genetic services for those at risk of developing breast cancer become increasingly available, daughters are likely to make up a sizeable proportion of the potential users of these services. The results of this study can be used to guide the development of genetic services for daughters and their families, and to impact the education of those who will provide these services.

THE STUDY

A qualitative study, funded by the National Cancer Institute as part of the National Action Plan on Breast Cancer, was conducted between January 1996 and September 1998. Up to three in-depth interviews were conducted with forty-one women whose mothers had early (age fifty and below) breast cancer. Women who had been diagnosed with breast cancer themselves were not included in the study. The sample included a fairly even distribution of women who were children, early adolescents, late adolescents, and young adults at the time of the mother's illness. Sixty-three percent of the daughters had mothers who died from the disease, and 37 percent had mothers who survived. Twenty-seven percent of the sample were African American, and 26 percent were Jewish.

Themes were developed out of codes taken directly from the data, using "grounded theory" methods to guide data analysis. As concepts and themes were developed, they were taken back to the respondents for feedback and adjusted accordingly. An advisory board, made up of breast cancer activists as well as health and mental health professionals, also discussed and provided feedback on the concepts as they emerged during the course of the study. Other techniques to increase the validity of the study were peer debriefing, journaling, and audit trail. Case studies were developed for women in each of these age categories to illustrate the major analysis categories. (See Chapter 2 for a more detailed discussion of the study methodology.)

Mother's survival was the most important factor that shaped the daughter's experience with her mother's disease. The impact on daughters was far greater, and more catastrophic, in those whose mothers died. For those whose mothers died, daughter's age was the second key factor. The four age groupings that were used in this study were: children, young adolescents, late adolescents, and young adults. For women whose mothers died, the experience was divided into clear phases: the period before mother's illness (family background), the period after mother's diagnosis and treatments, the period after her death, and the long-term impact. In the cases of daughters whose mothers survived, daughter's age was not as important, although it did have some effect on the experience of the mother's illness. Time periods were less distinct, and these daughters were spared a major adjustment period following the mother's death. For these daughters, the critical phases were the period before the mother's illness (family background), the period when mother was diagnosed and had treatments, and the period following mother's illness and treatment. The study also identified key components affecting the daughters' perceptions of their own risks for breast cancer.

The sections that follow describe the key findings of the study. Following a summary of key themes in each phase, the results are compared with the findings of other researchers. Implications for patients, families, and practitioners are then presented. Because qualitative research is of unknown generalizability, women who have breast cancer, their daughters, families, and advocates should carefully assess the results and recommendations made here and use them only if they "ring true" to their individual situations.

FINDINGS

Experience of Daughters Whose Mothers Died

Women Who Were Children at the Time
of Mother's Illness and Death

Three themes were identified for the youngest breast cancer daughters (age ten and under) during the period of mother's illness and treatment: lack of communication, am I still safe?, and independence. The youngest girls (ages one to nine) were generally told very little about the mother's illness, but often sensed that something was wrong. This created anxiety, and at the same time, discouraged daughters from asking about their mothers' health or seeking reassurance. A second theme for this group was a concern for their safety. The youngest daughters were fearful when they experienced changes in their routines, and even more fearful when they were physically separated from their mothers. They were less upset by the symptoms of the disease and treatment (mastectomy scars, loss of hair), accepting the explanation given to them by their parents. Those daughters who were children at the time of the mother's illness often were aware that their mothers were attempting to make them more independent.

The mother's death precipitated major changes in the family situation. Fathers tended to remarry shortly after their wives' deaths, requiring major adjustments by the daughters to life in a stepfamily, with a new "mother," and possibly new siblings, new homes and different, often more conflictual, relationships with their fathers. At first, most daughters were numb, but they typically adopted a tough, protective exterior, trying to appear unaffected, and did not share their loss or their pain with adults or other children. They focused on their survival, determined to make sure their most basic needs were met. These children did not engage in traditional grieving activities. In the new stepfamilies, they were often deprived of any reminders of their mothers, including pictures, sharing of memories, and mementos. They did not have access to support groups or counselors. (Fortunately, such services are more common today. See Appendix IV.)

As adults, women whose mothers died when they were children tended to search for information about the mother and her illness. Having long repressed their feelings of loss, they often entered therapy for an outwardly unrelated problem, and were surprised to find themselves finally dealing with the long-buried grief for their mother. These women described themselves as strong and independent, while at the same time, they mentioned problems such as low self-esteem, insomnia, and depression.

Women Who Were Young Adolescents at the Time of Mother's Illness and Death

Young adolescent daughters (ages eleven to seventeen) focused on physical deterioration when their mothers were ill, and were very disturbed by it. Also during the illness period, a conflict often developed between the young adolescent daughter's need for separation from the family and the demands of the home, especially if her mother was unable to function normally.

Relationships with fathers became especially problematic after their mothers died. Young adolescence is normally a difficult time in the father-daughter relationship, as fathers tend to detach when daughters develop sexually. Although this group was less likely to need to adapt to a stepmother, they experienced instead a sudden absence of all parenting. The peer group was especially important for this group as a potential source of support. Although adolescents are thought to be capable of conventional grieving activities (Christ, 2000), the young adolescent girls in this study did not want to appear different from peers or to lose control in a counseling situation.

Some young adolescent daughters experienced excessive anxiety long after the mother's death. This may be a kind of PTSD, a diagnosis that is increasingly recognized in survivors of traumatic life stress. A mother's death from a disease associated with female sexuality, accompanied by a visible bodily deterioration, may constitute a traumatic event for a young adolescent girl who is just forming her feminine identity. Another long-term consequence may be difficulty forming intimate attachments.

Women Who Were Late Adolescents at the Time of Mother's Illness and Death

When their mothers were diagnosed with breast cancer and entered treatment, late adolescent (ages eighteen to twenty-two) women suddenly found themselves carrying major responsibilities in the home, often for the first time. A positive outcome for some was seeing their relationships with their mothers shift from a more contentious adolescent relationship into a more satisfying adult relationship.

Daughters took on many of the mother's roles and responsibilities in the period after her death, including caring for fathers and (possibly) siblings. This may have led to a replay of oedipal tensions; when fathers began to date, the daughters often felt resentful and unappreciated. Because of their many family responsibilities, daughters were cut off from peers, and from others who had similar life experience and/or similar losses. As a result, they tended to be very lonely. (Some of those who were in college changed schools to be closer to home, losing contact with friends who may have been able to provide support.) Perhaps because of their isolation, and because of their household responsibilities, they generally did not grieve, and if they did, they did not derive comfort from traditional rituals.

For these daughters, the long-term impact was a chronic type of grieving. Although literature on grieving suggests that late adolescents are capable of normal grieving (going through the steps of denial, grieving, and restitution), the women in our study generally did not do so, in part, because they took on so many family responsibilities following the mother's death. When they did return to activities common to their age group (e.g., education), they had a difficult time finding friends who could understand their bereavement. The result may have been a long-term depression. As adults, these women focused on the loss of the mother's support, such as help with children/ grandchildren, financial help, access to old recipes, help in emergencies, or simply support when the daughter felt overwhelmed.

Women Who Were Young Adults at the Time of Their Mother's Illness and Death

Women whose mothers had breast cancer when they were young adults (ages twenty-three and up) were likely to have jobs, to be married, and in some cases, to have children. During the period of the mother's illness, role conflict was common as daughters tried to balance their mothers' care with the demands of work and their own families' needs. Young adult daughters took an active role in their mothers' illness, including in some cases direct communication with the physician. They experienced adult relationships with their mothers, including, open communication about death.

In contrast to younger daughters, young adults grieved heavily, benefiting from traditional rituals and the support of friends and therapists. After the mother's death, young adult daughters assumed many new roles, trying to mother their younger siblings and, in some cases, to care for grandparents. However, they were not likely to take on a "wifelike" role with their fathers, because they had their own lives, with husbands, jobs, and sometimes, children. They were not very invested in the caregiving role, but did it out of a sense of responsibility. Despite their efforts, they were not always successful in keeping their families of origin together. Fathers of young adults were likely to remarry, although not as quickly as fathers with young children (perhaps feeling less desperate for immediate help). Although young adult daughters' feelings were similar to those of younger daughters (anger at father, rejection of stepmother), the father's remarriage was not as traumatic for them. Already independent, they did not have to spend time in the new family if they chose not to. Some were successful in changing their relationships with their fathers and/or stepmothers. Loss of the family home may have been painful, but it was not devastating for them, because they often had their own homes. As young adults, they also had more understanding of their fathers' needs, and even of the difficulty in their stepmothers' roles.

Young adult women whose mothers died often changed life priorities. Many gave more attention to their families, found more meaningful work, and became advocates for breast cancer or other causes. Although not depressed, some reported having a periodic "big cry" to deal with life stress.

Experience of Daughters Whose Mothers Survived Breast Cancer

Those whose mothers survived breast cancer experienced the same issues during the illness and treatment phase that were discussed in the previous section. After the acute phase, both daughters and mothers continue to move through life stages and family events together. As a result, the analysis does not identify separate themes for different age groups. The themes identified here apply to daughters of survivors, regardless of their ages.

Among women whose mothers survived breast cancer, worry was the most common theme; another was closeness to mother. Some daughters of breast cancer survivors also delayed developmental tasks of adulthood, such as independence, intimacy, and procreation, perhaps in order to be available in case the mother has a recurrence. In addition, these daughters were more likely to change their priorities, placing more emphasis on family, meaningful work, and advocacy. The mother's way of coping with the illness, the level of communication with the daughter, and the extent to which she maintained a protective role in spite of the illness were also important factors. (See Chapter 8 for a more detailed discussion of this group.)

Risk of Breast Cancer

This book also has discussed the genetics of breast cancer, focusing on how daughters think about their risk, and how they react to it (see Chapter 9). Basic themes identified were fear, assessment of risk, actions to prevent breast cancer, actions to detect breast cancer early, genetic testing, and coping. Many of the daughters had an intense fear of getting breast cancer, far greater than could be explained rationally. Not surprisingly, the fear was highest in women whose mothers died.

Fear was also intensified by events such as finding a lump or approaching the age at which mother was diagnosed or at the age at which she died. For adolescents, fears were especially high during breast development.

Daughters are involved in an ongoing process of assessing their risk. This process involves the development of an "explanatory model" (Kleinman, 1980) to explain the reason for the mother's breast cancer. Using these explanatory factors, daughters then assess how similar or dissimilar they are to their mothers.

Daughters commonly used diet, exercise, and stress reduction to try to prevent the disease. However, activities to detect breast cancer early, such as breast self-examinations (BSE), were extremely anxiety provoking, and many daughters were unable to perform them. They were more accepting of mammography and clinical breast exam. Daughters approaching the age at which their mother was diagnosed were frustrated when their insurance companies did not cover mammography.

The daughters in this study had little interest in genetic testing. Some were not aware of the possibility, and others had explored it and found that either they could not get the information needed for a thorough family history or tissue samples; others did not want to face the possibility of a positive test result, or feared insurance discrimination. Overall, the benefits of genetic testing were not seen to outweigh the risks.

Women used a variety of psychological mechanisms including fatalism, spirituality, and hope to cope with fear of breast cancer. In addition, they tried to "do the right thing," and not let their fear or fatalism prevent them from monitoring their breasts and practicing a healthy lifestyle.

Summary of Themes by Phases of Experience

An analysis of the phases of experience regardless of daughter's age allowed for the identification of overarching themes for each phase. Overarching themes for Phases 1 and 2 apply to all daughters, while those for Phases 3 and 4 apply only to those whose mothers did not survive. This analysis also made visible patterns that clarified the impact of age.

In the period prior to the mother's illness, three factors in the family background were identified: "family configuration," "family communication style," and "prior family problems." These family background variables structured the context of a daughter's experience.

During the period of the mother's illness, three overarching themes were identified: "communication," "increased responsibilities," and "more mature relationship with mother." Daughter's age was related to each of these. Communication tended to increase with daughter's age: youngest daughters were given the least information. Increased responsibilities were greater as daughter's age increased, and were greatest for oldest daughters. Daughters of all ages tended to shift to a more mature relationship with mothers. These issues were affected by family background characteristics and by the nature of the mother's treatment.

For women whose mothers died, the period after the death was especially difficult. The two themes for this period were "family changes" and "survival." All daughters experienced major family changes following the mother's death, but these were most traumatic for the younger daughters. These young daughters feared for their survival after losing their mothers. Older daughters focused more on the survival of the family unit, or the survival of the mother's legacy.

The overarching themes found in the long term for daughters whose mothers died were "mental health" and "relationships." The youngest daughters tended to suffer from insomnia, anxiety, depression, and low self-esteem. Those who were young adolescents often mentioned symptoms similar to PTSD. Late adolescents were more likely to experience depression. In contrast, those who were young adults when their mothers died did not have problems with mental health. Problems in relationships were also common in the three youngest age groups, and tended to be more profound in those who were youngest when mother died. The themes for each phase were found to be related to those of the earlier phases.

Study Limitations

The study design was retrospective, and therefore the results are based on the memories of adult women about their earlier experiences. These memories may be inaccurate, as they are highly selective and possibly distorted. Similar to most qualitative research, the extent to which the results of this study can be generalized is not known. The study population was small, and reflects the population in the area where the research took place, with fairly large representation of African-American women and Jewish women compared to national figures. Groups such as Asian Americans, Latinos, and Native Americans were not represented in the sample.

A conflict between representativeness and quality of informants in research always exists in in-depth interviews. Because the study was done in a school of social work, a high proportion of the respondents were social workers or other mental health providers. Others were clients or members of support groups who were referred by therapists. This may have skewed some of the results (e.g., the high proportion of women who changed priorities and sought meaningful work). At the same time, it resulted in a group of women who had a high degree of self-awareness—an important quality of an informant in this type of research.

I suspect that the sample contained a high proportion of women who were either older daughters or only daughters. It is not surprising that daughters who were most affected by their mothers' breast cancer would be most interested in a study like this one, and most likely to participate. The study results are probably most relevant to these daughters.

It also is important to note that although some of the study informants' mothers had only recently been diagnosed, many of the women were sharing stories from ten, twenty, or thirty years ago. As a result, some of the treatments and practices described are no longer relevant. The level of open communication has most likely increased since the times of some daughters' experiences. However, this remains a difficult issue, and still needs attention.

Because of the potential contribution of this research to the development of genetic counseling for breast/ovarian cancer, this study focused only on women whose mothers were diagnosed at fifty years old or younger. This means that the daughters described here are younger than the typical breast cancer daughter, as breast cancer strikes older women predominantly (American Cancer Society, 2002).

Finally, my own experiences as a mother and as a daughter colored how I perceived and interpreted the data. As with the fish that tries to describe the environment and omits any mention of water, I have overlooked much that a researcher of a different background would find interesting. Also, there were many "mini-themes" that time and space would not allow me to develop.

IMPLICATIONS FOR RESEARCH

Research on the Impact of Parental Death on Children

Early studies on the impact of the death of a parent sought, and often found, a relationship between death of a mother and later mental health problems such as depression (Bifulco, Harris, and Brown, 1993; Freud, 1917; Saler and Skolnick, 1992; Tennant, 1988). More recent research has presented a more sanguine view. For example, Worden (1996) and Silverman (1987) studied children for two years after the death of a parent in the Harvard Child Bereavement Study and found that most children do not need special intervention following parental death. Christ (2000) studied children whose parent had terminal cancer and was being treated in a tertiary cancer center. These children's families were involved in a psychosocial counseling intervention during the terminal and bereavement periods. In contrast, my study found that for daughters whose mothers died, the effects were profound and long-lasting, especially if they were children or adolescents at the time of the mother's death. Although the findings did not suggest that the bereaved daughters developed serious psychopathology, the loss of their mothers constituted a major defining event in their lives.

On the surface these findings may appear to conflict; however, the differences may be due to differences in methodology. For example, a major difference is that this study included only girls who had lost their mothers, while Worden's (1996) and Christ's (2000) studies included both boys and girls who had lost either mother or father. When Worden (1996) looked specifically at children who lost mothers, he concluded, "It is clear that the impact of mother loss was in many ways greater than the loss of a father" (p. 76).

> We found that mothers tended to be more sensitive to their children's needs than were fathers. In fact, even depressed women were more likely to be aware of their children's needs than nondepressed men. . . . They [fathers] rarely talked about helping children with their feelings. . . . At one year [after the death]

children who had lost mothers had the most difficulty talking about their dead parent and were also having more emotional/behavioral problems. (Worden, 1996, p. 46)

One reason mother loss may be more profound is that men (widowers) are more likely to remarry than are women (widows), and remarriage may occur very quickly. Because all of the women in this study lost mothers, most experienced major family changes after the mother's death, including quick remarriage of the surviving parent. Worden (1996) found that bereaved fathers were the most likely to begin dating quickly, and that "children whose parents were dating during the first year experienced more emotional/behavioral problems, including somatic symptoms, withdrawn behavior and delinquent behavior" (p. 82).

Worden (1996) and Christ (2000) also found that parental loss was more problematic for girls than for boys. Worden (1996) concluded,

Girls, regardless of age, showed more anxiety than boys over the two years of bereavement. This anxiety manifested itself in concerns about the safety of the surviving parent, as well as their own safety. Girls, more than boys, were sensitive to family arguments and fights that occurred in the early months after the death. . . . Girls were more likely to be crying throughout the first year of bereavement. . . . Girls tended to be more attached to the dead parent than boys, and, after 1 year, were more likely to idealize the deceased. (p. 91)

Christ (2000) too found different patterns for bereaved boys and girls.

The process of renegotiation [relationship with surviving parent] seemed to be less complicated for boys than for girls. . . . Many parents had come to rely on their older daughters during the patient's terminal illness. As single parents who were struggling with their own grief, they tended to turn to these daughters for comfort and support. As a result, the parent-child boundaries and roles became blurred at times. (p. 208)

Given these patterns of more distress in bereaved girls than in boys, and less support when the surviving parent is a father (rather than a mother), it is not surprising that this study, which included only girls who lost mothers, found more distress than did the studies of Christ (2000) and Worden (1996), which did not look specifically at the impact of mother loss on daughters.

Other reasons for the differences in findings between this study and other research on the impact of parental death may include the following:

1. The timing of this study was very different. A retrospective view of daughters, many years after mother's death, may be very different than the view of a child going through the experience. The finding (see Chapter 4) that children focused first on their survival, putting on a tough exterior, could contribute to an overly optimistic view of how children are progressing in studies that rely on observations of children recently after the parent's death.

2. Studies in which surviving parents or guardians are asked to rate their children's distress after a cancer diagnosis or death tend to show little or no distress, while studies on the children themselves are more likely to show "greatly increased psychological symptoms" (Kroll et al., 1998). A possible explanation is that the children are successful in hiding their distress from their parents, whom they do not want to further upset. Research methods that are better able to get beyond these tough exteriors may be needed before researchers will be able to truly understand bereaved children.

3. The population in this study represented women from a wide range of socioeconomic backgrounds. In contrast, the population in Christ's (2000) study was almost exclusively upper-middle class. The population in that study was also undergoing a psychosocial intervention, necessitating a possible self-selection bias toward well-functioning families who communicate well. Christ and colleagues (1993) reported that the highest anxiety period for the children was during the terminal phase of the illness, and not after the death. This was not so for most of the daughters in this study, many of whom did not realize that the mother was dying until after the fact.

4. Because my study population was made up of volunteers, there may have been selectivity toward a more negatively impacted group of women.

Research on Mitigating and Risk Factors in Parentally Bereaved Children

Mitigating factors identified in this study were the "family background factors" such as family communication style, presence of other family problems, and family configuration. Also, daughter's age at the time of mother's death, the family changes she experienced after her mother died, and the kind of support available to her were identified as important mitigating factors. These results were quite consistent with the findings of other studies with respect to these factors. For example, Worden (1996) identified a high-risk group of children, based on age of child, preparation for death, predeath relationship, dysfunction of the surviving parent, ability of surviving parent to perceive how the child was feeling, dating and remarriage of surviving parent, family size, family cohesiveness, family stressors, family style of coping, and family solvency.

Christ (2000) identified characteristics of cases with poor outcomes as

> situations in which the parent's death played a secondary role to the cascade of other stressors related to the death and the presence of unrelated but significant additional stressors, or both. What was apparent in most of these families was the multiplicity of stressful situations and events that added to the compromised or symptomatic outcomes: For example, the surviving parent's parenting skills were minimal or absent; other family members were ill or had recently died; the family was impoverished, had recently immigrated, or both; or the child had pre-existing problems. In short, the entire ecological system of the child and family conspired to add stresses and reduce supports. (p. 239)

The factors identified by Christ are very similar to those identified in this study, such as prior family problems, family communication style, and family changes after the mother's death. The major difference in outcome between this study and Christ's is that these outcomes were relatively rare in her population, and were very common in this one.

Other Research

Unfortunately, research on the impact of mother loss to women, whether from breast cancer or from other causes, has been very limited. Nor have the dynamics of mother-daughter relationships during the illness period been studied. Although the themes developed in this study are consistent with those described by researchers (Lichtman et al., 1984; Wellisch, 1981; Wellisch et al., 1991, 1992, 1996) and by women describing personal experiences (Edelman, 1994; Quindlen, 1995; Tarkan, 1999; Spira and Kenemore, 2000; Weingarten, 1994), much more research is needed in this field before firm conclusions can be drawn.

The following suggestions for future research are made:

1. Researchers should study separately the impact of parental death by gender of the child and gender of the parent who died. When this is not done, the profound impact of mother loss on girls is obscured.
2. Researchers also should separate women whose mothers survived and those whose mothers died in studies of the impact of breast cancer on daughters. When this is not done, the profound impact of mother loss (as opposed to mother's illness) can be obscured.
3. Researchers should recognize that the experience of mother's breast cancer is greatly affected by the phase of the experience. Researchers need to make clear which phase was studied, and limit generalization of results to that (those) phase(s). Thus, a researcher whose study is based on the phase of "illness and treatment" needs to be careful to generalize results to this period only, and not to the long term.
4. Researchers should pay more attention to the issues of family changes and survival in the period after a mother's death. While the child's grieving has been studied intensively, these issues have been largely ignored.

THEORETICAL IMPLICATIONS

The goal of any grounded theory study is the creation and development of theory. The results of this study—that is, the themes developed and the suggested relationships between them—can be considered a theory of the experience of breast cancer daughters. The study results also can be compared to other relevant theories, and implications can be drawn. Although not the primary focus of this book, the study results do suggest the following:

1. Our theories of life-course development have not done justice to the life-course development of girls, particularly to the nature and importance of the mother-daughter relationship for women.
2. Our theories of the impact of illness on children have not recognized the special status of daughters in the family, particularly older daughters, and the impact of illness on them.
3. Our theories of bereavement have not recognized the importance of the family changes and fears about survival that occur following a mother's death.
4. Our theories of bereavement have not incorporated the special nature of the mother-daughter relationship. New theories may be needed to understand how women mourn the death of a mother.
5. Our theories of understanding perceptions of risk and health prevention behavior may be too heavily based on rational cognitive models, and may underestimate the role of fear.

The findings of this study were supportive of the theoretical work being done on mothers and daughters at the Stone Center (Jordan et al., 1991). However, these theories have not yet been integrated with theories of illness and death in women.

RECOMMENDATIONS FOR PRACTICE

Because of the study limitations discussed in Chapter 2, practice implications from the findings must be developed with caution. Qualitative research is not easily generalized, because the samples are small and are not selected to be representative of broader populations. Some argue that it is inappropriate to draw any practice implications from this type of research. Instead, they suggest that larger studies, using traditional quantitative research methods, be done first, to test the qualitative results. I heartily agree that my findings should be subject to rigorous testing. However, I think to omit practical implications would shortchange the daughters who participated in the study, as well as this book's readers: The daughters, because many participated in the study out of a desire to have their experience benefit others; the readers, because it is likely that many of them are practitioners of some sort, and I trust them to assess these findings and to decide which of them are "trustworthy" and applicable to the populations with which they work. In cases where their practice populations differ in major ways from the population in this study, I am confident that they would not blindly apply the recommendations.

As a professor in a practice profession (social work), I feel that it is important for researchers to develop practice implications. Were I to wait for definitive proof of the validity of my results before doing so, women might be harmed, because women are being diagnosed with breast cancer in large numbers every day. Practitioners who work with these women must do their best to help, based on what is known now. The following recommendations are presented in full recognition of their limitations. I hope that they will be tested, by researchers, practitioners, and women, and discarded or modified if not valid. I also urge practitioners to consider the nature of the study and the population on which the results are based, and to use those recommendations that apply to their settings and populations. I hope that they, too, will write about their experience, so that the knowledge base of the field will be expanded and refined.

Recommendations Based on Family Background Factors

1. Consider family background factors of "family configuration," "prior family problems," and "family communication style" to identify families "at risk" for later problems.

Health and mental health providers who work with women who have breast cancer, and women who are diagnosed with breast cancer, can use the family background factors to identify those most likely to have problems. Because older daughters are most likely to take on major caretaking responsibilities, it is possible to identify which daughter in a family will likely need extra support early in the process and to make arrangements for family caregiving in advance. In addition, family communication style can be assessed early on, and resources can be identified to help families improve their communication skills. By assessing prior family problems, such as previous illness and deaths, history of abuse or neglect, dysfunctional patterns, and alcohol or drug problems, these issues can be identified, addressed, and dealt with early in the process. By resolving these prior problems early, women and their families will be in a better position to communicate openly, and support each other during difficult periods in the course of the illness.

Recommendations Based on the Period of Mother's Illness and Treatment

2. Improve communication in the family.

Communication is mentioned again and again by the women in our sample. Families with younger daughters were especially likely to need help with communication about the disease, since communication tended to be more open in families with older daughters. Women who have breast cancer need to learn how to share information with their families, especially children and young adolescents, without frightening them. Because mothers feel responsible for protecting their children, health professionals may need to help women with these tasks. Providers should educate breast cancer patients about the dangers of keeping information secret. They can help women share information by modeling how to do so, developing and sharing written materials for family members, holding information seminars for family members, and holding family meetings where the whole family receives information together, in a format where questions are encouraged.

Women must help daughters anticipate the side effects of the breast cancer treatments, understand why these are occurring, and deal with their reactions. Young adolescents, especially, were very frightened to see the physical manifestations of their mothers' illness.

It also is important to emphasize that the shared information should include emotional as well as physical aspects. The emotions a woman with breast cancer is likely to feel (shock, fear, anger, and sadness) are well known, and it is appropriate to discuss these with family members. This can help daughters understand how their mothers are feeling, and what they might be able to do to help. It is especially important that children and young adolescents be encouraged to express their own feelings, and to learn that these feelings are normal.

Some excellent materials (booklets, videotapes) are available to help parents discuss a cancer diagnosis with children. The Internet also can be a good resource for children to learn and to share their feelings about their mothers' treatments. Appendix IV contains examples of materials which can help women to improve communication with their children about breast cancer.

3. Prepare daughters for increased responsibilities.

It is common for health and mental health providers to focus on the patients and overlook the impact of the illness on the family members. Cases in which daughters, especially late adolescents and young adults, have had to interrupt their lives and become caregivers, their needs should not be ignored. These daughters need support, both emotional and concrete. Unfortunately, most existing support services are directed to caregivers of the elderly. Hospices are particularly good at extending services beyond the patient and providing support to caregivers. Some women who do not want hospice services may accept them if they see them as supportive for their daughters rather than for themselves. Support groups for young caregivers might also be of value.

4. Provide support for changes in relationships between mothers and daughters.

One theme of the study was that breast cancer led to changes in the mother-daughter relationship. These changes may be welcome, but they also may be disturbing to mother, daughter, or both. Open discussion of these shifts may help, as would family counseling.

Recommendations for Terminal Illness Period

Although our study did not identify themes related to the terminal illness phase, the tremendous disruptions that occurred in the lives of daughters following the mother's death suggests that some services in the terminal illness phase may be of value. For example, Christ and colleagues (Christ et al., 1991) tested an intervention during the terminal period and showed that they could work effectively with spouses and children prior to the death of a parent with cancer.

5. Encourage mothers to talk with daughters about what will happen after the mothers' deaths.

Daughters especially appreciated having mothers tell them what they might feel after the mothers' deaths, and that these feelings would be normal. If consistent with their beliefs, mothers may be able to tell daughters that they will still be with them in spirit, supporting and listening to them. Mothers should be encouraged to express their unconditional love. Daughters often feel guilty for having behaved badly, having said mean things to their mothers, or even having wished for their deaths. If possible, women can use the dying period to forgive their daughters for these real or imagined sins, and to help their daughters accept the death and move on with their lives.

6. Encourage mothers to provide a legacy for daughters.

Women whose mothers died were eager for information, especially if they were young at the time of the mother's death. Daughters were interested in learning about mothers' medical histories, including the breast cancer and its treatment. Those who might someday be interested in genetic testing would appreciate a frozen tissue sample.

Daughters also missed knowing family stories. They wanted especially to hear about the mother's childhood, and about their own childhoods. Women may be able to tell these stories on tapes (audio or video). Making a list of names and addresses of relatives and old friends also would be helpful. Some daughters wished they had their mothers' favorite recipes. Daughters held very dear any possessions of their mothers', such as pictures, jewelry, even clothing. If women can provide this type of legacy for their daughters, it will be very appreciated.

7. Refrain from admonitions to daughters.

Some practitioners encourage mothers to tell their children to accept a new stepmother after their death. In this study, quick remarriage only exacerbated the problems daughters experienced following the mothers' death. Daughters almost universally maintained a loyalty to mothers that precluded accepting a stepmother. Advising a mother to encourage her children to accept a future stepmother may be unwise; it could make the postdeath adjustment more difficult.

Some of the mothers of older daughters left daughters with a list of expectations before they died (e.g., "Keep the family together"; "Take care of your father/siblings/grandparents"). While extracting such promises may make the dying woman feel better, it can be detrimental for the daughter later. She may be unable or unwilling to fulfill these expectations, and feel guilty about it. She may alter her life, postponing getting married and having children, in order to fulfill the promise she made. Open discussion between mothers and daughters may clarify expectation (or wishes), and prevent later guilt.

8. Prepare daughters if a home death is planned.

Many younger daughters were traumatized by their mothers' death, especially if they died at home. Sights, sounds, and smells of the terminal period and following the death (e.g., seeing mother's body being carried out in a body bag) were especially difficult for children and young adolescents. If a home death is desired, it is important to prepare children for what will happen, to support them during the process, and to provide opportunities for them to talk about it after the fact. Organizations such as hospices have expertise with these issues, and can help families avoid traumatizing a child or adolescent.

Recommendations Based on Period After Mother's Death

Two overarching themes emerged for the period following mother's death: "family changes" and "survival." Family changes were especially difficult for the youngest daughters.

9. Provide family-focused services for widowed fathers and reconstituted families.

Services for widowed fathers and stepmothers are needed to teach them to support the newly motherless daughter. Services such as support groups, individual counseling, and family therapy all would be appropriate. Bereavement programs must be targeted at the family unit, similar to the family camps now being offered to AIDS families in bereavement. Bereavement services also are needed for daughters of all ages. These can be school-based support groups, Internet support groups, after-school programs, college counseling department services, and outreach services. After a mother's death, special support may be needed to help fathers deal appropriately with their early adolescent daughters. Intensive counseling services, such as those offered to trauma survivors, may be appropriate for the women who were early adolescents when their mothers died.

Many women in this study lost contact with their maternal relatives and with the mother's friends after the mother's death. They felt that their loss was multiplied by their inability to share stories and memories, as well as the loss of love and support. It can be very difficult for family and friends to maintain contact with children after the mother's death. However, it is possible that before her death a mother could make arrangements with her extended family members (grandmother, aunts) to reach out to her children. Perhaps the children could be included in a holiday celebration that occurs every year. If a close friend will agree to be a kind of "big sister," it could make a real difference to the young daughters who experience the loss of a mother to breast cancer.

Recommendations Based on Long-Term Impact for Daughters Whose Mothers Died

10. Provide mental health services for motherless daughters.

Because many daughters identified mental health problems, it is important for mental health providers to be especially sensitive to the issues that motherless daughters experience. They need to know that despite their cognitive ability, daughters who were children and adolescents did not necessarily experience grieving, but may have concealed their feelings after the death. Therefore, as adults, they may need to mourn for their mothers and express long-buried anger, guilt, and sadness before they can successfully move forward with their lives. (Insurance providers should recognize the importance of these issues. Mother loss for a daughter should not be lumped with other bereavement services. More intense mental health services may be needed by these daughters.) Specialized services also may be needed for women who were children or adolescents at the time of the mother's death.

11. Provide services that improve relationships.

Many daughters identified problems with relationships, long after their mothers died. Mental health providers such as family therapists, marital therapists, and family counselors, should develop special services that target these problems. Relationship problems in these women may be related to their failure to develop the empathy and mutuality that women learn through their relationships with their mothers (Jordan et al., 1991). Services that recognize the source of the problem are needed.

Recommendations Based on Findings on Women Whose Mothers Survived

Recommendations discussed earlier on family communication and role shifts are appropriate for daughters of survivors. Because a recurrence is always possible, services that provide support for open communication are appropriate at any time. In addition:

12. Help mothers to communicate emotions with daughters.

In some families, women take a strong, protective role. They minimize the seriousness of the illness, and provide reassurance to daughters. As daughters get older, they may realize that their mothers are vulnerable to recurrence, but fear discussing it. This leads to excessive worrying about the mother. Health and mental health providers could help these families by facilitating open communication about the likelihood of recurrence, and the family expectations of the daughter were this to occur.

13. Help daughters who are "stuck."

In some families of survivors, daughters' concerns about mothers' health lead to an unusually strong closeness between mother and daughter. Some daughters were reluctant to leave their mothers and form committed relationships, and some were afraid to take on the responsibilities of children, in case their mothers might need their care. These families would benefit from open discussion. When open communication is not possible, daughters may need help in separating from their mothers enough to move forward with their lives.

Recommendations Based on Findings on Risk

14. Provide accurate information for daughters of all ages about the causes of breast cancer, its prevention, and the benefit of early detection.

This study reveals that many daughters are misinformed about the causes of breast cancer. At the same time, their fear makes it difficult to gather this information. Educational materials which are targeted to daughters and which are sensitive to their fears are needed.

15. Help daughters gain an accurate idea of their level of risk.

Many daughters vastly overestimate their risk of developing breast cancer and of dying if they are diagnosed. Educational materials that target daughters are needed to help them understand their actual risk. These materials need to be sensitive to daughters' high levels of fear.

16. Develop strategies for communicating with daughters that reduce anxiety without demeaning daughters.

High anxiety in the daughters can interfere with good medical care. Health providers must learn to communicate in a way that respects daughters while reducing their anxiety.

17. Support mammograms and clinical breast exams for daughters, instead of breast self-examination.

Mammograms and clinical breast exams should be provided for daughters beginning five years before the age of their mother's diagnosis. Breast cancer advocates should pressure insurance companies to provide these services. Breast self-exam should not be pushed excessively, because it may not be helpful in detecting breast cancers in younger women, and it is extremely anxiety provoking. When they are unable to perform it, some daughters feel guilty.

18. Provide sensitive genetic services.

As genetic testing becomes more common, providers of genetic services should be educated about daughters' experiences. Although they may look alike on a genogram, the very different experiences and outlooks of women whose mothers survived and those whose mothers died require very different counseling techniques. Also, genetic counselors must understand the differences in daughters' experiences depending on their age. They also must understand the mother-daughter dynamics of "mutual protection," worry, and closeness in families of survivors. This will allow them to provide services that incorporate the themes identified by this study, and serve as a referral resource for family and mental health counseling.

19. Support the effective coping of daughters.

Daughters do a remarkable job of coping with a very high level of fear by using a variety of mechanisms. Health providers need to explore these techniques with daughters, and support them, recognizing how difficult it can be for them to "do the right thing."

SUMMARY

This qualitative study of those breast cancer survivors who are daughters has focused on a population that often has been overlooked. It is important that breast cancer advocates and health providers pay attention not only to women with breast cancer, but to the needs of these other survivors. New ideas that have emerged from this study include: age of the daughter at the time of the mother's illness is critically important, especially if the mother dies; the period after the mother's death is profoundly traumatic, especially for younger daughters; issues of adapting to family changes and fear for survival were more important, especially for youngest daughters in this period, than was grieving; loss of a mother may be a more profound experience for daughters than is reflected in literature on parental death; daughters of women who survive breast cancer may have problems separating from mothers and moving on with their lives; and daughters have exaggerated fears that may interfere with their health care—

especially those whose mothers died. Recommendations for research-ers, health providers, advocates, and women with breast cancer and their families were identified based on these findings.

By allowing yesterday's daughters to voice their experiences, I hope that the daughters of tomorrow will face a more sympathetic world—one that has more understanding of their needs. By reading the stories of women who have had similar experiences, tomorrow's daughters may feel less alone, and advocates and providers may be able to prevent and treat problems that have been too long ignored.

Appendix I

Interview Guides and Other Pertinent Material

Interview #1

Complete informed consent procedures before beginning interview.

1. Could you start by telling me a little bit about yourself? (Probes: age, marital status, work, children, family, education)
2. How would you describe your relationship with your mother before she had breast cancer?
3. I understand that your mother had breast cancer. Could you tell me about that? (Probes: age of mother, age of R (respondent), family involved, mother's diagnosis, treatment, illness course)
4. What was that like for you? (Probes: How did you learn about your mother's illness? What do you remember about how you found out? Who else knew? What were you told? Do you remember what you thought at the time? Do you remember what you felt? [Repeat these probes for major events: e.g., diagnosis, treatments, death.] Do you feel your mother's illness affected your relationship with her? Who took over your mother's roles in the family? Do you remember any reactions or behaviors that you went through at that time? What happened after that? [Changes in family living situation])
5. How do you feel that this experience has affected you? (Probes: Effect on your personality? Your emotional health? How you face life? Your relationships? Your plans for the future? Are there special times or events winch are particularly difficult for you? How have your thoughts and feelings about your mother's illness changed since then? Have you had opportunities to discuss your experience with others? Who? Was that helpful?)
6. How did your mother's having breast cancer affect the other members of your family? (Probes: Fathers? Siblings? Grandparents? Family roles? Family dynamics?)

7. (Ask only if brought up by the informant) How about the impact on your (future) children? (Probes: Knowledge of genetic testing? Interest in genetic testing? Thoughts—pros and cons. Worry? Concerns about children?)

8. Any other important *things* about this experience that we haven't covered? Thank you for sharing your experience. Give project phone number if further concerns come up. If informant is upset, refer to mental health or support groups.

Sample Interview Summary

Case #8
Interview ftl
Reviewed by Susan

I. Summary of interview #1

1. *Demographic Information:* R is 33 years old, married with no children. She is the oldest sibling and has a younger brother who resides in another state. She and her brother appear to have a strained relationship. Parents divorced when R was in college. R was 19 years old when mother was Dxed. Mother was 39 at the time of Dx and was 45 when she died. R first became involved in breast cancer organizations when she ran in the Race for the Cure in October of 1995. R found out about the study at the Komen Symposium. R is close to her maternal grandparents and has taken on some caretaking responsibilities for them.

2. *Relationship with mother before breast cancer:*
   • Throughout her childhood and teen years, R and mother were very close prior to the breast cancer.
   • Mother instilled a sense of confidence, optimism, and self-esteem in dtr.
   • Mother instilled the importance of community service in dtr.
   • Father is an alcoholic and mother tried to shield children from this.

3. *Dx of mother's breast cancer:*
   • Parents separated in the fall of R's sophomore year in college.
   • Mother told R that she had a lump in her breast and was Dxed with cancer during a December holiday break. Mother told R that she would be just fine and not to worry, that it was only a minor inconvenience.
   • R remembers her mother having a partial mastectomy with some lymph nodes removed. Mother had chemo and radiation for about a year and did lose her hair (losing her hair did not appear to be "that

big of a deal," according to R). R thinks it was a bigger deal than Mo. let on.

- Mo. started a support group in her area for other women who had BRCA.
- Mo was in remission for apx. 5 years.
- Relationship between R and Mo. became strained after mother remarried and R began dating a Bahamian man of color. R was surprised when mother voiced her disapproval. R notes that she was not raised to be prejudiced. R feels strongly that Mo. was influenced by her 2nd husband's prejudice beliefs.
- R expressed a strong dislike for the 2nd husband, indicated that he had multiple problems and was financially exploiting Mo.
- R and husband dated for 5 years and married after mother's death.
- Mother had a reoccurrence of breast cancer in June and R indicates that she and Mo. became close from that point on.
- R acted as Mo.'s caretaker until Mo.'s death in October.
- R left an unhappy job situation immediately following the recurrence of Mo.'s BRCA.
    —R commuted to care for Mo. a significant amount and acted as Mo.'s caretaker as well as advocate (when she was hospitalized).
    —Mo.'s cancer metastasized to the brain and she began experiencing neurological difficulties and had greater difficulty caring for herself.
    —Mo. refused hospice care and thought it was for people who had "given up on hope," and she wasn't ready to give up even up until the very end of her life.
    —R and Mo. would talk about how Mo. was not afraid to die and how Mo. wanted to die. Mo. said that she wanted to die at home.
    —Mo. ended up dying in the hospital.

4. *How was it for daughter:*
    - R indicated that the experience was profound and heartbreaking.
    - She found it hard to talk to her friends and husband-to-be as they had not shared a similar experience.
    - R remembers trying to stay positive when her mother was sick and thinking, *Well, miracles do happen.*
    - R felt that Mo. received good care from medical staff at the hospital and from the in-home nurses.
    - Some time after R arrived to the hospital after Mo. died, R witnessed Mo. being zipped up in a body bag. R was very angry and regrets having seen this.
    - R had anger toward mother's husband for not visiting the hospital in the days before her death and for agreeing to pay the funeral expenses and not following through on this promise. She was also angry that he

did not arrange a burial service at the cemetery where her mother's ashes were being buried.
- R was grateful that Mo. had made a tape recording prior to her death. R has only listened to it twice and thinks that it would be hard to listen to it again, yet comforting at the same time.

5. *How experience has affected daughter:*
- The experience has helped R focus on her priorities in life, in recognizing who is important in her life, and knowing that life is an adventure, and that you only live once (her words).
- R has recognized the significance of important people in her life and cultivating and nurturing those relationships.
- R and husband went back to live in her mother's house (also the house where R was raised) a year after Mo. died. R indicates that it was a good feeling to be there and at the same time it made her miss her mother in a significant way.
- R had wished that her mother could have attended her wedding and she missed her Mo. being there.
- R misses her Mo. during significant times of the year (holidays, Mo.'s birthday, Mothers Day, etc.).
- R says that she feels less and less sad and more accepting of her Mo.'s death as time passes.
- R had never spoken to anyone about her mother's breast cancer in this much detail before this interview.
- She has never pursued counseling, though she indicated that running at the "Race" and attending the Komen Symposium had been very helpful/healing to her.

6. *How mother's breast cancer affected other family members:*
- This area was not covered in enough detail.
- I had asked the R this question but I now realize that the question was answered in a way she described the other relatives rather than discussing "how the experience actually affected other family members."

7. *Daughter's perception of risk/own health actions:*
- R does not feel that she is destined to get BRCA, however, she does think that she is at high risk.
- She has made it a point to be more knowledgeable about BRCA.
- An oncologist had recommended that R receive a mammogram every year from age 30 on, since R may be at high risk as her mother developed BRCA in her 30s.
- R notes that she is "acutely" aware of the need for breast self-exams, for a regular mammogram, and a GYN exam once a year.

II. Identify Any Areas That Came Up in the Follow-Up Call

R did not have anything to add about the interview. She indicated that she had received the information on the motherless daughters meetings that she had requested and that I had sent her.

III. Identify Any Areas Where Information Is Unclear, or Where Further Information Is Needed

- Relationship with father.
- Explore in more depth how the experience affected other family members (brother, father, grandparents, Mo.'s husband).

Is she choosing not to have children so that her children do not have to go through what she went through?

IV. Identify Any Areas Where Feelings May Not Have Been Explored

V. Identify Any Areas Where R May Be Different from Others in Similar Circumstances

- R cared for grandparents on a regular basis and provided financial support to them.

VI. Identify Any Concepts, Themes, or Hypotheses That Are Especially Relevant to This Respondent

- R acting as primary caretaker for Mo. while she was ill
- R providing support to grandparents
- Divorce

VII. Any Additional Areas That Came Up at the Team Discussion

Interview Instructions for Interview #2

    I. Prior to interview:
        A. A summary of the interview should be written by the interviewer, following the interview outline. It should provide brief, clear answers to the various questions asked.
        B. Interviewer should identify any areas for follow-up which came from the phone call.
        C. At least two people (interviewer and one other) should read the transcription and identify areas for follow-up:

       1. areas where information is unclear, or where further information is needed to fill in the picture
       2. areas where feelings may not have been fully explored
       3. areas where the individual may seem different from others in similar circumstances
   D. The case should be discussed at a team meeting prior to scheduling the second interview.
  II. Interview:
    A. Interviewer should ask respondent if there were any areas which respondent thought of since the interview that she would like to add, or to talk more about. Additional thoughts, results of talking with others since the first interviews, events since the first interview (such as attending a meeting, support group, therapy, thinking about or going to genetic testing or counseling, or reading). Check for any changes in life circumstances.
    B. Interview should review the summary of interview #1, and ask R for her reaction. Is this correct? Does it adequately reflect the interview? Are there things that were not emphasized enough, or that were overemphasized?
    C. Interviewer should ask for further information on the areas identified in the transcript review and follow-up phone call.
    D. Interviewer should identify from the list of developing concepts, variables which are relevant to this respondent, and then review them with her. Ask for her reactions as to whether these things are important to her, how they may have made a difference, how they might relate to other variables.

Excerpts from Journal

12/4/98

I am at Carolyn [Walter's] today, and we spent the day talking about many things. We started with my telling her about Kathy Weingarten's idea about the "good mother," and how I disagreed that it was good for the child for the mother to share her fears, panic, insecurity. Carolyn felt that it was good for her to share what she was feeling, but not to ask her child to "mother" her.

Also, daughter may feel she needs to protect mother—from having hurt her in some way. That is, mother has done badly by her daughter, and feels guilty that she has done her child harm. Or, this is what mother fears. So, daughter has to be careful—to protect mother from hearing this, and confirming her fear. So—daughter says that it has had no impact, or . . . no negative impact. So as not to hurt her mother.

Another facet would be that daughter may not know that mother was ill, or be able to separate out what was caused by the illness by what is just her mother's personality. If a woman did not have a mastectomy, and did not have chemotherapy, then her daughter is only going to know what her mother, or others, tells her. If they don't tell her anything about the illness, she is not going to see it as the cause of something about her or her relationship with mother. This, of course, relates to the younger daughters. But . . . breast cancer can be easier to hide than arthritis. It is not a chronic disease. So it is also related to the nature of the disease, and the issues around chronic illness, which is invisible, and disability, which is not. So, I think we ended up with more understanding of why the daughters felt that mother's illness had so little impact on them. Carolyn talked about invisible losses, like a very young child who loses a mother, or, as in one of her cases, a child whose twin died at birth. She feels that these are the hardest to deal with.

We also talked about the qualitative goal of presenting the insider's view, and so I was saying that I couldn't put in the analysis, for example, what [I just wrote], because they said it had no effect. But . . . a clinician would analyze them. I said I thought it broke my compact with them, and that if I wanted to do that, I should do a clinical study, where I discuss my cases. But I do feel I can discuss what other authors have said about the same situation or related situations, if it is directly relevant to the cases. Hard issue, this. Needs more thought. See Deborah Padgett's article on this.

We also talked about the mutual protection stuff that goes on between mothers and daughters. A lot of mutual protection. Not only when mother is dying, but around the genetics. (Daughter has to say, or insist, that she isn't interested in genetic testing, because mother can't handle the idea that she passed on the defective gene. Both agree that the breast cancer wasn't caused by genetics!) I was seeing that it is like the struggle for independence in the older women and daughters that we discussed in our book. It is, who is the protected one, and who is the one in need of protection? "The mutual protection society: Mothers and daughters (don't) talk about breast cancer."

We talked quite a bit about the issue of separating or integrating the women whose mothers died and those who survived. I tried it out both ways—that is, chapter on children, with survivors and motherless daughters in the same chapter. One main reason why I did not was that I imagined women reading it, and wanting to turn to the chapter that describes them and their experience. I still don't think that women whose mothers died want to read about women whose mothers survived, and vice versa. Carolyn also asked me to tell her what were my goals with the book. I said that my original goal was to draw implications for genetic counselors—this soon-to-expand field (blah, blah, blah). But then, as the study progressed, I was so moved by the experiences of these vulnerable daughters that I shifted focus, and a new goal became to expand services for this group.

We also talked about how the women emphasized that they wanted me to get the word out to doctors. At the final reception, they wanted doctors to be more sensitive and understanding, e.g., about how hard it is for them to do breast self-exams. So, I was thinking of how to reach doctors. Also, talked about how to disseminate to advocates, etc.

11/30/00

I am feeling a lot of time pressure now, but I am still working at the same pace. It is slow, but I don't really know how to (or really want to) speed it up. I will need to use January for a lot of the grunt work—editing, sending case studies out, references, etc. I hope I am up to it. But the work is moving along. I am working on the themes for the "young adult" chapter, now called the "late adolescent" chapter in my mind.

It occurs to me that there are two mistakes being made in the literature. One is the lumping of all kinds of parental death (mothers and fathers, daughters and sons, and sometimes, different causes of death—less of a problem, I think). But the other may be considering that there is only one model of grief. The modern thinking is very into the healthiness of long-term connection, but the type of grief is not distinguished. I am thinking that loss of a mother, for a daughter, at any age, is fundamentally different from other losses. I'm thinking that the crash that adolescents face—according to Gilligan's group—where they learn to "be nice" at the expense of "being honest"—the relationship with mother is probably the only one that is free from this. They express their anger at mother for allowing this loss of voice to happen. They also vent honest feelings to mother, knowing that the bond will not be broken. They don't have to be "nice" with mother. So when mother dies, or is so sick that she can't be attacked, the loss for the daughter is especially profound. Gone is support for the "voice" (if indeed mother was at all supportive of it—not always the case). It is almost like my own mother has always been something for me to push against. If she isn't there, I'm afraid I will fall down! The loss of the mother, for the daughter, is a loss of a part of herself, as she has never completely separated. We want to see our mothers strong and successful, even if this means strong in conflict with us. It means that we are strong too.

Another thought was on the loss of the caregiving role when mother becomes elderly. Although this role is perceived as a burden, for a daughter, it is meaningful in a number of ways. For one, it is a chance to be the strong and competent one in the relationship, and that is a boost to self-esteem. Also, it can be a chance to pay back for the mean things daughter did to mother in her adolescence. It is a chance for mother to forgive her daughter for this behavior too.

12/21/00

I originally thought my book was all about illness, and adapting to illness in the family. But then, it seemed to be all about grief, and death and dying. But now I am thinking that it is all about the mother-daughter relationship, and how death interrupts a necessary separation between mothers and daughters.

12/18/01

It's late and I'm tired. But just wanted to put a brief note here. I am working now on the "mother survived" chapter. It is difficult because I realize that I have put this one off—from the beginning, I found this material less compelling. I was surprised that the daughters seemed to be so little affected by their mother's illness. I interviewed less of them than I expected to—feeling how mothers successfully protect daughters so that daughters never realize how vulnerable their mothers are and unprotected they are. But now I am not so sure that I really saw what was going on. It now seems to me that there are effects, in that there isn't separation, and the mutual protection continues. These are the main themes. It isn't going to be as rich as the other chapters, but I think it will still be good.

8/26/02

I have to say again how ironic it is to be writing and reading about women who feel their lives have been ruined because they do not have a mother, and to contrast this to the attitude of the women whose mothers survived. I ran a word count on the word *alone* to see if the women whose mothers died used the term more than those whose mothers survived. It turned out that they both used the word *alone* about the same amount, but the daughter whose mother died was likely to say, "I feel so alone," and the daughter whose mother survived was likely to say, "I wish my mother would leave me alone." The "mother survived" women reflect how I used to feel about my mother—close but with an unappreciative closeness. Now, my feelings are close to the women whose mothers died, as my own mother moves more and more into herself. You can push your mother away, as long as you know that she will be there when she is needed. The reality is that someday, sooner or later, she won't. Still, this is hard for daughters to see. I think that perhaps the daughters whose mothers had breast cancer (survivors) use denial to keep up the original relationship, but underneath, they know that mother is vulnerable, and so they stay close by. Their actions belie their talk.

Project Analysis Outline (Coding Categories)

I. Base data
    A. Current age
        1. Teens
        2. Twenties
        3. Thirties
        4. Forties
        5. Fifties
    B. Mother's age at diagnosis
        1. Thirties
        2. Forties
        3. Fifties
    C. Mother survived
        1. Yes
        2. No
    D. Daugher's age at mother's diagnosis
        1. Child
        2. Adolescent
        3. Young adult
        4. Adult
    E. Daugher's age at mother's death
        1. Child
        2. Adolescent
        3. Young adult
        4. Adult
    F. Race
        1. White
        2. Black
        3. Other
    G. Religion
        1. Catholic
        2. Protestant
        3. Jewish
        4. Other
        5. None
    H. Marital status
        1. Married
        2. Single
        3. Divorced
        4. Other
    I. Children
        1. Yes
        2. No
    J. Career

II. Family background
    A. Members of family of origin
        1. Mother
            a. Relationship before BRCA
        2. Father
            a. Relationship with
        3. Older sister
        4. Younger sister
        5. Older brother
        6. Younger brother
        7. Grandmother
        8. Grandfather
        9. Aunt
        10. Other
    B. Family-of-origin problems
        1. Addiction
        2. Physical abuse
        3. Sexual abuse
        4. Verbal abuse
        5. Spousal abuse
        6. Marital discord
        7. Divorce
        8. Enmeshed
        9. Lack of open communication
        10. Other
    C. Strengths
        1. Role of religion
    D. Cancer experience
III. Breast cancer
    A. Discovery
    B. Treatment
        1. Mastectomy
        2. Radiation
        3. Chemotherapy
            a. Loss of hair
        4. Alternative medicine
        5. Mother receives MH Tx [mental health treatment]
        6. Tx other
    C. Recurrence or remission
    D. Preparing for death
        1. Mother preparing for death
        2. Family prepares for death
        3. End-stage symptoms
    E. Death
        1. Postdeath activities

F. How cancer was handled
  1. Mother protected
  2. Secrecy
    a. Minimized
  3. Shame
  4. Denial
  5. Openness
  6. Scientific
  7. Conflict
  8. Daughter protected
  9. Other
G. Daughter's role in mother's illness
  1. Caregiver
  2. Helper
  3. Distant
  4. Other
IV. Daughter's reaction
  A. Grieving
    1. Daugher supported
    2. Didn't grieve
    3. Rituals
      a. Funeral
    4. Significant dates
    5. Therapeutic cry
    6. Guilt
  B. Daughter's vague memory
  C. Denial
  D. Powerless
  E. Anger
  F. Isolation
  G. Anxiety
  H. Other
V. Impact
  A. Losses daughter experienced
    1. Unconditional support
    2. Best friend
    3. Discipline
    4. Help standing up to father
    5. Source of information about womanhood
    6. Loss of mother's role in family
      a. Buffer
      b. Peacemaker
      c. Glue
      d. Guidance
      e. Continuity
      f. Extended family
      g. Fun-loving, adventurous mother

       7. Adult relationship with mother
       8. Mother's friends
   B. Surrogate
       1. Yes
       2. No
   C. Daughter's role
       1. Takes mother's role
       2. Caregiver of grandparents
       3. Other
   D. Daughter shares role
       1. Yes
       2. No
   E. Daughter pregnancy
   F. Change in family dynamics
   G. Intimate relationships
       1. Positive
       2. Negative
   H. Children
   I. Femininity
   J. Mother-daughter relationship
   K. Long-term illness
   L. Other losses
   M. Mother's scar
   N. Other
VI. Daughter's mental health
   A. Problems
       1. Stuck
       2. Depressed
       3. Daughter isolated
       4. Separation anxiety
       5. Abandonment
       6. Anxiety
       7. Other
VII. Daughter's coping
   A. Change priorities
       1. Yes
       2. No
   B. Seek help
       1. Therapy
       2. Support group
       3. Mother-daughter group
       4. Other
       5. None
   C. Social supports
       1. Yes
       2. No

    D. Faith
    E. Postdeath contact
    F. Independent
    G. Daughter activist
    H. Reads mother-daughter book
    I. Other
VIII. Family impact
    A. Family effect
       1. Mother
       2. Father
       3. Older sister
       4. Younger sister
       5. Older brother
       6. Younger brother
       7. Grandmother
       8. Grandfather
       9. Aunt
      10. Other
    B. Family survives
       1. Yes
       2. No
       3. New family
       4. Father's remarriage
          a. Father's remarriage/family conflict
IX. Risk
    A. Risk factors
       1. Genetics
       2. Other
    B. Expects to get cancer
       1. Yes
       2. No
    C. Activities to prevent
       1. Diet
       2. Exercise
       3. Family planning
       4. Alternative medicine
       5. Other
       6. None
    D. Activities to detect
       1. BSE
       2. Clinical BE
       3. Mammograms
       4. General medical care
       5. Other
       6. None

E. Symptoms
   1. Yes
   2. No
F. Pedigree
G. Genetic testing
   1. Thought about it
   2. Wants it
   3. Doesn't want it
   4. Learned
   5. Insurance
   6. Other
   7. Mother survives
H. Fear
   1. Fear level
      a. High
      b. Medium
      c. Low
   2. When
      a. Lump
      b. Ages
      c. Development
X. Health care system
   A. When
      1. Mother's treatment
      2. Daughter's prevention
   B. Who
      1. Physicians
         a. Positive experience
         b. Negative experience
      2. Hospital
      3. Other

Follow-Up Letter to Participants

December 22, 1997

Dear Participants in the "Daughters" Research Project:

I am happy to inform you that the "Daughters" project is nearing its final phase. We have held interviews with forty-one women whose mothers had breast cancer. We have studied the transcripts of these interviews, and have completed our preliminary analysis. Now, we are turning to you again for your help. We would like to have your reaction to our ideas, and to be able to add your ideas into our final results.

I am sending you some material showing the current analytical model for women whose mothers died of breast cancer. There is an overall diagram, and then there are figures for each of the components in the diagram. For example, one section in the diagram is "Background Factors" and you will find that there is a page that shows what the "Background Factors" are. For each section of the diagram, there is also a "questionnaire," where you can indicate which of the various factors were important in your case. There is a place for you to identify whether each factor was "very important," "somewhat important," "not very important," or "not at all important" for you. There is also space for you to add additional factors, or to add comments. I hope that you will be able to review these materials, and if possible, complete the "questionnaire" before your final interview. (We are still working on some additional material that provides information on what women who were in your same age group experienced. These materials will be sent to you as soon as they are ready.)

We plan to conduct the final interviews in January (1998), and your interviewer will be contacting you soon to set up a convenient time for this interview. During the interview, you will be asked, as before, if you have anything new to add. Your interviewer will then review with you the "analytical model," and your responses to the checklist. We will again tape the interview, to be sure we have your comments, ideas, and suggestions for any changes in the model. As before, you will be given $25.00 as a small "Thank You!" for your participation in this project.

We want to thank you again for your contribution to our research. We are looking forward to the final interview, and to hearing your ideas about our analysis. Please contact the "Daughters Project" at (410) 555-5555 or (toll free 1-800-555-5555, ex 5555) if you have any questions or concerns. We look forward to talking with you in January.

Happy Holidays and Happy New Year!
Sincerely,
Julianne S. Oktay, LCSW, PhD
Professor

Questionnaire for Respondent's Feedback

Case number:
Interviewer:

Please rate how important the following factors were for you by circling or marking through the number that comes closest to your feelings and perceptions about how important each factor was in your experience of your mother's breast cancer. Examples of items which would fit into each category follow in parentheses.

Background Factors

	Very important	Somewhat important	Not very important	Not at all important	N/A
Social factors (class, race, ethnic group, religion)	5	4	3	2	1
Your age at time of mother's illness (child, adolescent, young adult, adult)	5	4	3	2	1
Family communication style (open or secrecy and denial)	5	4	3	2	1
Family problems (illness/ death of family member; alcohol/substance abuse; child abuse—physical/ sexual/psychological; other)	5	4	3	2	1
Other family factors (your relationship with mother before breast cancer; your birth order position)	5	4	3	2	1

Additional Comments, Background Factors:

_____

_____

_____

Actual Experience of Mother's Breast Cancer

	Very important	Somewhat important	Not very important	Not at all important	N/A
Characteristics of mother's illness (length of illness, effects on her appearance, effects on mother/daughter relationship; role played by daughter during illness)	5	4	3	2	1
Communication with daughter (open or secrecy and denial)	5	4	3	2	1

Family dynamics (family conflict, father's role, role of siblings)	5	4	3	2	1
Outcome of mother's illness (mother experienced frightening symptoms, pain, and suffering, whether mother survived or not)	5	4	3	2	1

Additional Comments, Actual Experience of Mother's Breast Cancer

_____
_____
_____
_____

Family Changes Following Mother's Death

	Very important	Somewhat important	Not very important	Not at all important	N/A
Your relationship with father (you assumed mother/wife role; felt abandoned due to remarriage)	5	4	3	2	1
Your relationship with your stepmother (how long before father remarried; loss of home, conflict with stepmother)	5	4	3	2	1
Your relationship with siblings (mothered them, became closer to them or more distant)	5	4	3	2	1
Your relationship with grandparents (assumed responsibility for grandparents; lost contact with mother's relatives)	5	4	3	2	1

Daughter's Coping and Social Supports

Your grieving process (rituals—funeral, visited grave, ceremonies/grief work—cried, sought info/contact with mother; memorializing mother)	5	4	3	2	1
Social supports available (mother/family surrogate; counseling/support groups; religion/faith/family support, friends, boyfriend/ husband)	5	4	3	2	1

Additional Comments, Family Changes/Daughter's Coping:

_____

_____

_____

Long-Term Impact

	Yes	No	N/A
Do you feel isolated and alone?	___	___	___
Do you have difficulty at life transitions such as marriage, graduation, childbirth?	___	___	___
Do you have difficulty with intimate relationships?	___	___	___
Are you superindependent?	___	___	___
Do you have separation anxiety?	___	___	___
Are you depressed?	___	___	___
Are you stuck?	___	___	___
Do you have low self-esteem?	___	___	___
Are you an unusually strong person?	___	___	___
Are you unusually compassionate?	___	___	___
Are you unusually self-sufficient?	___	___	___
Have you put off getting married or having children?	___	___	___
Have you changed your outlook on life or your priorities?	___	___	___

Additional Comments, Long-Term Impact:

_____

_____

_____

Risk

	Yes	No	N/A
Do you feel that you will get breast cancer about the same age as when your mother was diagnosed?	___	___	
Are you fearful about getting breast cancer?	___	___	___
Are you confused, frustrated, or angry that so much about breast cancer is not known or cannot be controlled?	___	___	___
Have you prepared yourself for breast cancer?	___	___	___
Have you taken actions to prevent breast cancer?	___	___	___
Do you find doing breast self-exams too difficult?	___	___	___
Are you uncertain about when to start, or how often to have mammograms?	___	___	___
Do you think genetic testing would be helpful to you and/or your family?	___	___	___
Do you think genetic testing would be harmful to you and/or your family?	___	___	___

Additional Comments, Risk:

_____

_____

_____

Final Results

We are considering how to present the final results of this study to the women who have participated in it. Which of the following would interest you? (Check all that you would like.)

___ 1. A written report which summarizes the results.
___ 2. A lecture which presents the results.
___ 3. A small group of similar participants for discussion of the results and implications.
___ 4. A small group of similar participants for sharing experiences possibly over a series of group meetings.

Any Additional Comments?

_____

_____

_____

_____

Appendix II

Typical Interview Description

Before leaving for the interview, I gather my supplies: the tape recorder, extra batteries and blank tapes, consent forms (two copies), the interview guide, a list of resources that I could use for referral, and a box of tissues. As per study procedure, I call the project number and leave information on the time and place of the interview. This interview was in an area of the city I am not familiar with, so I take my map, and leave plenty of time. When I arrive, it is a bit early, and so I wait in the car in front of the house until the scheduled time. The house is a small, two-story bungalow on a residential street just off of a major thoroughfare with lots of shops. The street is quiet, although the houses are quite close together. Each has a small yard with flowering bushes out front.

S answers the bell, and invites me into her home. She is an attractive woman who appears to be about 30 with a healthy glow about her. Her house is filled with comfortable, somewhat worn furniture. There are many pictures on the walls and tables—mostly of her three children. S sits on the couch and invites me to sit across from her in a large, comfortable chair. I give her the consent form to read over, and set up the tape recorder, glad that there is a plug nearby. (I am always nervous when I have to rely on the batteries.) An old, large dog flops down by our feet, and his deep sighs can be heard on the tape, as if moved by S's story. S tells me how she heard about the study, and signs the consent form; we settle back and begin.

I explain the purpose of the study and give her a copy of the interview guide, so she can follow along. (I find that this relieves anxiety, as there are no surprises or unexpected questions.) I begin with a typical identification question, "Could you tell me something about yourself?" and the interview is off and running. S is eager to talk, and she quickly tells me about her children, husband, job, sisters, etc. She provides a lot of detail, and I can see that this will be a long interview. I focus on her, and give her my full attention, although I occasionally flick my eyes to the tape recorder to make sure the red light is on. The interview lasts for about two hours, and I hardly say a word.

She tells me in detail about her mother's illness, about the family background, about her mother's death, and the aftermath. She is an animated sto-

343

ryteller, and both acts out the primary parts and provides commentary. The house is very quiet, and I find myself wondering at one point where the children are and whether they will be coming home at some point during the interview. I assume they are in school. At one point, S becomes tearful, and I offer a Kleenex. She is embarrassed, apologizes, saying something like, "This part is hard." I try to convey that it is okay to cry, and not to make her feel uncomfortable. The interview flows easily and the only interruptions occur when I hear the tape recorder click, and have to stop to put in new tapes. S is so eager to talk that even these short interruptions are frustrating, as they interrupt the flow of her story.

At the end of the interview, S and I look at the interview guide for the first time, and realize that we have covered all of the areas except "risk." She talks a bit about how she would like to have genetic testing, but her insurance won't cover it. She says that if she gets testing in a research setting, that she might be getting a "placebo"—which is not the case in genetic screening of research. I wonder if I should inform her of this, and decide to say something after the interview is complete.

At the end of the interview, I ask S if she would be willing to be contacted for a second interview. She indicates that she would, adding that her motivation is to help other women in her position. I gather up my equipment and return to my car. As I drive away, I turn on the tape recorder again and record some comments about the interview. I talk about S's religiosity, and also about her relationship with her sisters. As the oldest sister, she was very frustrated by her inability to keep her family together after her mother's death. I speculate that birth order is an important variable, and that perhaps the pattern in this family of three sisters is a common one. I note that the point where I was most uncomfortable in this interview was when S expressed a very Catholic worldview to explain what happened to her mother, since I am Jewish. I speculate about whether my nonverbal reactions may have affected the interview. I note that our "matching" system did not work here, and reaffirm that it is probably best if I interview the Jewish women.

I also identify the strong emotional moments in the interview: S's ongoing sadness about her mother's death, and her strong anger toward her father. I also note to discuss with the team the issue of how to handle respondents who provide information we know to be in error.

Appendix III

Additional Case Studies

Daughters Whose Mothers Died

*Marci (age at mother's breast cancer diagnosis: 1;
age at time of mother's death: 3)*

Background. Marci was born into a Jewish family, the third of three girls. Her father owned a small business and her mother stayed home with the children. Around the time of Marci's birth, her mother became ill.

Experience of mother's illness. Marci has few memories of her mother's illness, because she was only a baby. Her family handled the illness with great secrecy. Even Marci's mother wasn't told the diagnosis. "No one talked to her about it, about her illness or her death. My mother died in 1960. You didn't talk about death."

Marci's mother wrote a brief letter to each of her daughters from the hospital before she died. "The only letter I have from her directly is a one-line letter written to each one of us. In it, she promised to get well and come home."

Marci has no memories of anyone talking with her about her mother's death. She did not attend the funeral.

> You know, children were not considered humans [laughs]. I know my father did not tell me anything. But I think I may have been told by my grandmother or somebody that she went to sleep. I'm only assuming this because . . . I have terrible sleep problems.

Experience following mother's death. Marci's father was rarely home and soon began dating. Then his business failed, and he considered giving the three girls to their maternal grandmother. Instead, about a year after her mother's death, Marci's father married a divorced woman with two children. Marci never had a good relationship with her stepmother, whom Marci reports was very jealous. Marci's step-grandmother favored her stepbrother and stepsister. "That was painful. It was painful but I always just accepted it. I don't know. I've always felt like an orphan." At around age twelve, Marci became a part of a friend's family, spending more time in that home than in her own. "She [friend's mother] was like my mother. So I was certainly a part of that family. I just wanted to be away from that house [home with father and stepmother]."

Secrecy and poor communication continued in Marci's family after her mother's death. There was no mourning. "No grief. Not for us. And my father didn't grieve either. Basically, we didn't have anyone to turn to. My father was a mess. He was really not around for us. He was trying so hard to hide from his pain." Nor were memories of her mother kept alive. "She was like, her name, she was like a dirty word. She was never discussed. You know, it was like she didn't exist." Marci has sought contact with her mother through spiritual contact (readings) and dreams. She became a Reiki healer to develop her spirituality.

Marci and her sisters went to visit their mother's grave. Marci now goes to synagogue on the anniversary of her mother's death.

Long-term impact. As an adult, Marci has tried to obtain more information about her mother's illness. "I knew she had some kind of cancer, but not which kind. I would call around to family members to find out. Finally, I just asked my father, point blank, what kind of cancer she had, and he told us."

Marci attributes much of who she is today to her mother's death.

> I know that I have a real issue with self-esteem as an adult. I'm sure that that stems from not having a mother. Not so much the fact that my mother died, but that she was never replaced with someone that just gave me unconditional acceptance.

Marci has chronic insomnia that she attributes to her mother's death. After she had her first child, at age thirty (the same age her mother was at her death), Marci went into a very severe postpartum depression. "I was just terrified to go to sleep." After she had her second child, she again had severe depression and sleep problems. This time, she sought medication, accepting that she had chronic dysthymia (sadness).

Risk. Marci has feared that she would not live past thirty. "I used to be obsessed with death and the fear of death."

She recently had a lump removed from her breast. Every six months, she has a screening for ovarian cancer.

> As far as my health is concerned, I know what I need to look for and take care of, and I will. I want to be here for my children. It's very important for me. And I need to learn as much as I can about my mother's illness, so that I can help my kids. I mean, it's their legacy too. It's their genes.

Marci thinks that she will have genetic testing when it becomes available. "Not so much for me, but for them."

Current situation. Marci was married at twenty-seven, and at the time of interview (age thirty-eight) had two young daughters. Communication in the extended family is still very limited, especially concerning her mother. "Talk about the elephant in the living room, there was one then; it's still there. It's just grown bigger and bigger and bigger and bigger." Marci has only one picture of her mother, which was given to her by a relative. Her father is still careful to call her only at times when her stepmother is not at home.

Marci became a social worker to work with people who were dying. She trained in a hospice, where she worked with cancer patients. Before she completed her degree, her middle sister was murdered by an abusive husband. This event reawakened many of the feelings Marci had about her mother's death. Marci feels that her sister got into an abusive relationship because of her low self-esteem stemming from their mother's death. Marci has refocused her work around issues of domestic violence. Marci participated in a group for motherless daughters, and benefited so much that she now leads the group. She sees leading the group as a way to honor her mother's memory. Since she passed thirty, and especially since her sister's murder, she is no longer afraid or worried. She says she just wants to live the fullest life she can.

Mary (age at mother's breast cancer diagnosis: 11;
age at time of mother's death: 13)

Background. Mary was born the youngest of five children (four girls, one boy) in an Italian Catholic family. When she was born, her oldest sister was twenty-two. Mother stayed at home until Mary was six, and then returned to work full-time. One of Mary's early memories is how her mother took her to kindergarten for the first time. This was special because she had mother's attention all to herself. "[Youngest sister] and I always seemed to be lacking that time with her. We never feel like we had enough time."

Mary describes her family as "close-knit." "We were raised that every Sunday you spent with your grandparents and your family. That was family day."

Experience of mother's illness. When Mary was nine her mother found some lumps in one of her breasts, but her doctor told her not to worry. Two years later, Mary's parents asked the children to stay after dinner because they had something important to tell them. This had never happened before. The children were told that Mom had cancer and would be going to the hospital to have an operation. Mary didn't realize initially how serious cancer could be. "When you say it or tell somebody else, it hit home. So that was hard."

Mother's cancer recurred and the whole family spent a lot of time at the hospital during chemotherapy treatments. A painful memory from this time was when she overheard her father talking with mother's doctor. He asked the doctor what could have caused the breast cancer, and the doctor had answered, "It could have been having a child late in life." Mary realized that the child being referred to was herself.

The theme of Mary not having enough of her mother's attention continued for Mary throughout her mother's illness. When her mother came out of the mastectomy surgery, she wanted to see Mary first.

> So I went in the room. I was only eleven. She made me sit beside her and she said that she'd never had the time with me that she had with everybody else. I can remember that day like it was yesterday. I can tell you what I had on, the whole bit. I thought that things would change at that point, and it never did. She lived three years longer, so I thought there was going to be an opportunity for us to get to spend more time together. There wasn't, and that was a big disappointment. She realized that she wasn't going to be here, so why didn't she spend more time with me then?

Mary's mother's condition worsened; Mary became more involved in her physical care.

> It was harder toward the end when she was really dying 'cause she had changed physically. . . . The thinness of her skin, and you know, sunken-in face and weight loss. She really didn't lose consciousness until the day that she died, so we were very fortunate in that. She was alert. She knew all of us 'til the very end.

At her school, Mary did a lot of praying for her mother.

> You know, they tell you to pray for healing and pray for this and pray for that. I used to read the Bible to my mother. The priest would come over and do last rites. I don't know how many times they did that. I guess I was just always hoping that things would get better.

One day when Mary was fourteen, she came home from school and no one was home. She didn't have her key and didn't know what was happening. Her mother had been taken to the hospital, and she had died. Mary felt bad that she had not said a final "good-bye" to her mother.

Experience following mother's death. At the time of her mother's death, Mary's two older sisters no longer lived at home. Although she was the youngest, Mary took on many of her mother's roles after she died, including making everybody's lunches and completing most of the household chores. Mary's father also took on many of her mother's roles after her death. "He became both parents, essentially."

Mary's family got closer after her mother's death. "I guess [the family] was a support group. If somebody needed something, there was always somebody there—to borrow money, to run errands. We made an effort to be there for one another. That's just the way we were raised." It took Mary's father a long time to get socially active after his wife's death. "It was always clear that the children came first." Mary's father never remarried.

> He still loves her [mother] dearly and misses her. He talks about her on a regular basis and laughs at a lot of things that she did. He said he married my mother and she was his true love, his one and only, and that was it. He doesn't have a desire to get remarried at all.

Mary did not feel that she was prepared for her mother's death, because as the youngest, her family protected her from knowing how serious the situation was. She did not have a chance to say good-bye or fully prepare. "I was angry at God for what he had done to all of us. I mean, that's reasonable. For a while there after she died, some of us stopped going to church." Mary talked with her priest about these feelings, and he reassured her that her anger was normal, and that we can never understand God's plan. He told her to "have faith that it [mother's death] was for a good reason and that she's in a better place."

Although Mary had a good relationship with her father during this period, it was not without problems. Mary felt that her father did not understand her style of grief and her need to feel sad.

> With her dying when I was fourteen, I mean, your father's not gonna tell you the things your mother would tell you as a teenage girl. Self-esteem needs to be built up during adolescent years, and it just wasn't there. The mothers are usually the ones that do that as well. You can get it from your peers, but I think your mother is really the one that you rely on, and I didn't have that person to rely on.

Long-term impact. As a teen, Mary suffered from an eating disorder, and also had low self-esteem, which she attributes to her mother's early death. This also affected her relationships with boys. "Relating it to guys, I didn't think I was good enough for anybody, so I'd let them walk all over me." She got into an abusive relationship that she blames on her low self-esteem and her need to find love. Now, when her husband compliments her, she tends to dismiss it. "I'm always trying to undermine. I never can fully accept compliments." This carries into her work relationships.

> I'm not assertive. I never think I'm as good or as competent as my counterparts that do the same thing. I get walked over in every relationship. I'm usually the person that makes the time to do things, even when I don't have the time to do it.

Mary and her family miss her mother at important life events, such as her pregnancy, during which she was on bed rest.

> It has come to mind what it would be like with her there. I think that she probably would have provided a lot of support. . . . I still do wonder what my relationship would be like with her if she were still here. . . . I certainly think there's a void there.

When her sister recently had a baby, Mary

> stepped in and did the motherly role—went to the hospital, helped her out, took care of her son. I recognize that loss there and try to fill it for her. I know I can't be her mother, but I can be of help or assistance where our mother would be if she were here.

Risk. Mary is very careful about her diet and exercises regularly. She also tries to reduce her stress level, but feels less successful with this. She sees her doctor every three months for breast exams, but has not yet had a mammogram. (She has requested them, but her doctor has told her to wait.) Mary cannot make herself do breast self-examinations, although she doesn't understand why not. She was frightened during a pregnancy when she had a painful lump, but it was not cancer.

Mary worries about her sister, who is not as conscientious about her medical care. Mary tries to persuade her sister to take better care of herself, telling her that she needs to protect her children against losing their mother, as they did.

Current situation. Mary, thirty at the time of our interview, was happily married and expecting her second child. Mary is careful to take every opportunity to say "I love you" to her family, and to let them know how much she cares. She does not want to repeat the experience of waiting to say these important words until it is too late. She also is determined not to shortchange her children of her time and attention. She now works part-time; it is important to her to be able to take her child to the bus, and pick her up at the bus stop after nursery school. Mary's family still gets together every Sunday. The family also celebrates Christmas and Thanksgiving together. "There's twenty-five of us when we're all together, and that's a lot of people, but we're all together, and it's important for us." The family uses these occasions to share memories of Mary's mother.

*Ruth (age at mother's breast cancer diagnosis: 15;
age at time of mother's death: 17)*

Background. Ruth grew up in a Protestant family and has a younger brother. Her mother and brother were particularly close. Her grandparents lived in another state, where the family had a summer cabin. One of Ruth's fondest memories is spending time at the "cabin in the woods."

Experience of mother's illness. Ruth was sixteen when she was told that her mother was sick and had to go to the hospital. No one told Ruth of her mother's diagnosis. "It never occurred to me that she had breast cancer. It was never explained to me. In my family, you didn't necessarily question the information that was given to you." When her mother went in for treatment, her condition was too far advanced for a mastectomy. She was given radiation, only "the radiation was very debilitating for her. She spent a lot of time in bed."

While Ruth was in her first year of college, she took her mother for radiation treatments still not knowing her diagnosis.

> I had gone away to live on campus, so I didn't really spend that much time with her in the last few months of her illness. But I was haunted by questions because it just didn't seem right. So, I wrote a letter to her doctor asking whether I could make an appointment to talk with him the next trip I made home. I never heard from him.

In the spring of that school year, Ruth's father finally told her about the illness.

> I found out that my mother was terminally ill and wasn't expected to live through the summer. It turns out that [mother's doctor] had told him [father] about my letter, and my father told me that she was dying. The next morning, my grandmother said she and my grandfather would appreciate it if I would stay home and look after my mother. I said, well, of course, I would do that. Whatever is necessary. And that night, my mother died.

Ruth learned later that her mother was never told her diagnosis.

> My father had known for a little over a year, but my mother's doctors advised him not to tell her that she was ill because they felt that it would take away any hope that she may have had of recovery. So he kept that to himself. The only people that my father told about my mother's illness were her parents. It's inconceivable to me that she didn't know she had cancer. She never talked to anyone about it.

Experience following mother's death. Ruth did not find the funeral helpful.

> The whole experience was so [un]real, because we'd never experienced death before. We'd never been to a funeral. I remember when we got back to the house after the graveside ceremony, I thought, *All these people are laughing and eating and having fun and enjoying one another's company.* I just wanted to stand in the middle of them and shout, "Stop this! You have no business celebrating. This is a terrible, terrible thing that's happened." But I didn't, of course. That was my inexperience in these matters, and my youth, that made me feel so angry at them.

After her mother's death, Ruth's family came apart.

> When we returned home, we sort of crawled into our shells. We would come into the house from school or from work and we would go up to our rooms. There was no dialogue. There was no sharing. Within six months, he [father] was dating and within a year, he was remarried. When my father remarried, my stepmother made it very clear to me that she was not going to have a rival for my father's attention. I lived with them for four years until I got married.

Ruth also lost the close connection she had with her grandparents.

> It's almost as though the connection that we've shared died with her. I would go and visit her [grandmother] but neither she nor my grandfather were able to talk about my mother very easily. I think it was just too painful for my grandparents. My mother was the apple of [grandfather's] eye. The grief was not something that they could experience with me.

Ruth has very few memories of her mother.

> In the thirty-two years that my father was married to my stepmother, I wasn't allowed to talk about her and reinforce my memories. They are really faded. I don't have any pictures of her. . . . A lot of memories come from photographs, and there just aren't that many of her. I don't even have any recipes of the things that she prepared when we were growing up. When she died, my father cleaned house and he got rid of everything. So over the years, everything that was hers that has come my way has been very precious. [I have] some dishes that were hers and a couple of pieces of jewelry. My stepmother wanted to get new furniture, so a couple of pieces of furniture that my mother and father had bought together are now mine.

Ruth and her brother lost contact with her father. "[After that] we would see each other at Christmas but rarely at other times. I always felt that he loved us but she was making him choose between us and her. The rejection was the hardest part."

Ruth attributes her unfortunate marriage to her mother's death.

> I met my husband-to-be about six months after my mother died. I never dated anybody else after that. It was as if I needed somebody to talk to, somebody who could relate to what I was experiencing. He had just gone through his parents' divorce so he had some pain to deal with. I think you reach out to find whatever help and comfort you can, and someone that supports you at the period of time becomes very special. If I hadn't been as vulnerable as I was, I wouldn't necessarily have stayed in that relationship. We provided each other an outlet, an escape from what was going on in our home life.

Ruth also was attached to her husband's family. "My husband had lots and lots of aunts and uncles and even though he was an only child, they were a very close extended family and I liked that. I felt a part of something, I guess."

Ruth thinks that her problems in maintaining close relationships with women are due to her mother's early death.

> I've had some very warm and close relationships with men and women, but I've also lost close friends. Just stopped being friends. And I haven't really been able to sort that out, whether it has anything to do with my mother dying. None of these women have been motherless. I don't know very many motherless women.

Long-term impact. When asked about the impact of her mother's death, Ruth says,

> I'm amazed that it has made me stronger and more independent. I think a big influence on my life has been that I don't take people for granted. I never go to bed at night without telling my children I love them. It helps you get your priorities in order when you lose someone at an early age. I don't need very much to make me happy. I take happiness in my children's happiness, and in the company of friends. I really enjoy simplicity.

Ruth also talks about missing having someone to talk to about the "girly things," such as "decorating and cooking and shopping and clothes and things like that. It was difficult when my children were born not to have somebody close that I could ask questions."

Ruth tries to imagine what her mother would be like had she lived.

> A difficult thing for those of us who lose our mothers early is not having that picture of what it's like to grow old. I don't know what my mother would have looked like with gray hair, or at what age she might have gone through menopause. I'll be store shopping and I'll see women my age who are in the company of older women who are obviously their mothers, and there's such give-and-take between them. It's sometimes a little feisty. But you can tell it's a mother and a daughter. There's just some kind of bond that I envy them for. It isn't necessarily the things like Mother's Day and Christmas and graduations. It's not that so much as it is the simple things that I miss, like calling your mother up and asking her how to prepare pickled eggs. I really feel a void there.

Risk.

> It certainly makes me feel very responsible about my own health and I take very good care [of myself], making sure I have checkups and annual [mammograms] and whatever. Mainly because I want to be around for my children and my grandchildren. If I had a daughter, I think I might be even more religious about my health. People don't realize how precious life is and how precious people are. Knowing that everything can be taken away from you so quickly, I treasure every single day and every single moment.

At the time she was interviewed, Ruth had passed the age at which her mother died.

> I guess growing older myself, and perhaps passing the age that she was when she died, I don't have a fatalistic attitude, but I sort of feel as if, if I was struck by a bus, that I've had a very good life. I wouldn't have any regrets that I had left some things undone. I think that if you live each day to the best that you can, that's all you can really achieve. It doesn't matter how many days you get on Earth. It doesn't matter if you're successful and wealthy and whatever. Your happiness is the most important thing. The hard thing about dying, I believe, is the people that you leave behind. It's much harder for them than it is for you. Your life is complete at that point.

Current situation. Ruth was fifty-two at the time of the interview. She had recently completed college, and worked in journalism. She was divorced, with two grown children. Ruth is an active volunteer in her community, and has participated in a breast cancer support group.

After Ruth's stepmother died, she and her brother immediately attempted to reconnect with their father. During a couple of vacations with her father, Ruth saw a very different side of him.

> I really got to know the man much more intimately. He was very absorbed in his need to find another companion. He more or less used my brother and me to help him with his social life. I don't have the same thoughts that I used to about my stepmother. The estrangement that existed while he was married to her wasn't necessarily all her doing. It was his choice.

Holly (age at mother's breast cancer diagnosis: 16;
age at time of mother's death: 19)

Background. Holly's parents were Holocaust survivors, as were her aunt and uncle. Holly and her older brother (by three-and-a-half years) lived with both parents in an Orthodox Jewish home. Her father was ill for a long time, and he died when she was eleven. Holly remembers feeling

> very scared about the future, about our financial stability. There's a sense that this rug has been pulled out from under you. I think that every kid who loses a parent worries about the subsequent loss of the other parent.

After that, her mother started working. Holly describes her mother as an "independent person—feisty—a "pistol."

Her aunt and uncle [father's brother] lived nearby. "They were European and they survived the Holocaust. They were in concentration camps. Their life was very different." Holly says that her older brother was allowed to study and excel, while she had more responsibilities in the home. "Like I couldn't make their lives more difficult, because their lives had been so difficult already. I had to be good."

Experience of mother's illness. When Holly was sixteen her mother found a lump. "I remember her saying that she felt something." Holly thinks now that her mother may have waited for some time before having the lump checked out. "Two months, or three months, or even up to six months could have made a difference." Holly does remember her mother telling her that it was cancer. "I was scared. But I think that there was a part of me that was hopeful. 'All right, she's going to go have this surgery and it's going to take care of the problem and then we'll go back to normal.'"

Mother did return to normal after her mastectomy, and Holly started at a local college two years later, as a commuting student. "I remember thinking, *Well, five years is the magic number, and she's gonna make it to five years and everything will be fine.*"

When Holly was a college sophomore, her mother noticed a swelling in her abdomen.

> She was a very small woman, and thin, and she just started having this big stomach. Her cancer had metastasized to her liver. That was pretty much the death sentence, knowing that it was the liver. I remember feeling like, *How could this be?* She was doing so well. Maybe that was her hiding from me. I don't really know, but I remember thinking, *My goodness. How could somebody be well one day and then be deathly ill the next?* And then the decline was pretty dramatic from that point on.

From the recurrence to her mother's death four months later, Holly became her mother's primary caregiver.

> It became hard for her to breathe, so they were draining the fluid. She was also getting some other kind of radiation treatment. She was pretty sick from that, and weak. She had to stop working, and became progressively more housebound, and then, kind of tied to the bed. I remember changing dressings, and doing stuff I never thought I'd be doing, certainly not at that point in my life. Just getting stuck with a lot of stuff. Obviously, her appearance changed. She lost a lot of weight. Became skeletal. Hair loss. It probably wasn't as startling for me as it was for somebody else coming in, but clearly, it was difficult to see those changes.

During this period, Holly continued at college as a commuting student. Her aunt cared for her mother while Holly was at school.

> That was a tough time. My brother, who is older chronologically, was out of town [in graduate school], and he wasn't really that involved with the caregiving, so my aunt was doing a lot. He was emotionally kind of distancing himself from things so I was dealing with all the day-to-day care, along with all the emotional stuff. So there was a feeling of resentment. I'm sure there was anger, and probably a little guilt. My feeling was, "Hey, wait a minute!"

As Holly cared for her mother, she noticed that their relationship changed.

> When she was no longer completely self-sufficient, there was almost a role reversal. I became more of the caretaker. I don't think she liked it much at all. She was by nature a very independent person, and I think this was really tough on her.

The family did not openly discuss the impending death.

> I don't think we talked that much about how it was going to be if she died. I don't think that enough was brought out in the open and discussed. So that was difficult. I have a lot of loose ends.

They had a caseworker to help out toward the end.

> We were working through this agency that was supposed to be helping us. They assigned her a caseworker. I'm not really sure if she was supposed to be helping emotionally, but she was absolutely useless. I was kind of hoping for someone who could help us get through this crisis, and we didn't get that kind of help.

Shortly before her mother's death, the doctor "just kind of went like this [gesture of hopelessness]. She went to the hospital on a Friday evening and she died on the Sabbath." Holly was not with her mother at the time because she did not drive on the Sabbath.

> I did speak to her on the phone and she sounded good. She sounded stronger, positive, and not like someone who was on their last leg. That was the last conversation we had. It was like she mustered up all of her energy. When the call came, it struck me: *How could this be?* Because she [had] sounded so good.

Experience following mother's death. The period after her mother died was a very difficult one for Holly. Her major source of support was her boyfriend, who later became her husband.

> I probably did a lot of crying. My boyfriend at the time got to deal with a lot of my emotional reaction. He was probably the biggest support. There were a couple of friends. It wasn't quite enough but it did help. I don't think there were too many people that I talked about it with because it's an issue that makes people uncomfortable. When somebody starts to squirm, it's like, "Better not talk about this."

Because her father died when she was young, at age nineteen, Holly was an orphan.

> It's hard enough to lose one parent, but then to be left with no parent. When it happened to me the second time, I knew I just had to pick up and move on. Do what I had to do. Make the best of it. In some ways it was a whole lot scarier the second time around. It's almost like there was something inside

pulling me along. I would have to find a job, or quit school, or stop going full-time. In my head I thought, *I have to either pull it together or lose it completely.* So I just fortified myself with the knowledge that I was capable of doing it. Maybe that was a piece of my mother in me. I considered briefly trying to stay in the house by myself, but everybody said, "You can't do that!" So I had to close the house down. Basically, I did that myself. Got the house up for sale. Packed up the house. When I wasn't working or doing whatever I had to do for school, I was back at the house, closing things down. That was hard because I was putting away my former life.

Holly moved in with her aunt and uncle, but this proved even more stressful, and after one semester, Holly obtained financial support from her college which allowed her to live on campus and enroll full-time. At school, Holly found herself in a different place than other students.

My whole attitude about college was a little different. Here I'd had this experience that most of the people around me were not having to deal with. It was difficult. There were some feelings of isolation. But when I moved onto campus, that was really a positive thing in terms of integrating me more into college life, and helping those feelings of isolation disappear.

Religious rituals were of little help to Holly.

As far as rituals go, obviously the funeral was very difficult. In the Jewish tradition, there are certain times of the year when one might go to visit the grave, but I found it difficult. It's just not something I relate to. It's more of a formality. On the year anniversary, we light a memorial candle. When I do that, it's much more symbolic. It helped.

Religion played an important role in Holly's adjustment to losing her mother.

I became more religious. I became more ritual oriented because I needed to find something that could help me pull things together, and it gave structure and some kind of connection. I became stricter in observing the Sabbath, for example. I think if I hadn't done that, the complete and total other end of the spectrum might have been the result. How could God let something like this happen? Here I am and I have nobody. I just didn't feel like I could do that. My mother had come from a very religious family in Europe. For both of them, it was very much a part of who they were. I had the motivation for not going in the opposite direction, that, "How could I do this to their memory?" To toss it out the window would have dishonored their memory. It would have made all of what they went through seem so wasted and futile.

Long-term impact. Holly feels one effect of this loss on her personality is a strong sense of independence. "When we have a family crisis, it's hard for me to say to somebody, 'I need you to help me do such-and-such.' But also, we don't have that many people available to us. So it's partially out of necessity." Holly now puts a "heavy emphasis on family and children, 'cause that's what really counts."

Risk. Holly sometimes worries about her risk of breast cancer but

> I find myself on occasion thinking, *Wow. I just had another birthday. I'm that much closer.* It's like the clock ticking. So there's an element of that. But I also know intellectually that my lifestyle is different. There are enough other things that are different about the way I've lived that might impact me in a positive way.

Holly has great difficulty doing breast self-exams.

> I'm not saying I couldn't learn how to do it. I'm just not able to do a breast exam. I'm sure that every place I touch, there's a lump. I try to be at least diligent about getting my annual exam, and I have been getting yearly mammograms since I was thirty-eight. The first time I went, I needed someone to go with me. I was shaking and everything. I was just a wreck. Now I'm more laid back. I'm still not where I need to be, though.

Holly participated in a support group for women at high risk for breast cancer, where she encountered other women who had difficulty doing the self-exam. Holly faults medical professionals for not being more understanding and providing more help with this exam.

> The doctor I had was a male, and he was the first person who validated my feelings. "I understand what you're saying. Why you're having so much difficulty with this." I appreciated that approach. But he didn't take it a step further and say, "Let me show you how."

Her new physician, a woman, has

> taken the time to show me how to do it. Used her fingers and her hands and then had me do it. It was helpful, and I tried it a little bit shortly after that. But you know, standing in the shower, actively doing the manipulation to see if there's something there. [With the mammogram] I'm taking action but I am somewhat passive in my action. My physician is actively taking control of the discovery. I don't think this is rational.

Holly is aware of genetic testing, and expressed concern about "how this will affect the health insurance piece of it if you have the gene." She also is aware of the difficulty in interpreting the results.

> Is it 1 percent or 10 percent of the women who carry the gene? It is a relatively small percentage. The fact that you carry the gene means you have a higher risk, but it doesn't necessarily mean you're going to get it. The fact that you don't carry the gene means you're not at higher risk, but it doesn't mean that you won't get it either. In terms of prevention, you could do some of these things and they wouldn't make a difference. It's kind of a crapshoot. Now, researchers are showing that maybe there isn't a good con-

nection between the fat intake and breast cancer, which was the big thing. Make up your mind. Take your pick. They jerk you one way and then they jerk you another way. This woman had a T-shirt that said "Eat carefully, exercise, die anyway!" So it seems like no matter what you do . . .

Current situation. Holly was forty-two at the time of the interview. She was married with two young children, and works as a librarian. Looking back on her life, Holly is sorry that she did not have bereavement counseling after her mother's death. Also, she wishes that family counseling had been available to help her reconcile with her brother. "I find myself now . . . I'm at the age . . . It's been a very strange thing to be watching my friends go through what I went through a long time ago."

Sally (age at mother's breast cancer diagnosis: 19; age at time of mother's death: 20)

Background. Sally was the youngest in a large African-American family of six siblings, with four sisters and one brother. She says,

> I pretty much stayed stuck under my mother being as I was the baby. We had a pretty good relationship together for a mother and daughter. It seemed like we was more sisters than mother and daughter. We went everywhere together, and did mostly everything together. She was there for me when I had my first two children.

Although Sally was married and had two children, she still lived with her mother, as did all of her siblings except one sister. When Sally was seventeen, her aunt died from breast cancer. "She had breast cancer in her right breast and before she passed away, she had caught pneumonia and it took her away real quick." Sally had completed eleventh grade, and was attending nursing school.

Experience of mother's illness. When Sally was nineteen, her mother noticed a lump near her underarm. Sally was in the room at the time, and remembers that "she really didn't pay it any mind because she thought maybe it came from her deodorant." Her mother ignored the lump, but

> as the months progressed, she noticed that the lump had come back again. She got worried and went to the clinic. She never received a mammogram from the clinic, and she went to Planned Parenthood, and that's when she found out that she had breast cancer.

Sally remembers how her mother told the children.

> She pulled us all together. We was all sitting downstairs in the living room, and she told us that she had something to tell us and she didn't want us to get upset about it. That's when she told us that she had breast cancer. Of course, everybody got upset and started crying and didn't want to accept the fact that she had it. Everybody was in denial for a while.

About her own feelings, Sally said,

> I felt sad because, as a child, I always thought I was gonna have my mother forever. Never thought that my mother could get sick. The day she told us that she had breast cancer, it just seemed like my whole life just ended at one time.

Sally's mother was treated with chemotherapy for about a year. She had to be hospitalized at one point because her "blood cells was real low" and later, she was hospitalized for pneumonia. Sally stopped going to school the day she learned of her mother's diagnosis, so that she could be with her mother. Sally was the primary caregiver, taking her mother to chemotherapy appointments, and visiting in the hospital. "I was always there with her." Sally describes this period as

> very hard. It was hard seeing my mother suffering the way she was. She was a good lady and it seemed like she shouldn't have been the one that was going through it. I kept asking God, "Why her? Why not me?" It was painful for a long time.

After her hospitalization, Sally's mother moved in with her oldest sister. "One week after she had just got out of the hospital, she was doing fine. She was walking around and going outside to the store, you know, her daily routine." Then suddenly, her mother took a turn for the worse.

> Then that following week, she had got real sick. I guess the cancer had got up in her throat. Me and her always was together, and I was the baby girl, and she didn't even know who I was no more. That was a hurting feeling. That was a hurting feeling.

Her mother's nurse came to Sally's sister's house and "she gave my mother six months." However, at the end of the same week, "she didn't expect for our mother to make it through the weekend." Her mother died that same day. "She passed so quick. It was quick. It seemed like she had waited for my brother to come home before she decided to leave, and she passed away."

Sally's major supporter during her mother's illness was her husband. "My husband, he was pretty much understanding what I was going through. He had just lost his mother the year before. So he knew what I was going through."

Experience following mother's death. Sally's mother's death was a major crisis for the family.

> It was terrible. It seemed like a dark cloud just came over our family. Everybody just went crazy. Just crying, didn't want to accept the fact. When the funeral directors came to get her, we didn't want to let them take her away. We kept telling them that she wasn't dead. She was just resting. We just couldn't take it.

Sally had a difficult time explaining her mother's death to her daughter, who was three years old.

> I told my daughter, and she was like, "Where's Grandma?" I said, "Grandma's gone." She says, "Is Grandma coming back?" And I said, "No." She was like, "What happened to Grandma?" And she kept asking me over and over again, "Will she ever come back?"

After the funeral, Sally's oldest sister arranged a group counseling session for the family.

> We supposed to have had an appointment for group counseling. We had an appointment after the funeral and didn't nobody keep it. I guess because everybody just felt as though they didn't want to talk about it right then and there.

Sally feels that her personality changed drastically as a result of her mother's illness and death.

> Before my mother got sick, I was the nicest person in the world. Now I'm just evil. I don't cut nobody no slack. I just yell and just fuss at people all the time. Once I found out my mother had got sick and before she passed away, I just totally changed. I just started being real evil and mean to people.

Other changes have occurred in Sally's life since her mother's death.

> It seemed like I knew that I wasn't gonna have my mother anymore. Now it was time for me to get out on my own. It was time for me to get out and start taking care of my own family and everything.

Sally did not continue with school. "Things wasn't the way I planned for things to be. Things just seemed like, once I found out my mother got sick, my life just started going downhill. Downhill completely."

Long-term impact. Sally does perform some grieving rituals.

> I go to the cemetery and put flowers on her grave if I can get a ride. I just sit there and talk to her. I don't want to be going to the cemetery 'cause I just can't stand talking to the ground instead of talking to her face to face.

Sometimes her whole family visits her mother's grave. Mother's Day, birthdays, and holidays are particularly difficult, "because I be expecting to see her and expecting to go to the house and give her stuff." The family has not been able to discuss the loss of Sally's mother. "Every time me and my sister get to talking about my mother, she get up and she'll walk away and get to crying, and I'll just be sitting somewhere just looking crazy."

Sally continues to be depressed, four years after her mother's death.

> See, it's like really still basically the same. Still with the crying and everything. Still thinking about some of the things that we went through with her. Some of the things she went through. Things will probably pretty much be the same *forever*. 'Cause seem like when my mother passed away, a part of my life was just taken from me for no apparent reason. It was just snatched away and it's not coming back. So I'll probably pretty much have the same emotions and the same feelings for the rest of my life.

Risk. Sally has talked about breast cancer risk with her oldest sister.

> She was telling me that she can also be a candidate for having breast cancer being as she's the oldest child. She said she haven't went to the hospital yet to get her mammogram to make sure that she didn't have it. And I was just thinking to myself, I just couldn't take it, not another family member going through the same thing that my mother went through.

Sally tries to learn about breast cancer, reading brochures and watching television programs, but this is difficult for her.

> I'm basically always trying to read up on it and I watched a program on it the other day about these women talking about they had breast cancer, and it just made me so upset. I just turned the TV off.

Current situation. Sally was twenty-three at the time of the interview. She was unemployed, and regretted that she had dropped out of school in the eleventh grade. Sally is married and now has five children.

She said she was interested in grief counseling.

> We need to find us another counselor so we can bring our children so they can have a better understanding about how their grandmother passed away and what was the reason why she passed away. I do think we need to all just stop acting so crazy and just go find a counselor and find somebody to really talk to.

*Linda (age at mother's breast cancer diagnosis: 18;
age at time of mother's death: 22)*

Background. Linda lived with her parents and an older brother in a Jewish neighborhood. Her father ran a small grocery store, while her mother stayed home to care for her home and children. Linda's father was very strict; Linda and her mother became especially close, often banding together to deal with his endless restrictions. In some ways, Linda's mother was more like a best friend than a mother.

Experience of mother's illness. The summer before she was to enter college, Linda's mother went in for a breast biopsy, and came out with a mastectomy. She had had the "one-step" procedure. Linda remembers hearing the doctor after the operation tell her father that the cancer was already in the glands. She had never heard the word *cancer* before. "Nobody talked about cancer. It was a terrible word, and you just didn't say it." She remembers, too, the "look of devastation" on her mother's face as she awoke from her operation and realized that she had had a mastectomy. After the operation, Linda's mother would no longer let Linda see her naked. For the first time, she turned her back when she was dressing. When Linda did see her mother's scar, "it was very scary. Her whole chest was concaved in. And she wasn't dealing with it. I knew that it scared her."

Linda did not want to go to college, but her father expected her to go, so she went. Once there, she had difficulty adjusting to being away from her mother, and she found herself constantly worrying. She wanted to call her mother to ask if she was all right, but her father had strictly limited the number of calls she could make, because of the expense. One day her father called and told Linda that she needed to come home to get a gamma globulin shot, which would strengthen her immune system. She still remembers riding the bus home, rain pouring down, feeling overwhelmed with sadness, loneliness, and worry. Linda did not do well at college. She dropped out after her second year, returned to live at home, and got a job. Four years after the original diagnosis, her mother began to have stomach pain. During exploratory surgery, the doctors found that the cancer had spread. Linda's mother was never told. She was told that she would be better soon. Linda's father told her, but insisted that the news be kept a secret from her mother.

When Linda's mother came home from the hospital, Linda became the primary caregiver. She learned to give her mother morphine shots. This period was very difficult for Linda, because not only was she losing her mother, but she could not be honest with her. Instead, she had to pretend that her mother would soon be better. She was forced to hide her true feelings. When her mother said, "I am getting better, aren't I?" she had to smile and say yes. She often had to run out of the room to hide her tears. This period also was difficult because her mother was in a lot of pain.

> Her room was right next to mine. I used to lay in bed and I would hear her moaning. I remember running to the basement to sleep because I couldn't stand to hear it anymore. In that house, the walls were breathing in pain. Sometimes I wanted to take a pillow and put it over her head. I just have these memories of her suffering.

Although the period before her mother's death was difficult for Linda, she is grateful to her father for hiring nurses so that her mother did not have to die in a hospital.

> It was good because I got to be with her as much as I chose to be. I would hope that it helped her that we went through it with her. I know she was comfortable. It's comforting to me that at least she was safe when she died.

Experience following mother's death. After her mother's death, Linda took on many of her roles. Even at the shiva (Jewish mourning period) she was busy preparing food, and therefore was not able to mourn. She took on the responsibility of caring for her father, making his lunches and doing the housework. Linda's father started dating very soon after her mother's death. She felt bitter and angry as she found herself taking care of some new clothes her father bought to wear on his dates.

Linda's father remarried a year and a half after his wife's death, and shortly afterward, Linda got married to a man she had known for many years. Soon, Linda was pregnant. She missed her mother when the baby was born, and after, when she did not have a "grandmother" to help her or to spoil her children. Linda never became close to her stepmother, but helped both her father and stepmother when they became ill later in life. Both died about six years after Linda's mother's death.

Linda had little opportunity to grieve after her mother died. "Her life ended, and I thought my life ended too." Linda saw a psychiatrist after her mother's death, but did not find his approach helpful. She then joined a transactional analysis group, and enjoyed the sense of connection it gave her. She has since gone to a number of psychics, attempting to make a connection with her mother's spirit. She feels that two of these people were able to make contact, and says that those were very good experiences.

Long-term impact. Linda has always felt different from other women, and is sometimes jealous when she sees them with their mothers. She often feels alone. "I'm no one's child. It's just that when your mother goes, you're alone, and that's it. Whether you have a husband, whether you have children, you're alone." She says that she does not dwell on these feelings, and that she has learned to be independent and strong due to losing her mother at a young age. Linda is always the "strong one" in her family. "I sometimes wonder where I get this strength." She also feels that her mother's death "took a lot of the fun out of my life," and is glad her husband is able to fool around and be playful with her children—something she cannot do easily.

When Hope Edelman's book on motherless daughters came out, Linda immediately bought a copy. "I was working out at the gym. I couldn't read it there, because I opened it up and started reading it and the tears were just streaming down my face." Linda realized that she had repressed a lot of feelings about her mother.

When Linda got a small dog for her children, she found that she benefited in ways she never imagined.

> I should have had a dog sooner, because of what this dog has done for all of us. It's just an unconditional love that's always there. You come home and its there. She's a dog that just loves you and you're not alone. It's very

> nice. . . . It's really weird but I think there is part of my mother in her. It's ridiculous, but this animal will give love to me all the time and never ask me for any back; and that's what my mother would do.

Risk. For many years, Linda was under the care of her mother's doctor, in whom she trusted completely.

> He was a god to me, and that's why when I had a lump removed, I was not a mess because he said to me, "I'm ninety-nine percent sure this is fine and I don't want you to worry about it."

Linda went to this doctor for breast exams every four months since she was eighteen. "I was devastated when he retired."

When Linda's new doctor recommended that she go on birth control pills, she researched the subject and decided not to. Linda has tried to get the best breast surveillance available, but she was frustrated when her doctor told her that she would have to wait about two weeks to have a biopsy if a lump was found. She felt that psychologically, a two-week wait would be very difficult for her. "He's the top guy in the world and he's so insensitive."

Linda has mammograms annually, but she stopped having frequent clinical breast exams. Nor does she do breast self-exams. "I can't tell what I'm feeling. It all feels the same. So I don't. I have done it but I can't tell, so I'm finished. It's out of my hands." When her health maintenance organization (HMO) would not pay for a radiologist to examine the mammogram right away, Linda arranged to have her test somewhere else, and paid for it herself. Although she has decreased her surveillance, Linda is confident that she will detect any breast cancer early. "As much as I think that I'm gonna get breast cancer, I also think that I'm gonna be early enough to catch it."

Linda initially was interested in genetic testing. However, she attended an educational seminar and decided that the risks (loss of insurance, confidentiality) outweighed any potential benefits.

> I am curious, and it would be something that I want to know, because the kind of person I am, I could handle it. But nothing is absolutely confidential. Anybody can get into anybody's records. And then, what if I had the gene, what would I do? More examinations? Have a double mastectomy? I'm not interested now.

Current situation. At the time of the interview, Linda was forty-seven. She and her husband ran a small business together. It was important to her to be home with her children. Linda's husband, who she described as a "workaholic," recently had a heart attack. Linda continues to feel isolated and alone—an outsider in other people's families. "The recurrent theme for me, without a mother, you've got this loneliness. There's just a void."

Linda was approaching the age her mother was at diagnosis. Her daughter was in her first year of college—as Linda was at the time of her mother's mastectomy. Linda's greatest fear is not being alive when her daughter has her own children. "I don't want her to go through that with having a baby and not having me around. That scares me more than the thought of getting breast cancer."

*Nancy (age at mother's breast cancer diagnosis: 15;
age at time of mother's death: 25)*

Background. Nancy was the oldest in a Jewish family with two daughters. She was close to her grandmother (mother's mother), and to an aunt and uncle (mother's brother) and her cousins, who lived nearby. Nancy's mother had a number of health problems while Nancy was growing up, and although they were not serious, they made Nancy and her sister more independent than other children their age. Nancy and her mother had a good mother-daughter relationship, but Nancy relied on her mother more for practical advice or help than for help with personal problems. "She just had difficulty communicating with us on that level. As I became older, I relied on her less for the deeper teenage kind of problems." Nancy explains that when confronted with a problem, her mother was more likely to give simple advice than to talk through a complex issue through with her children. Both Nancy and her sister were "good kids," and neither used drugs or alcohol or had trouble with school as teens.

Experience of mother's illness. Nancy came home from school one day when she was fifteen and found her mother

> sitting in her room—my parents' bedroom—and she was just sitting there and she was crying. I went up to her, and I said, "What's wrong?" And she didn't tell me and I think I left her alone.

Nancy says that in her family it was normal to leave someone alone if they were feeling bad. "It wasn't always the right solution, but that's the solution we [had]." When Nancy's father came home, she asked him not to tell her what her mother's problem was, but to write it down instead.

> I was hoping that he'd write down some really long, medical, technical thing that I wouldn't be able to figure out. And I remember opening it [father's note] and reading it, and all he had written was CANCER. I was mad at him because he had made it so easy for me to understand. Really, since that point, with a few isolated exceptions, almost every communication about the cancer was through my dad.

At first, Nancy's mother cried a lot. She had a mastectomy and chemotherapy. "I remember we were all flabbergasted because we were expecting her hair to fall out and things to happen after her chemo treatments, and none of that happened. She bought a wig and it stayed in the corner."

Nancy's father took responsibility for managing her mother's medical care, taking her to appointments, and informing the girls on how she was doing. "My father was the one that gave us the updates. He wasn't very technical. He'd be like, 'Your mom's doing a little better.' Or, 'Your mom's doing a little worse.'"

After her treatments, Nancy's mother returned to work. "For the first five years, it was fine. She went back to work. She did okay." Nancy entered a nearby college and later went on to law school in another state. "At that five-and-a-half-year mark is when it came back. Then things kind of snowballed downhill. We had ups and downs. Eventually, my mother quit her job." The period after her mother's recurrence was very difficult. Nancy's mother went through a period when she was not sleeping well.

> She was very upset and she would sleep during the day and cry during the night. Everybody was getting irritable because you'd hear crying at three o'clock in the morning, and you'd have to get up the next day for school or work. Everybody was mad at everybody.

While Nancy was in law school, she was out of town—except during the summers—so her younger sister was affected more than she was.

> A lot of that time I was away. I was in college. I was in law school. [Sister's name] was there and it was 100 percent harder on her than it was on me. I would come home and I'd deal with it all at once, but she dealt with it on a daily basis.

Nancy feels she is being "nasty" or disloyal when she says that her mother's personality was not changed by her illness, and that this made life difficult for the family.

> TV movies and such, I think are very off base. Because it [cancer] didn't change her. It just kind of reflected her personality. She became very self-absorbed. I mean, like, "I'm sick and you don't know what I'm going through." It was very difficult sometimes to deal with her twenty-four hours a day. I have to give my father a lot of credit because she became very dependent on him. He would take off during the week so he could go with her to the doctors, and then when he went to work overtime to make money, she would get mad at him. I understand that I wouldn't want to be left alone either, but it was just very difficult to feel bad around her. Our reaction [to her] was sometimes very nasty, verbally.

One day, Nancy's father called her at school. "I remember him saying, 'Things don't look good. We're concerned. You might to have to come home.'" Her mother had a second round of chemotherapy, and this time she lost her hair.

> She started losing weight and she got very depressed. She started seeing a psychologist or a psychiatrist. I think that helped her to a certain extent. At some point, she kind of mellowed out a little bit and things got a little easier.

One of Nancy's memories is from her law school graduation, four years after her mother's recurrence. Nancy was talking with a friend about where their families were going for dinner, and found that they had both chosen restaurants very close to the campus. Nancy learned that her friend's mother had Parkinson's disease, and Nancy then shared that her mother had cancer.

> It was one of those things where it was this instant simpatico. So we just looked at each other and we were like, "So, for the past three years we could have been talking about this or at least sharing certain experiences."

After graduation, Nancy moved back to her hometown to be closer to the family. "I felt a little guilty that I hadn't borne my share of the burden. I felt my sister had been here through most of it. My father was certainly here through all of it. And I wasn't." After passing the Bar exam, Nancy took a job at a law firm. She did not share information about her mother's illness with her colleagues, but she told the secretary, so that she would understand why Nancy got so many phone calls from her father. Her mother had a bone marrow transplant, and when this was not successful, she entered a hospice.

Before her mother died, Nancy had an opportunity for some meaningful conversations with her. She particularly remembers one of these. "It was like one of the only times I think we actually had a heart-to-heart. I had a chance to go over some of the really fun [family] stories." As she approached death, many family members came to visit Nancy's mother, including her siblings, nieces, and nephews. The day her mother died, Nancy's father called the law firm, and the secretary took Nancy out of a meeting to give her the news.

Experience following mother's death. Before mother's death, Nancy had given a friend a list of the phone numbers of her friends. Many friends came to the funeral and supported Nancy. Even so, Nancy felt somewhat lost after her mother's death.

> I feel like I've lost an arm in a sense. Not only did I lose my mom, and that's a big thing, but all the doctor's appointments, it was a part of my life. And it was a huge part of my dad's life. I always had to remember that or check on that or call to find out what was going on, and the fact that that's not there anymore is taking some adjustment. It was just part of my day, and it was part of who we were as a family.

Nancy expects her wedding day to be difficult without her mother, and she regrets that her mother never got to be a grandmother.

Nancy's interview was fairly soon after her mother's death, and she and her family were experiencing the first holidays without her.

> Her birthday came, and my sister and my father and I were actually all together that day, but we didn't talk about it. I felt kind of strange that we didn't bring it up. But I didn't want to ask, "What are we going to do?" and be really morbid. So I didn't, and it was uncomfortable. I'm hoping I can address it better next year.

She was more satisfied with their Thanksgiving celebration; they had a small dinner and spent all day cooking together. "My dad said something, you know, sentimental, and then we ate and it was really nice." On New Year's Eve, Nancy wanted to go to a party, but was concerned about what her father would do. "He went to visit family, and the next day, he went to an event at the hospice. So it turned out fine."

Nancy and her sister are each other's main sources of support. "If something were to happen and it was the middle of the night, she would call me in a second. And I would do the same for her. We're very close." Nancy also has used the bereavement support services of the hospice, as has her father. "I was invited to go to some of the group counseling things, but I don't think that's for me. The times when I really break down and need someone to talk to are, like, four o'clock in the morning."

Nancy's father recently started dating.

> He's trying to find things to do twenty-four hours a day. He joined a couple of museums. He started dating [laughs], which doesn't thrill me. Not so much because I think it's too soon, but I'm just concerned that he's jumping without looking. Like he has a master list: "Here are eighteen things I should be doing in the next couple of years." The counselor at the hospice said to me that she thought he genuinely missed my mother; missed coming home and talking to her or calling her on the phone in the middle of the day. That hadn't occurred to me because that hadn't happened in a couple of years. That was the old mom. And I think she was right. But I do think we're all still in an adjustment period.

Long-term impact. Since the interviews were conducted soon after Nancy's mother's death, it was too early to assess long-term impact. However, Nancy emphasized that the fact that her mother was ill for such a long time period had a major effect on her.

> It was such a large part of my life. I think that the fact that it was such a long period of time probably shaped me in ways that I don't see right now. But it had a stronger impact on me than if it were to have happened in a short period of time.

Nancy also recognized that the long period of illness had some positive aspects. "I got a chance to go over some of the really fun stories before she got very sick. So there was some closure."

Risk. Nancy has not given a lot of thought to her own risk of breast cancer. She mentioned her mother's illness to her physician, and he did not make any recommendations. "I'm just twenty-five. When I start hitting late thirties, early forties, I'm going to be . . . 'Let's go for a mammogram every year.'" She has not changed her diet or other health behaviors.

> It's not like I have a death wish, and it's not like I think I'm immune. It's just that I'm of the generation that is so jaded by this managed care system that I don't want to deal with it. Like, I'll go to the doctor when I don't feel well, is my attitude. I know that's not a good one, but I'm just not past that yet.

Current situation. At the time of the interviews, Nancy was twenty-five. (The study took place within a year of her mother's death.) Nancy mentioned that she is often upset by how illness is portrayed in movies and on TV.

> They always present the person who has an illness as this person who goes out of their way to be selfless to everybody else and that kind of thing. And that was not my experience. Now I'm more aware of the impact that it can have on a family. It was not just the fact that your mother died, but how she coped with the illness, which, in my case, I don't think was very good. It kind of permeated everybody's life. Which also wasn't very good. But then, we are still standing, which is pretty good.

Cheryl (age at mother's breast cancer diagnosis: 19; age at time of mother's death: 25)

Background. Cheryl was the older of two children. Her mother was very active in the church, and encouraged her children to be involved in community service. She shielded the children from the fact that their father was an alcoholic. During Cheryl's freshman year at a nearby college, her mother came to tell her that she and Cheryl's father were separating.

Experience of mother's illness. The next year, Cheryl was home from school on a break when her mother told her she had discovered a lump. Her mother said it had been caught early, and that she would beat it. Cheryl did not realize how serious the disease could be. "I tried not to worry about it, because at that point, I really didn't know anybody else who had ever been in that situation before." Her mother had a very positive attitude. Cancer did not slow her down. After losing her hair in chemotherapy treatment, her mother would come to her softball games with "that little duck hair that came up."

Her mother's treatment was not discussed at the time, but Cheryl now knows from reading her medical records that her mother had a partial mastectomy, radiation, and chemotherapy. During the three years after Cheryl graduated from college, she and her mother were fairly estranged. Her mother remarried someone Cheryl did not get along with, and her mother did not approve of Cheryl's boyfriend, who later became her husband. "We just didn't have the same relationship that we had earlier."

During this time, Cheryl's grandparents told her that her mother was having headaches. Thinking that it was not serious, Cheryl sent her mother a poster that said THINK POSITIVE. Her mother went to the hospital for some tests, and learned that the cancer had returned. At that point, Cheryl moved to be closer to her mother and took a job working with her father so that she would have the flexibility to provide the needed care. Cheryl and her mother became closer than ever before.

Cheryl was frightened, and tried to hope for the best. She did not have people to talk to, since neither her husband nor her friends had had a similar experience. Her grandparents visited every week, but did not want to talk about the emotional aspects, or about the possibility of death. Her mother was in and out of the hospital for about four months. Cheryl's new stepfather was not very helpful during the illness. During that period, Cheryl became a companion and an advocate, making sure her mother was properly cared for and also that the physician treated her as a person. Her mother could no longer work, and she began to worry that she would lose her house. Cheryl began making her mother's house payments. Cheryl also set up a trust so that she and her brother could take ownership of the house. Cheryl cared for her mother's pets—a beagle and several cats.

The cancer eventually metastasized to her mother's brain. She began treatment. When the treatments were no longer effective, the doctor told Cheryl her mother would live for about two weeks. In fact, she lived for a couple of months. "She was willing to try any type of treatment, but, if that [death] was the outcome, she wasn't afraid of that. She had a very strong faith."

Remembering the end of her mother's life, Cheryl comments,

> Some good things came out of it. This forces you to deal with each other on a level that's not superficial, but to confront really how you feel about a lot of different things. Everything from death to religion to relationships. It was not a time that I would choose to relive, although my grandmother would say that it builds character.

In the end, her mother returned home, and Cheryl arranged for a home care service to help her. She talked with her mother about where she wanted to die.

Three days before her death, Cheryl's mother began to have hallucinations. When she could no longer be cared for at home, Cheryl took her back to the hospital. Her mother took the sacrament, and slept a lot. Although

Cheryl tried to be with her mother as much as she could, she was not there at the time of her death. When she got to the hospital, she saw her mother's body being closed into a body bag. This was very upsetting for Cheryl. "That's the one thing that I wish I hadn't seen. Because that's something that sort of sticks in your mind for a long time."

Experience following mother's death. Cheryl's stepfather made the funeral arrangements. Although Cheryl would have preferred a more informal, uplifting service than he provided, she did not get overly upset about it. At the funeral, she was more worried about her grandparents and their being able to handle the loss than her own needs. Her mother was cremated, as she had requested. Cheryl was the only one who attended the burial of the ashes, and she was left with the bill for her mother's funeral expenses.

Immediately after her mother's death, Cheryl set up a scholarship fund in her memory. Her mother had made tapes for Cheryl and her brother, grandparents, and stepfather. "It was several days after the service before I had the nerve to listen to it. But it's something that I still have and I will certainly be eternally grateful that she made it [crying]." On the tape, her mother told Cheryl how much she loved her, and was proud of her, and she thanked Cheryl for taking such good care of her. She also asked her to stay in touch with her brother, and to take care of her grandparents. Although it is difficult for her to listen to her mother's voice on the tape, Cheryl finds it comforting.

Cheryl needed a long time to get past remembering her mother as a sick person. Only recently has she been able to remember the good times. Cheryl and her grandmother send flowers to the church on the anniversary of her mother's death. She feels especially sad at Christmas, and on her mother's birthday, Mother's Day, and anniversary of her death.

After her mother's death, Cheryl and her husband moved into her house and renovated it. Living in her mother's old neighborhood was difficult for Cheryl, because it triggered many memories of her mother, but at the same time, she enjoyed the sense of connection, and keeping her mother's memory alive.

Cheryl's grandfather had a stroke and has Parkinson's disease as a result, so Cheryl moved to be closer to her grandparents. She helped them maintain their home. She also helped them financially. Cheryl organized a sixtieth wedding anniversary party for them. "Sometimes I feel [as if] I took Mom's place as their daughter."

Long-term impact. Thinking back on her experience, Cheryl reflects,

> You just realize all the sacrifices that she made, and you wish you had that time to get to know her as an adult. It's a time when you can really reflect back and appreciate everything that she has done for you.

Experiencing her mother's death has made Cheryl realize the importance of expressing how she feels toward people. She has trouble sympathizing with people who get upset about trivial things such as getting a flat tire. Also, she has realized that

> you can't go through life just saying yes to everything and to do everything and become close friends to everybody. You can only invest so much in relationships that you have. . . . I'm just not interested in superficial relationships [anymore]. It certainly helped me focus my priorities on who's important to me, and that life is an adventure. You have to recognize that you may not always be here, so appreciate what you have and share that with the people around you, and hopefully leave the world a better place.

Risk. Cheryl's mother was diagnosed with breast cancer at the age of thirty-nine, and Cheryl is in her early thirties. Although she doesn't believe she's "destined" to get breast cancer, she believes she needs to be more knowledgeable about it because of her mother's illness. Cheryl's doctor discovered a small lump around the age her mother was when she was first diagnosed, but it was not cancer. When Cheryl turned thirty, her doctor suggested that she begin annual mammograms. "I guess that the side effects of having mammograms every year would be outweighed by the advantage of finding something early." Cheryl's doctor found another lump during our study. Her doctor thought it was not significant, but Cheryl wanted to be sure.

> So on my own initiative, I made arrangements to see a breast specialist . . . who did a mammogram and a sonogram. It turned out to be nothing. I guess for a woman my age, it is more difficult to detect lumps. I don't have a lot of faith in mammography. For women my age, it's a poor tool. I just find it unacceptable that that's the best diagnostic tool for women!

Current situation. Cheryl was thirty-three at the time of the interview. She was married, had a very responsible job, and also was active in sports and community activities. She continues to carry major caregiving responsibilities for her grandparents. Last year, Cheryl participated in the Race for the Cure, in memory of her mother. She found this to be a profound experience.

> I went by myself. I didn't know what it was going to be like. It was just a great experience. It was so wonderful seeing these ladies in the pink hats, doing great. But on the other hand, there were a lot of people with the cards on their backs that said "in memory of," like me. It was just a strong feeling of sisterhood.

At the final interview, Cheryl was pregnant, and very happy to be starting a family.

Lily (age at mother's breast cancer diagnosis: 20;
age at time of mother's death: 25)

Background. Lily grew up in a divorced family with a younger sister.

> In our family, you always looked to my mother for the emotional [stuff]. My
> father was a weekend dad, and we went on vacations with him, but he was
> not there for the day to day. She [Mom] worked full-time, and she really did
> her best as far as getting involved in our activities—Brownies, Girl Scouts,
> ballet, things like that.

When Lily was nineteen, her mother remarried, and the family moved to her
new stepfather's house. Lily, who had just completed an associate's degree,
got a job and moved into an apartment with a friend.

Experience of mother's illness. Lily's memories of her mother's initial
diagnosis and treatment are blurry. She first heard about her mother's lump
from a phone call she received while at work. Her stepfather told her that the
test results were not good, and that her mother would have to have a mastectomy. Lily remembers feeling "emotional" and "scared." After the surgery,
Lily's mother told her that they got all of the lymph nodes that had cancer in
them, and that that was a good thing. "She showed me her mastectomy scar
once, and it was very upsetting, although she somehow felt better for showing me." Lily's mother lost her hair when she had chemotherapy, and was
very sick. Lily asked many questions, and her mother would say, "Well, I
don't know. They said, 'It's nothing to worry about.'" Lily attended one of
her mother's treatments, and sat with her while she received chemotherapy.
"My mom always tried to stay positive, and I think she knew how sensitive
[sister] and I were. I think she kept that guard up for me."

After the chemotherapy ended, her mother's hair grew back. "Things
were looking pretty good and I think we all were kind of like, 'Okay. Well,
that's it.'" But just as her mother was starting to become hopeful, two unusual spots showed up—one on her neck, and another on her thigh. The cancer had returned. Lily's mother had radiation treatments. "She looked like
she belonged in a concentration camp. From then on until she died [it] was
just one thing after the other." This was a very difficult time in Lily's life,
because at the same time, she was having trouble at work and problems with
her apartment roommate.

Around this time, Lily cornered the physician and asked him, "Is she going to make it?" He said, "six months." After only one week, Lily's mother
went into respiratory arrest. She never regained consciousness.

Lily feels bad that neither she, her sister, nor her stepfather visited her
mother the night before she went into the coma. However "she didn't know
that it [coma] was going to happen either. It wouldn't have made any difference at all, just to have one more night."

Experience following mother's death. Even though Lily knew that her mother was very ill, her death came as a shock. "It was just like, oh, the rug was just, *shwoomp,* ripped out." Lily received some support from her sister, her father, and her church. She also had a close friend who was especially important at that time. Her grandfather was particularly helpful.

> My mother's father has made it a point to take everybody out for Mother's Day. The first one was awful. You know, age teaches people so much. He knew that he could show [us] that you still have family and there are other people to celebrate.

Lily said her mother's death changed her. "After my mom got really sick and died, there was more of a neediness that I didn't have before." Although she had support from older people, she wished she could talk with other young people who had lost their mothers. "I don't think there was anyone to relate to for a while. A year later, a very good friend of mine lost her mother. So she and I shared." Lily also sought out individual counseling with a social worker and attended for about two-and-a-half years. More recently, Lily read Hope Edelman's account of her experience with losing her mother to breast cancer (Edelman, 1994), and then attended an eight-session group for motherless daughters.

After her mother's death, Lily realized that she did not know many of the details of her mother's illness. Five years later, she tried to get information from her stepfather and from her mother's physicians. "I need to do things in pieces because it's too upsetting. I have to spread it out." Although talking about her mother brings tears, Lily very much wants to keep the memories, especially the good ones, alive.

> My sister and I talk about silly things a lot, like growing up, and the things Mom used to say. So I have a lot of pictures around, especially pictures of before the time she was sick, because those were good times.

Lily also seeks out information about her mother from her mother's friends and her grandparents. "I like to talk about how she was growing up and how she was when we were little. It validates who I am."

Lily has taken on a "subsitute mom" role with her younger sister. Lily also took on some of her mother's roles with the rest of the family. "My mother was the glue. She was the communicator between everybody. Now I'm kind of the one who calls the cousins together. I kind of feel like I stepped in my mother's shoes in a lot of places."

Lily's stepfather recently remarried. He was devastated by her mother's death, as was one of Lily's mother's cousins, and they grieved together. "Sharing their grief together over my mother, they fell in love. It was from out of left field! It just happened! So my stepfather married my mother's cousin. They had a rose up there [on the altar] in memory of Mom."

Long-term impact. Lily is not depressed, but

> I will always and forever feel I have a "hole" in my life where my mother once existed. You have a long-term feeling of sadness and loss. It comes and goes with life's experiences. When there's something negative going on, it almost makes it easier to reach out and feel the grief again for my mother.

Despite this saddness, Lily has learned to make positive occasions out of situations that remind her of her grief. For example, Mother's Day is close to the anniversary of her mother's death.

> When Hallmark says it's time to celebrate mothers, it's like, "Okay." That's great! I love it! I love getting together with my grandmother. I'm glad she's still here. And my aunts. I'm so glad I have somebody to celebrate it with.

Lily puts her sadness aside, but has a good cry periodically.

> I stick things in the back of my mind so that I can be happy for [others] and then I deal with it later. I think I store it up, and think, *I'll cry about it one day.* Sometimes the dam is full. Then I'll cry for a couple of hours. I'm talking about a good cry. Like a heaving sob. Disabling. Not the kind of cry where you can wipe your face off and go out in public soon afterward. It's a "cry-yourself-to-sleep" kind of thing. A cleansing. Sometimes it produces a headache for me. But the next day, I'll feel better.

Sometimes, these crying spells are associated with anger. She wants to scream, *"She is not here!"* Lily at first had a very negative attitude about her mother's death. "I was very angry about it." Lily does not want to direct her anger toward God, or toward her mother.

Lily's philosophy of life has changed since her mother's death.

> I felt like I had to do something positive and I think, too, I felt like life is too short, so I bought a house and got a new job [laughs] at the same time. Not all things last. I guess it changed my views about a lot of things, like not to take people for granted, because they may not always be there.

Lily also feels that she has gained strength from her mother's death. "I kind of use my mother's death to weigh things against. I think, *If I can get through losing my mother, I can get through this.*"

Risk. Thinking about her own risk for breast cancer, Lily says, "I try not to be pessimistic. Sometimes I think, *Well, if I think about getting it and facing the fact that I may someday, maybe I won't.*" She thinks that stress may have played a role in her mother's illness ("When my dad left and that whole thing"), so she tries to avoid stress in her own life. "I've tried to take 'time out' when I know that there is no way that I can deal with it anymore. I usually try not to let it get to that point." In addition, Lily monitors her eating habits, exercises, and tries to be more balanced in her life. "I think life's a lot about learning happy mediums. I wish that my mother had been able to do that."

Lily has a physical exam every six months. "I just go for my own peace of mind." Recently, Lily had her first mammogram.

> And they called me back and said, "There's an area we want to make sure is okay." And they called me for a sonogram. So I was very nervous. It's fibrocystic breast disease, is what I have. So I have to go every six months for a mammogram.

Lily is uncomfortable with the radiation of the extra mammograms. She thinks about her mother every time she has breast examinations. "I can't go through these things and not think about my mother. It's really scary. I have to tell myself, *You're not in her shoes. You don't have breast cancer.*"

Although we did not discuss it in our interviews with Lily, she wrote about genetic testing on the final questionnaire.

> I've read a lot recently about the genetic testing. I am choosing at this point to believe I am not destined to get breast cancer, although I admit that there are times fear gets in the way. It is a very scary disease. But I don't believe that just because my mother had it, I'll get it. I can't fathom the fear and disappointment of getting a positive result for being predestined to get breast cancer. Therefore, I'll never be genetically tested.

Current situation. Lily was thirty-one at the time of the interviews. Her sister was about to get married, and this brought up many feelings about her mother's death. "My mother would have been, no question, very involved in the planning. Mom would have been a big part of it." Lily is to be the maid of honor, and she feels uncertain about her responsibilities. "I was looking at a whole big section of wedding gifts, and I was just feeling so overwhelmed. Like, what am I supposed to be doing? Part of it all is Mom not being around."

Lily is not married, but she does anticipate having children one day.

> I already miss my mother for raising children. I think about the scenario of not being able to pick up the phone and say, "Mom, Joe's got a fever. What do I do?" The first person I would want to call is my mother. People don't realize how lucky they are to have a mother around to do that.

Lily's cousin is now pregnant, and she watches how she shares "every detail of her pregnancy" with her mother.

> Then I'm feeling the pain of knowing that I'll never know what that's like. I think the mother-daughter relationship is very instinctive. Carrying on from one generation to the next one, down to the next one, and on down. I'm glad my [maternal] grandmother is still around.

Wendy (age at mother's breast cancer diagnosis: 26;
age at time of mother's death: 29)

Background. Wendy is an African-American woman whose family con-
sisted of mother, father, older sister, and younger brother. Her mother
worked in a hospital as a nursing assistant, and enjoyed many activities with
friends and neighbors. Wendy graduated from high school and attended
technical school. Wendy was close to both parents, and loved to go shopping with her mother. Single and living alone, she worked in a medical office, often dealing with women with breast cancer.

Experience of mother's illness. When Wendy's mother found a lump and
had it biopsied, Wendy only knew about it because of her job. Her mother
had not yet told her.

> I can't recall her sitting down and discussing it with us too much. I think she
> was probably retaining it and just trying to deal with it herself. I already
> knew, so I started kind of preparing myself so it wasn't a major shock.
> When it came back positive, she didn't say anything. She made the deci-
> sions herself. Nobody [family members] went to any visits to anything with
> her. She really kinda kept it basically to herself, until surgery time.

Wendy's mother chose to have her surgery at a different hospital from the
one where Wendy's boss practiced. Later, she had chemotherapy. "I do remember the sickness that she went through with that." Wendy usually went
with her mother to chemotherapy visits.

Her mother had breathing problems after her treatment, and was forced
to stop work and go on disability. She relied increasingly on Wendy for information about the disease, and for care and maintenance of the household.
"Everything pretty much falls on me anyway. I've always done it. And that's
just the way it was. Like running the household as well as dealing with trying to help her out and, then, my own life too."

Wendy was disappointed with the medical care that her mother received,
and felt that she should have gotten care from the center at which Wendy
worked. "I was a little upset, to say the least, with her decision, without discussing it with anybody." Wendy also describes the frustration she sometimes felt trying to care for her mother, who would say,

> "I'm really starving. I want a pizza." And then you get it and then it was like,
> "I don't have the appetite to eat it." She took one bite and wanted no more.
> But I knew it was the stress. You can't be hostile because they can't help it.
> They're sick.

One day, Wendy visited her mother, and "she was standing there holding a
wig up off her head because her hair had completely come out. And she
would just laugh. 'Look—I'm totally bald!' She kept it lighthearted."

Her mother returned to work following the chemotherapy, and maintained her good spirits. "She could have been internalizing it, but she really didn't talk about it too much." However, about the third year postdiagnosis, "it started getting to a point." Wendy knew what to expect, due to her experience at work. The doctors had told her mother she would live for about four years.

> It got progressively worse. One time, we were leaving for a doctor's visit or something. She was complaining about her hip. So the next thing you know, they put her in the hospital. It had metastasized to the bone. She went into diabetic ketoacidosis. Next thing I know, a few days later, it's labored breathing all the time. I was like, "Oh man, it's getting close. It's got to be getting close."

At the end of her life, Wendy's mother had support from her oldest daughter, her sisters, sisters-in-law, and husband, in addition to Wendy. Within five days, she passed away.

Experience following mother's death. Wendy's mother had told her her wishes for a funeral. "She just kept on saying, 'I just hope everybody gets together as a family unit and I'd like everybody to go to somebody's church. Anybody's church." At the funeral, Wendy was numb. "I was sitting there at the funeral and I kept on saying 'Okay, you really have to cry now.' But I had to be together, because I had to do everything." She mostly remembers looking at her father, who was having a difficult time, and thinking about her grandmother's funeral, which had been only a year before.

Since her mother's death, Wendy has become very close to her father, who has had a heart attack. She calls and visits him frequently.

Long-term impact. Wendy feels that she is more empathetic to women with breast cancer because of her mother's experience. When patients are very anxious, she tries harder to fit them into the schedule. However, she has little patience with "the ones that are basically, 'Feel sorry for me!'" Sometimes, work is difficult for Wendy, because

> you get people that come in here [doctor's office] and they're really, really nice people. You get comfortable with people, and a lot of times you see their results before anybody else sees them. It's a little bit hard sometimes, particularly the younger patients. You're thinking, *That's right there in my age group.* It's always in my face, always. Constantly. But it helps to be around other people and to know that, even though I have this problem, I can still go on with my life, as long as it works out that way.

Wendy relieves her stress by listening to music and by talking with girlfriends.

She continues to miss her mother.

> You miss people; you know, they are a part of you. I mean, a mother is just, a mother! That's really special as a person you cannot replace. I'm not going to fall apart, but I might not be as happy or smiling all the time like everybody else.

Wendy has never really allowed herself to grieve. "I totally have to take charge of everything. Deal with this, push that back."

Although she participates in a support group for African-American women organized by her employer, she rarely shares her own feelings.

> I don't really even know myself what I really and truly feel. . . . It isn't going to change the outcome, so . . . what's the sense of talking about it? It's not going to change. Everything is the same, so . . . move on to the next thing. Which is not good. I worry myself into an ulcer.

Risk. Wendy has had annual mammograms since she turned twenty-eight. "For a while, they were monitoring me every six months, because I'm extremely cystic and because of the history." Wendy lists her risk factors: "Now, I'm over forty, overweight, the mother with breast cancer, never having any children. . . . All right, it's time to check this out."

Wendy experiences anxiety whenever she has a cyst. "That does kinda wreak havoc in the old brain sometimes. It is probably my biggest fear." Wendy says it is difficult to locate information on extended family's history. "I don't know who else [had breast cancer]. Her [mother's] mother could have died from that for all I know. Or another aunt of hers. But I have no idea, because those people never talked about this stuff."

Wendy contacted the hospital where her mother was treated to obtain her records, but she did not pursue the matter after learning that the records were in a vault. She indicates that she would be interested in genetic testing, but has not initiated the process.

Current situation. Wendy was forty-one at the time of the interview. She got married during the course of the study. She remains very close to her father, and continues to work with women with breast cancer in a physician's office. Wendy had no health insurance at the time of the interview, and was having clinical exams done by her employer to substitute for mammograms and regular health care.

Daughters Whose Mothers Survived

Chloe (age at mother's breast cancer diagnosis: 6)

Background. Chloe, the youngest of three children and the only daughter, lived with her family in Europe. Her father was alcoholic and abusive to his wife and children. Chloe has few memories of her mother before her breast cancer, but she remembers that she used to take the children to the swimming pool in her motorcycle's sidecar. Her mother was the soft, calming influence in the family.

Experience of mother's illness. Chloe's parents told the children that their mother was going to the hospital and would be home that night. This took place in the time of the "one-step" procedure. Instead of the expected biopsy, Chloe's mother had a radical mastectomy. The hospital was not far from her elementary school; when she visited, her mother was in a high bed, and Chloe couldn't reach her.

> I was always somewhat of an impulsive kind of child. I ran into the door and I was trying to jump on her bed and give her a big hug. And she said, "No, no, no! You just stay down." They took the lymph nodes and the breast, and she had her arm all bandaged up.

When her mother pulled away from her due to the surgery, Chloe felt rejected.

However, Chloe also has happy memories of her hospital visits.

> Every day I went over to the hospital. I did my homework at a table, which was filled with flowers. I remember all of the wonderful smells of the flowers. I must have spent all afternoon there. I tried to make her laugh, and do things for her. I would go and get her water.

Although cancer was never discussed, Chloe could sense that something was seriously wrong with her mother. "We knew there was fear in the household. You're just terrorized, but you can't do anything about it. I mean, you're completely out of control. You're powerless about it."

Experience following mother's illness. Chloe's mother changed after her surgery. "For me, the main thing I noticed was that she was not available." She became an invalid, resting much of the time. "She sat in her chair a lot. There was something very fragile and not accessible about her in that chair. We had to leave her alone." Chloe's mother began to accompany her father on weekend trips, and visited a spa for several weeks every year. Young Chloe sensed a change in her mother's personality: while she had once been fun-loving, now she seemed sad all the time.

After her mother's operation, Chloe had little supervision. "We spent all our time in the woods. We grew up in a very free, kind of unsupervised way. I remember being very independent." As a young adolescent, Chloe was sexually molested by someone who worked for her father. She never told her parents about it.

Chloe was angry that her mother would not stand up to her father, and would not defend her to him. At seventeen, she left home, and eventually married and moved to the United States.

Risk. Chloe has very cystic breasts, and has had several lumps, but these have always gone away without medical attention. She never has needed to have a biopsy. Instead, she uses alternative health remedies to treat her breasts (castor oil). She also uses a cream made with sweet potatoes to treat menopausal symptoms. She has an annual mammogram and does breast self-examination. "For all I care, I might have breast cancer tomorrow, but I'm doing the best I can to avoid it."

Current situation. Chloe was forty-seven at the time of the interview. Her father was deceased, and her mother was in a nursing home and had Alzheimer's disease. She is married and has no children. She creates artwork now, some of which is based on the themes of her early childhood. She also works with the elderly as a social worker.

Jody (age at mother's breast cancer diagnosis: 17)

Background. Jody's parents were divorced, and her mother was remarried. Jody had a stepsister and a stepbrother who were considerably younger than herself. When Jody was twelve, her mother had some lumps removed, but cancer was never mentioned. "'Well, your mom is just gonna go in and have a little surgery and that's it and come back out.' And then everything was fine. I really wasn't that concerned and they didn't say cancer. They didn't say anything."

Jody lived with her mother and stepfather. She was rebellious, and used to run away to visit her biological father. As a young adult, Jody moved out and lived in a nearby city. She had a job in food services.

Experience of mother's illness. When Jody was seventeen, her mother had a mammogram, and told her, "Well, I have breast cancer, and it's pretty bad. It went to the lymph nodes." Her mother blamed herself because she hadn't been getting mammograms. At this point in her life, Jody had little contact with her mother and stepfather. "I was working constantly, so I really couldn't be there for her. I just had my own life by then and they had never helped me." Jody was angry with her mother for not supporting her education.

Her mother had a mastectomy followed by chemotherapy. "She did real bad with it, she would just cry and cry and cry. She was sick and weak." Her mother did not tell her younger children (Jody's stepbrother and sister) she had cancer; however they were still upset because they knew she was ill. Jody sometimes cleaned the house for her mother.

When her mother had reconstruction (tummy tuck), Jody helped change the bandages. She had a second reconstruction operation, and Jody helped with the children when her stepfather could not be there. However, Jody did not feel obligated to help, she says, because her mother and stepfather were not particularly nice to her. "She never really helped me out," she said.

Experience following mother's illness. Jody did not worry about her mother, because "she told me it wasn't serious. I guess if I would think about it, I'd get really upset and really sad. Like now, I just don't think about it really." Jody indicates that she never allows herself to think that her mother could die, because that might bring her [mother] bad luck.

Risk. Jody attributed her mother's cancer to poor health habits.

> She always ate awful. She's always eating fat foods. She is a big woman, but she's never been obese. I grew up on cheese and crackers, no vegetables. She's always ate junk food. No one else in our family on either side has breast cancer. She doesn't exercise. She's got a treadmill, and it's a clothes rack.

Jody tries to eat a healthy diet with lots of fruits and vegetables. She also uses olive oil instead of other types of fat, and has reduced her caffeine intake. "I read everything, and everything I read, I do. Anything that says, 'Prevent breast cancer,' I do." When Jody had fibrocystic disease, her grandparents paid for her sonograms because her health insurance did not cover them.

Jody worried about getting breast cancer ("I just always wonder what's gonna happen. Like when I'm dating a guy, I always mention, 'Well, if I had cancer, would you stay with me?'") but at the same time, she felt confident that she would not have her mother's experience. "I know that I would definitely catch it early, if I would get it."

Jody was not interested in genetic testing, because she was concerned about the impact on health insurance. Also, she felt that she was not at high risk, because she attributed her mother's cancer to her health habits, and not to genetics.

Current situation. At the time of the interview, Jody was twenty-four. She worked in the food service business, and was single but lived with a boyfriend.

Tina (age at mother's breast cancer diagnosis: 14)

Background. Tina lived with her mother, father, and younger brother. She describes her father as "nasty."

> [He] didn't speak to me and my brother and was nasty to Mother and stuff. [There was] a lot of slamming. Slamming the door, slamming the glass down on the table. He didn't talk to us at all. I've been hit maybe twice by him.

When Tina was thirteen, her mother got thyroid cancer, which was treated successfully. "She didn't say it like it was anything tragic. She tried to act like, you know, you would have thought she had a cold or something." The family had other problems, including financial difficulties, and Tina and her brother had trouble in school. Her mother tended to deny these problems.

> My aunt [a social worker] says she's [Tina's mother] got a personality disorder. That she's been a little strange since she was young. We didn't get along that well growing up. You know, screaming, constant fighting. It was a free-for-all in the house.

Despite these problems, Tina says, "We were always close, my mother, my brother, and I."

Experience of mother's illness. Tina was not told very much about her mother's breast cancer.

> I didn't really understand it. I was so young. I think she told me she had a lump and that she was going to get it checked. She didn't really like to dwell on it. She had a mastectomy. Then she had reconstructive surgery on both [breasts]. So she was in and out. I think she was in for a couple of days. And then she had her nipple reconstructed and that was, like, outpatient.

Tina was more worried than her mother.

> I don't really remember her being that sick or anything. I used to say, "You're probably going to die" and stuff. I used to watch those medical shows like *St. Elsewhere* and *20/20*. I used to think she'd die under the knife. So I worried about that. I remember when she came out the one time she said, "I'm still alive!" because I'd freaked out so bad, you know. I used to go and visit her and sit with her in the hospital and stuff. I guess [an aunt] used to take us to see her in the hospital. She'd bring food to us and stuff. [My father] never went to the hospital, I know.

After her mother came home from the hospital, she continued to take care of the house.

> She never had a nurse come to the house. She hated anybody to do dishes, because my mother's, like, a clean freak. She wouldn't let anyone [help]. Like cleaning or anything like that. And she was always there to drive and stuff like that. Pretty much the same as always.

A pattern of secrecy about illness exists in Tina's family.

> I'm not sure [my brother] knows. It was never really spoken about in any kind of way, really. I wouldn't be surprised if she never talked about it with him. I'm lucky I knew, the way she is. You know, it's just that whole keeping it to yourself and being strong thing.

Tina's mother never told her husband's family about her illness. "Imagine, we went there every Sunday for dinner, and they knew not one thing. She wouldn't let him tell them. She didn't want them to know."

Tina continued to worry about her mother's health. "I think I worried about her a lot more. I worried and worried and worried to death and asked her about it all the time." After Tina missed three months of school, she was not allowed back. She transferred to a different school, but her attendance there was poor, and she was eventually expelled. She tried to enter school one last time, but got pregnant, had a miscarriage, and was too ashamed to return to school. "I was so embarrassed about it because everybody knew." After this, she said, she became "wild."

> Imagine not having a curfew and being able to do whatever you want and drinking and stuff. And my mother. I drank with my mother. Partying and stuff. My mother would drink rum and Cokes, and I'd do it with her. My friends always said, "Oh, you got a cool mom!" She was always really like that. She wanted to be our friend more than be our parent.

Soon, Tina entered counseling. "I was depressed. I felt like I couldn't work and stuff. I had gained, probably like sixty pounds at that point." Then, Tina's parents' marriage broke up, and her father moved out.

> Her mother [Tina's grandmother] died in January and then her father died in December of that [same] year. So we had both of her parents, breast cancer, and my father leaving all in the same year. Then, my aunt had a miscarriage too. It was, like, everything.

Experience following mother's illness. Tina worries about her mother's cancer recurring.

> Because she lies so much, I worry that stuff will happen and she won't say it. She doesn't like to talk about it. I guess she'd have to tell me if she has to go in the hospital. But sometimes I worry that she'll have stuff wrong and be afraid to go to the doctor. I ask her from time to time, just to make sure. I always think—it's been twelve years now—and I always feel it's going to hit again. They always say you have remission for ten years and then your chances of getting it get more. But she never talks about it. I think about that sometimes.

Risk. At age twenty-three, Tina was diagnosed with fibrocystic breast disease.

> I got really scared and I said, "Well, I want a mammogram." Because she [doctor] found this one lump she kept focusing on. She was brushing it off and acting like I was stupid. I said, "Well, my mother was only thirty-six years old. It's not a very comfortable feeling to be told that you've got lumps all over your breasts when your mother was really young when she had it." [I was concerned] that I had cancer or something.

She eventually had a mammogram, but she had to pay for it herself. "Some people say it's bad for you because of the radiation that you get. So it's like I don't know what to believe. You have to be fifty to even qualify for a free program."

Tina has thought about having prophylactic mastectomy.

> I watch all the talk shows, and I heard this one woman say two of her sisters had gotten it young, and she went and had a mastectomy without even having anything, just because she was so afraid of having it. And I said to Aunt [name], "That's what I feel like doing now that I have this fibrocystic breast disease. Just to get rid of it all and get implants." Not that I could ever afford it or anything. I did think about that. That sounded like a good idea to me. Just cut them off and start over.

Tina also was aware of genetic testing. "I'd love to know. I mean, I guess it would be bad in a way, but I'd love to know."

Tina tries to do breast self-exams, but "You don't really know what you're doing. You know, I've got them [lumps] all the time. So I could just freak myself out and think, *What's this?*" Tina has taken vitamin E and reduced her caffeine intake in an effort to prevent cancer. "But I couldn't stand it anymore because I felt, like, dead, you know. So I've been back on caffeine, but I do take vitamin E every morning." She also lost a significant amount of weight, on her doctor's advice. She has avoided birth control pills.

> My mother was on the pill for, like, twenty years, and it made me wonder if maybe that was it. They say if you smoke, if you drink, if you're fat, if you don't get enough exercise. I mean my mother went to exercise classes. My mother never drank. She never smoked cigarettes. My mother was like the exact opposite of everything that they say you shouldn't do.

Current situation. At eighteen, Tina moved in with a man seventeen years her senior. They were still living together, but not married, at the time of the interviews. Tina was twenty-six. Tina continued to suffer from health problems and depression. She also was frustrated because she could not get treatment for her health problems due to lack of medical insurance. She was unemployed.

Tina and her mother were still close, but her mother had an abusive boyfriend, and this put some strain on their relationship. This man has abused and stalked Tina. Her mother once tried to leave him, but then went back to him and kept this from Tina. She continued to have financial problems, and recently had been evicted. Tina helped her out periodically.

Betty (age at mother's breast cancer diagnosis: 18)

Background. Betty lived with her mother, father, and a brother four years older than Betty. "I had the good, happy childhood surrounded by friends and parents. A great family and lots of friends." Betty's mother had been a teacher, and Betty describes her as having a "laid-back" personality. She returned to part-time work when Betty was in the fourth grade, working as a secretary, and then at a local university. Betty's parents were active in sports, and when Betty and her brother played on various teams, her parents served as referees. Betty and her mother had a difficult time during her teen years. "I was more of a typical adolescent. I knew everything. I had the mouth. It was just flip back talk." As a teenager, she began to confide more in her friends than in her mother. Betty's family members always were very healthy, although her grandparents and several other relatives were deceased.

Experience of mother's illness. One day when Betty was seventeen, her mother was upset as she unloaded groceries from the car.

> I mean, I could tell she was crying. And she said that they had found a lump. She told me right then. She told me first, and I hugged her and cried. I think just when you hear the "C" word, it's just automatically, like that's it, that's the end. Like death. The worst.

Her mother had a mastectomy. "She told them, if it was cancerous, just remove it. That was kind of her idea." Betty's main reaction to her mother's surgery was fear. "Here they are. They're cutting something off, they're removing a piece of her. It was, like, very real. You know, it's scary." Betty said her mother's breast cancer was unexpected. "I've been going to funerals from when I was real little. It's just kind of something [that goes] with the aging process. But it just doesn't happen to someone forty-eight years old. It doesn't happen to your mom, who's strong and healthy and so full of life."

Betty never saw her mother's scar, but she remembered seeing her "all bandaged up." She helped out at home after her mother came home from the hospital. "It was my mom, and it was [happening] right in my house. I had to be there, and I had to be the one to talk to her and be strong. It really hit home." However, the burden did not fall on Betty alone. "We all kind of pitched in and did stuff around the house that she normally did. In my house, we weren't really big on separating jobs." Her mother maintained a very strong and positive attitude.

> She accepted it. She'd say, "It's in God's hands." I mean, I remember her crying and I remember her being upset. Who wouldn't be? But I don't remember her becoming bitter or going into a shell. We were raised Catholic, and she wasn't an astute Bible scholar by any means, but she was spiritual. She seemed at peace with what happened.

Betty's relationship with her mother changed after the diagnosis. "She confided in me, more so than my dad. It just brought us closer, because I wasn't, like, this kid or this teenager. I was becoming more of a woman, and this was, like, a woman kind of issue." Betty's mother told her "how she felt, emotionally, losing her breast. How it's gonna reflect on her as a woman. Emotional things." In the past, Betty and her mother shared "girl-talk stuff," so when her mother began to confide in her, "I didn't really know how to respond. She was talking to me like I would talk to her, you know. Kind of reversed." Although her husband was supportive, Betty's mother relied more on Betty. "This was something that women experience. It's a woman thing. And it was hard because your mother is always the supportive one. Your mom has traditionally been like the backbone of the family. She takes care of everyone, and here it is, she needs to be taken care of." Betty had a friend who supported her during this period. "I had a best friend that I was real close to, and I told her what was going on."

Experience following mother's illness. Betty began attending college, but she soon dropped out. "That didn't work. I just wasn't ready. I had no interest in it." After that, Betty lived for a while at the beach with friends, and she was living in a nearby state when her mother died suddenly of a heart attack.

> It was such a shock. It happened so fast, and it was, like, so much to do. I had to kind of take over her role. I had to be the one to make the arrangements for the funeral. I had to pick out what she was going to be laid out in, and then to make arrangements for the little reception afterwards. It was just not something I was used to doing. It seemed like such an adult role that I had to do, and I wasn't even the oldest. I guess it was just because I was the female and I kind of got stuck with doing all that.

Although her family and her mother's friends tried to support her, Betty did not find it helpful.

> Some of her friends I had known all my life. They were just like family to me. But I just didn't feel like dealing with them. The phone would ring a lot. "Is there anything I can do?" "Can I help you?" "Do you need anything?" [I said] "No! I don't need anything. I just want to be left alone!"

After her mother's death,

> everything just fell apart at the seams. I think that Mom kind of, like, was the binding of the family. After she died, it was just like, a lot of her friends weren't around anymore. I didn't really see my brother that much anymore, 'cause we would kind of meet over there to see Mom and Dad.

It took Betty a couple of months to get over the shock of her mother's death and begin to grieve. The death had a devastating effect on Betty's brother, who later had problems with alcohol and drugs. "I know it devastated him. He never really talked to anybody, but he would talk to her. Mom always stood up for him. Him and my father never got along that great. [After mother died], my brother just kind of fell apart."

Betty lived "like a gypsy" for a time, and had a short marriage. At one point in this period, Betty tried living at home with her father.

> It lasted about three weeks. He had a girlfriend, you know. And he was used to living on his own. We just did not get along. He was just particular about things. I can't really describe it. I was an adult, and here I am living back under my parents' roof, and it was just hard. And I think that there was anger too, with the new girlfriend. No matter how old you are, when your dad starts seeing somebody that's not your mom of thirty-two years, it is just different. I was angry at him. It was like he wasn't there for me. I was seeing him in a different way. He was a man with his own life, rather than just my father. I wasn't number one anymore. You know, "How dare you have your own life?"

Later, Betty put herself through college by working as a waitress. She entered a new relationship and then had a baby. She had no financial help from her father, and worked to pay her expenses.

Betty missed her mother especially around her pregnancy, and her baby's birth. "I think of her a lot at Christmastime, but a specific day does not set me off." She wishes her mother had been there to tell her about "when she was pregnant with me, what I was like as a baby." She also wishes her mother could to baby-sit. "You know you can always drop the kid off with your mom. I mean, everybody does it. Moms are different. You don't have to call first. You can just call up and say, 'You got to take him.'" She also felt that her mother would have helped her with school, financially, and with a place to live when she needed one. "I would not have struggled half as much had she been around. I would have had a roof over my head, and could have worked part-time. I wouldn't have had the day care problems. I mean it may sound selfish. But my life would have been a lot easier."

Betty said her mother's death had one positive impact on her: "It made me stronger and more independent."

Risk. Although her mother died from heart disease, Betty is more fearful of getting breast cancer. "I think the heart attack could have been prevented. She was a heavy smoker and her cholesterol was high, whereas I think cancer is more genetic." Because of this, Betty worries about getting breast cancer herself. "I don't know the statistics but I know that daughters are more likely [to get it] if their mothers had it." She is more aware of her health, and tries to take care of herself. "I try to run every day, try to eat right, don't smoke, don't drink that much. I mean, it makes you a lot more aware of just how important health is." Betty also does breast self-exams. "She [doctor] doesn't feel that mammograms are right for me now. My breast tissue tends to be, like, tougher, or dense, and a mammogram this young isn't gonna really show anything."

Betty hopes that, if she does get breast cancer, she will have a supportive husband. "I know my dad was very supportive of her [mother]. I guess I would be hopeful that if I were ever married and this would happen, I would have a husband that was that way."

Current situation. Betty was twenty-nine at the time of the interview. Betty and her baby's father were having relationship problems. "He and I have not been getting along real well these days, but that's kind of normal. That's kind of been normal for the past two years. That happened with my first husband also." At the time of our last contact, Betty had begun a new relationship with a man whose mother had died when he was six. Betty's father was being treated for lung cancer at the time of the interview.

Charlotte (age at mother's breast cancer diagnosis: 20)

Background. Charlotte was the oldest of five children in a close-knit African-American family. Her family lived near her grandmother and two aunts, and the cousins grew up as siblings. Her father was "not in the picture." After high school, Charlotte moved away from home to attend college. "You know, older daughter. I just couldn't wait to get away from home."

Experience of mother's illness. When Charlotte was twenty, her mother called the family together and told them that she had breast cancer. "That was the last thing, really, that we expected to hear." She had already had a biopsy when she told the children, and had decided to have a mastectomy, chemotherapy, radiation, and reconstruction. Charlotte was not involved in her mother's treatment, and was only marginally aware of the effects.

> We didn't really go through the treatment. I mean, we saw the stages. Saw the hair coming out, and then she eventually started wearing a wig and all. At the time, I wasn't living there. You know how you know it's something, but you don't acknowledge it. That's what it was.

Only later did Charlotte realize that her mother's life was threatened. "I think the realization came through, because the next-door neighbor's wife had had breast cancer, and then she developed a tumor on the brain that killed her. It could happen to your mother." The family never openly discussed the breast cancer. Watching her mother go through the illness made Charlotte respect her mother more. "I mean, she was a brave woman. I admire my mother a whole lot more today than I did before. She is a strong person. . . . I think I actually felt closer to her."

Experience following mother's illness. Although no major change has occurred in the mother-daughter relationship since the breast cancer, Charlotte feels that the family as a whole is closer.

With stuff like this, it tends to bring . . . We are a pretty close family anyway and it tends to bring you a little closer. I think it may have opened our eyes a little more. You know, people don't think about death, and when that happened, it made you realize.

Risk. Only a few months after her mother was diagnosed, Charlotte went in for a routine physical, and her practitioner detected a lump. A biopsy was scheduled, but, in the meantime, the lump went away, and Charlotte did not follow up. "It was a rude awakening."

Charlotte tried to take care of herself, and did breast self-exams. "I'm still not very health-conscious when it comes to the food part."

Current situation. Charlotte was thirty-six at the time of the interview. She was married, and had three children. Her mother was working and also was working on an advanced degree. Since her mother's diagnosis, Charlotte's grandmother and grandfather have both been diagnosed with cancer. Both are survivors. Charlotte contributed money to breast cancer research weekly through her work.

Tomasina (age at mother's breast cancer diagnosis: 21)

Background. Tomasina lived with her mother, stepfather, sister, and brother. She was a college student, and returned home to stay with her family on weekends. She is African American, and described hers as a family in which people hide illness from one another. The family lived in a rural area with many close relatives nearby.

Experience during and following mother's illness. One weekend, Tomasina and her brother overheard relatives talking about their mother and realized that she had had breast cancer. They discussed it with their stepfather, and found out that he knew. Then, they confronted their grandmother and aunt. They were extremely upset not only because of the diagnosis, but also because their mother had not trusted them. "We're your children here and you should have informed us so we could prepare each other for, you know, when things get worse." Tomasina's brother stormed out of the house and, later that evening, totaled his car. Her sister also was very upset, screaming and acting out. Tomasina herself was in total shock. "I didn't know what to do, what to say, or where to go." Her mother told Tomasina and her siblings that she was just trying to find the right time and place to tell them. They were especially upset because their mother had always told them to be open and honest with one another. "It's like a two-sided thing."

After learning of the illness, Tomasina and her siblings tried to piece together the past. Tomasina remembered that her mother was away for a long time; their grandmother had told them that their mother was on a trip. Tomasina also learned that her grandmother had also had breast cancer. "[I was] puzzled, scared, had a lot of questions. It makes you feel depressed—especially when you don't know and it's more scary than knowing."

It took a long time for the family to be able to openly discuss her mother's illness. Tomasina's aunt noticed the negative impact on the family, and encouraged them to get counseling. Tomasina's grades were falling, her younger sister became very rebellious, and her brother had problems at work.

> It was not overnight that we got at the stage that we are. It took a lot of arguments, almost fistfights, you know, between me and my sister and my brother. It took a lot of, wow, nights and days of us waking up realizing that we only have each other so we have to stick together and, you know, respect one another.

Tomasina initially did not want to share her inner feelings with a counselor. She had many questions, but wanted answers from her mother. "That's what stunned us the most [that mother kept the diagnosis secret], because it had separated the family for a while. We felt as though we couldn't trust her."

Shortly after Tomasina and her siblings learned of their mother's disease, Tomasina's grandfather died. This loss made the adjustment to her mother's illness even more difficult.

> At nighttime, it really dawns on you because you are by yourself. . . . You're alone. The noise is quieted down and you're thinking about what is happening in your life. I never imagined nothing like that. Never. To have to deal with it two times. Me and my mom was close and we did everything together. I guess I felt as though I was losing my better half, my best friend as well as my mother, and about me also losing my grandfather. And I didn't talk about that because they was asking me, "Are you all right?" and I was like, "Leave me alone!"

In addition to pastoral and psychological counseling, the family had support from the community. "Something like in a little fairy tale. A little community, and everybody came together. [The extended family became] our arms and our shoulders to cry on and stuff like that."

The diagnosis also changed Tomasina's relationship with her stepfather, because he began to discuss with her his emotions. "'Oh, who's going to listen to my problems? . . . Who's going to listen to what I'm feeling?' He dealt with it, almost drinking his self away . . . because he didn't know what to do. He didn't want to lose her." Around this time, her stepfather died from a sudden heart attack.

Risk. Tomasina went to a support group, where she heard stories of breast cancer in other daughters.

> My head was like, *Oh my God, let me go get tested!* And they're telling me, it was like, there's no sense worrying about it. And I'm like, this kind of runs in my family a little too strongly. For now, they're saying everything is fine. I

went the whole nine yards. I went to get my sugar done, and so everything came back negative.

Tomasina and her sister both did breast self-exams.

My sister, her fear was that she might find something, so she didn't want to do it. But her doctor talked to her, one on one, and told her that it's best if you give your own self breast exams, as well as when you come in to see me. So she got better [at it].

Current situation. At the time of interview, Tomasina was twenty-eight. Her mother was participating in family outings, and the family had returned to church. Tomasina's brother had been diagnosed with HIV, and the family was keeping this information secret from her mother.

Tomasina had a son, and this helped her and her mother reconcile. The baby is now Tomasina's mother's pride and joy.

That helped a great deal because I guess my mother was experiencing new life all over again. It was like she was carrying him. She was more excited than I was. And she wanted to do everything, so I allowed her to do everything.

Recently, her mother's doctors saw signs of a recurrence. "It may be coming back, getting larger or going into her left breast." She may need more surgery. Tomasina's brother became her major caregiver, going with their mother to all of her appointments. Tomasina was still in school.

Soon after the study was completed, Tomasina's mother died. The family never discussed the possibility of her death openly, and kept the prognosis a secret from her mother.

Laura (age at mother's breast cancer diagnosis: 24)

Background. Laura came from a very poor, African-American family and grew up living in housing projects. She is the middle of three sisters and has a stepsister from her father's previous relationship. Her father was an alcoholic who was not involved with her family when she was young. Much of the time she was growing up, he was in jail. Her mother's boyfriend sexually abused Laura and her sisters. As a teenager, several men tried to exploit her sexuality, including some of her friends' fathers.

Laura was close to her mother, but not to her sisters. Because she was mechanically inclined, her mother called her "the son she never had." When her mother joined the Jehovah's Witnesses, Laura did too; this provided her a supportive community.

Laura's sisters both had children as teens. Laura graduated from high school and got an advanced degree in a technical field. Laura's father reentered her life when he got out of jail, and he and Laura's mother were married for the second time. (Laura was twenty-two at the time.) The reunion of her parents was stressful for Laura because her father was violent. She moved out and then moved from place to place, looking for a stable home. Although she wanted to leave the family, and "spread my own wings," she was the most stable person in her family, and they relied on her support. Laura's family had an ethic to "be strong" when dealing with life's problems. "Everything that comes along, you just deal with it."

Experience of mother's illness. Laura was twenty-four and temporarily living at home when her mother was diagnosed with breast cancer. Her mother had told the family she needed to go to the hospital to find out about a lump in her breast. She said she did not think it was anything serious. She had found the lump herself, by doing BSE. Some time after that, her mother cried as she told the family, "It was malignant. I have cancer." Her mother then called her other family members.

She had a mastectomy. "I can't even remember which one it is. The right. I'm pretty sure it's the right removed." Laura, her father, sisters, and other family members went with her mother for the mastectomy. "I can remember them coming in and saying it was okay. And I was delirious." Although her mother often cried about losing her breast, she maintained a positive outlook.

Following the surgery, her mother had chemotherapy. Laura drove her to the appointments, as she was the only one in the family with money for transportation. Her mother's hair thinned with the chemotherapy, and her fingernails turned black. Although Laura helped out in an instrumental way, she did not provide emotional support.

> I guess [when] you are dealing with poor folks who are just limited, or don't even realize they have resources, everything that comes along, you just deal with it. My mother probably needed more of a shoulder to lean on . . . I did things, like buying her [nonaluminum] cookware, but really just putting my arm around her, I just didn't do much of that. I didn't know how.

Laura's mother considered reconstruction, but Laura was worried about the potential dangers of silicone, and also feared her mother having more surgery. "I don't want that to happen to my mother, and thinking, all because she wanted another breast, she died. I would be so upset and thinking that I encouraged it too."

Laura's father was very supportive, and used humor to help her mother during her illness. "They didn't do much surgically to make it look appealing to the eye, so it was good that my father had a sense of humor and their relationship wasn't tied up in her breast." Laura had hoped that her father would continue to be

> the man that he was supposed to be, so that my mother could lean on him. Because she always leaned on me a lot. And I didn't mind, but I sort of

wanted to spread my own wings. And I really couldn't so I felt, now, I just have to stay that much longer. I had to be committed and take care of my mother.

Laura became very angry at God after her mother became ill, and this anger led to her leaving the Jehovah's Witnesses. "I was angry, but what can we do?" Her boyfriend also was a Jehovah's Witness, and she broke up with him when she left the church. "Don't be bitter," he told Laura. "You know it's not God's fault." However, Laura could not understand why, since

> This is Your [God's] world, and You can run it the way You see fit. We learned that You take it out on everybody because Adam and Eve sinned. . . . That seemed childish to me. I had that attitude with my mother being sick. I just told Him, 'Look, if she dies . . . I don't want to hear anything about You!" If I had the power to fix problems and make everything just hunky-dory, I would. It doesn't make sense to me, it doesn't sit well, to see people suffer. I don't understand Him.

Experience following mother's illness. After her treatment, Laura's mother's life returned to normal. "I mean, what is normal for our family." Three years after her mother's diagnosis, her father died from complications from alcohol. "He asphyxiated himself."

Concerned about her mother's health, Laura bought her glass cookware and reminded her mother not to consume caffeine. She bought her mother detoxifying tea. Laura feared that her mother's cancer was just in remission, so she worried whenever she had any pain or unusual symptoms. She read all she could on breast cancer, and encouraged her mother to practice good health behaviors. "I just try to keep my mother healthy. Pass on information to her, so we don't have to go through this again, where we may not be so fortunate."

Laura wanted to focus more attention on her own needs, instead of always trying to please others. "I don't even know what makes me happy. I'm always concentrating on other people's happiness." She sought out therapy, and learned that she was depressed. She realized that she needed to make her own choices in life, and not just do what others want her to do.

Looking back, Laura considered her mother's cancer as just one in a lifetime of tragedies.

> It didn't change my life. It really didn't. It's just another tragedy. That's basically what it was. My life was filled with tragedies. I know that my mother could have died. I've known many women to die. So I'm just thankful that she's alive.

Risk. A doctor told Laura, "There is a ninety percent chance that one of the three of you [sisters] will eventually have breast cancer." Laura was certain that she will not be the one, because her sisters smoked and did not eat healthy diets. Laura herself was very careful with her diet, eating no sugar, flour, or meat. She also took vitamins A and E. She exercised regularly, and tried to reduce the stress in her life. (Laura attributed her mother's breast cancer to the stress caused by her father's alcoholism and abuse.) When she has aches and pains, the first idea she has is, "It must be cancer."

Laura has not had any breast cancer symptoms, but she has had an abnormal Pap smear. She fears her mother's illness.

> Cancer is going to kill me. Sometimes I think if it comes, it might be a relief. That's the way I think. I don't want to sound suicidal, but sometimes it gets rough and I say, "Jeez, death wouldn't be so bad now."

She has had breast exams, but has not yet had a mammogram and does breast self-exams only casually.

Current situation. Laura was thirty-one at the time of the interview. She was unemployed. Her mother worked as a day care provider, and Laura helped her with this. She often was frustrated with her family, because they "are just stuck, and they don't seem to want to get better because they keep doing the same stuff over and over again. Making the same mistakes. They don't want to see it differently." Laura has set up a savings plan for her family to provide for them in case of an emergency.

Dora (age at mother's breast cancer diagnosis: 26)

Background. Dora, the older of two children, was raised in a middle-class Jewish family. Her parents separated when she was in the tenth grade, and divorced a couple of years later. Her father remarried and lived in another state. Although she had been close to her father when she was young ("Daddy's little girl"), the separation left them estranged. "I was bitter. I was angry with my father and my mother." Although she wanted to live with her father, she and her brother stayed with their mother. She and her mother did not get along well, and sometimes, Dora would experience the "silent treatment" from her mother. When Dora returned to live with her mother after several years of being away at college, their relationship improved. "We finally got all our stuff out in the open and we resolved any kind of issues from the past, and ever since then, we've become much closer."

Experience of mother's illness. Just before leaving for a vacation, when Dora was twenty-six, her mother told her that she had breast cancer, and would have a mastectomy right after they returned home. Her mother had had a number of cysts, and the doctors had always reassured her that they were not problematic. "And finally, she just got fed up with it and she's like, 'Look, take it out and see what it is.' And so they did and they found out that it was cancer." Dora remembers that when her mother told her, "It upset me a lot 'cause, you know, *cancer;* you hear *cancer* and then you hear *death.*"

Because the cancer was detected at such an early stage, Dora's mother did not have any chemotherapy or radiation. After doing extensive research, she decided to have a mastectomy to prevent future problems.

> She didn't care that she didn't have a breast. It wasn't the most important thing to her. I know that some women , when they find out they're going to lose a breast, they think they're just losing their whole femininity, and it wasn't like that for her, which was good.

Dora's mother decided not to have reconstruction, because she did not want to miss any work.

Dora went to the hospital the day of her mother's surgery. Her brother, grandfather, and mother's friend also were there. When the surgery took longer than expected, Dora left to play in a softball game. When she returned to the hospital, her mother was "loopy." "It really upset me because this is my mother, this is my solidarity here. You know, she is my grounding force a lot of the time, and here she is, she's just—she's not with it." Dora went home after visiting hours, feeling quite worried. "At about eleven, the phone rang, and it was her [mother]. 'I'm back! Get me out of here!' and I'm like, 'Oh, it's nice to see you are back.'"

After the surgery, Dora stayed at her mother's house for a couple of nights and helped her bathe and wash her hair. Dora was bothered by the surgical tubes, but "I handled it okay." Dora did not want to look at her mother's scar, but her mother wanted her to see it.

> I couldn't look at it, and she's trying to make me look. I said, "Look, I don't want to. I'm not ready to." At one point, she practically forced me. She made me look at it. So I took a quick look and I'm like, "Fine. That's it."

She told her mother, "I looked at it, now don't do that to me anymore."

Seeing the scar made her more aware of her mother's cancer. "I was thinking, you know, *My mother does not have a boob now. She's missing an appendage. It's a part of her body.*" Dora would even cry herself to sleep some nights. The surgery seemed to bother her more than it bothered her mother. However, she did not want to express her feelings. "I keep my emotions inside."

Experience following mother's illness. Dora's mother never told her father about the breast cancer, and asked Dora not to tell him. This put some stress on Dora, because she did not like to keep secrets. However, she respected her mother's wishes.

When Dora's mother had another lump on the other breast, she made a deal with Dora: If the lump was not cancerous, the two would go on a vacation together. "So the next day, we made our travel plans and we went." Although Dora and her mother live near each other and see each other frequently, their relationship is sometimes conflictual.

> We still have our moments. I mean, I still get on her nerves and she certainly still gets on my nerves. We are very different. She's a lot more outgoing than I am, and I don't like to draw attention to myself. . . . I get uptight about things, but I hold it all inside. If she has a problem, she'll verbalize it. I'm just like, "Whatever."

Dora did not think that her mother's illness has had any effect on her personality or life.

Risk. Dora was aware of a strong family history of cancer.

> Well, I have resigned myself that I am going to die of cancer, one way or another. My mother has it. She has skin cancers too. Her mother died of ovarian cancer. My father's mother died of some kind of cancer. So, it's inevitable.

In spite of this certainty, Dora did not do breast self-exams.

> The doctor asked me if I do breast self-exams, and I said, "No, not really." She's right, but I haven't. I know that's something that I need to do. But I'm not a pursuer. It's the passivity. If someone will give me a breast exam, that's fine. I'm more apt to do that than if I have to do it myself.

Another reason she does not do breast self-exams is,

> If you happen to feel something that you're not so sure of what it is, then you start to panic and you start to think bad things, and until you make it to the doctor to get it checked out, you're freaking out.

She has not yet had a mammogram because her physician told her she is too young.

Dora also paid a lot of attention to her health. She did not smoke or drink, and she was very athletic. "I played sports all my life." She was not interested in genetic testing. "That'd probably be something that I wouldn't want to know at age twenty-nine."

Current situation. Dora was twenty-nine at the time of the interview. She was single and shared a townhouse with her younger brother. Her mother lived nearby, and they frequently spent time together. "We usually do dinners on Wednesday night, and on weekends, we go to baseball games, go shopping, or go to movies together." Dora worked in accounting, but she was not happy with her job, and hoped to find a more satisfying career.

Dora learned only recently that her grandmother passed away from ovarian cancer—the same year that her parents separated. "So I know what cancer does to someone and the thought of that happening to my mother, I just couldn't imagine. So I'm glad things turned out the way they did."

Appendix IV

Resources

General Web Sites

<www.cancer.gov>: The National Cancer Institute's Web site. Includes resources for talking to children about cancer.

<www.cancer.org>: The American Cancer Society's Web site. Includes information on talking to children about cancer.

<www.oncolink.org>: Web site about cancer provided by the Abramson Cancer Center of the University of Pennsylvania.

Resources for Children Who Are Dealing with Parents' Cancer

Books

Cancer in the Family: Helping Children Cope with a Parent's Illness (2001) by Sue P. Heiney, Joan F. Hermann, Katherine V. Bruss, and Joy L. Fincannon (Editors). Atlanta, GA: American Cancer Society.

Moms Don't Get Sick (1990) by Pat and Ben Brack. Aberdeen, SD: Melius Publishing Corporation.

Videos

Kids Tell Kids What It's Like . . . When Their Mother or Father Has Cancer. Los Angeles: Cancervive. Available at 310-203-9232 or 800-4toCure, 11636 Chayote, St., Los Angeles CA 90049.

My Mom Has Breast Cancer. Interviews with seven children and four mothers who have experienced breast cancer treatment. Available in the community service section of Blockbuster video stores, at public libraries, or through <www.kidscope.org>.

Talking About Your Cancer: A Parents' Guide to Helping Children Cope. For more information, call the Fox Chase Cancer Center at 215-728-2668 or 800-Fox-Chase.

Web Sites

<www.kidscope.org>: A nonprofit organization dedicated to helping families and children cope when a loved one has cancer.

<www.komen.org>: The Susan G. Komen Breast Cancer Foundation provides lists of books for children.

Resources for Women Regarding Loss of Mother/Mothers with Cancer

Books

Her Face in the Mirror: Jewish Women on Mothers and Daughters (1994) by Faye Moskowita (Editor). Boston: Beacon Press.

The Kitchen Congregation (2000) by N. Seton. New York: Picador Publishing.

Letters from Motherless Daughters: Words of Courage, Grief, and Healing (1996) by Hope Edelman (Editor). New York: Dell Publishing.

Motherless (2000) by Lynn Davidman. Berkeley: University of California Press.

Motherless Daughters: The Legacy of Loss (1995) by Hope Edelman. New York: Dell Publishing. Also available as an audio book.

My Mother's Breast: Daughters Face Their Mothers' Cancer (1999) by Laurie Tarkan. Houston, TX: Taylor Trade Publishing Company.

One True Thing (1995) by Anna Quindlen. New York: Random House.

Web Sites

<www.circleofdaughters.com>: A nonprofit organization in New York offering support to women who have lost their mothers.

<www.motherlessdaughters.org>: Hope Edelman's Web site, developed from her book *Motherless Daughters: The Legacy of Loss.*

<www.motherlessdaughtersbiz.com>: Web site for motherless daughters of Los Angeles.

Bibliography

American Association of University Women (1991). *Shortchanging girls, short-changing America.* Washington, DC: American Association of University Women.

American Cancer Society (2002). Breast Cancer Facts and Figures 2001-2002. <www.cancer.org>.

Apter, T. (1990). *Altered loves: Mothers and daughters during adolescence.* New York: Ballantine Books.

Apter, T. (1993). *Altered views: Fathers' closeness to teenage daughters.* In Josselson, R. and Lieblich, A. (Eds.), *The narrative study of lives* (pp. 163-190). Newbury Park, CA: Sage.

Armsden, G.C. and Lewis, F.M. (1994). Behavioral adjustment and self-esteem among school-age children of mothers with breast cancer. *Oncology Nursing Forum, 21*(1), 39-45.

Atwood, M. (1996). *Cat's eye.* Prescott, AZ: Anchor Books.

Baider, L., Rizel, S., and De-Nour, A.K. (1986). Comparison of couples' adjustment to lumpectomy and mastectomy. *General Hospital Psychiatry, 8,* 251-257.

Balk, D.E. (1996). Attachment and the reactions of bereaved college students: A longitudinal study. In Klass, D. and Silverman, P.R., and Nickman, S.C. (Eds.), *Continuing bonds: New understandings of grief. Series in death education, aging, and health care* (pp. 311-328). London: Taylor and Francis.

Balk, D.E., Lampe, S., Sharpe, B., Schwinn, S., Holen, K., Cook, C., and Dubois, R. (1998). TAT results in a longitudinal study of bereaved college students. *Death Studies, 22*(1), 3-21.

Bassoff, E.S. (1987). *Mothers and daughters: Loving and letting go.* New York: New American Library.

Becker, M.H. (Ed.) (1974). *The health belief model and personal health behavior.* San Francisco: Society for Public Health Education, Inc.

Belenky, M.F., Clinchy, B.M., Goldberger, N.R., and Tarule, J.M. (1986). *Women's ways of knowing: The development of self, voice, and mind.* New York: Basic Books.

Berlinsky, E.B. and Biller, H.B. (1982). *Parental death and psychological development.* Lexington, MA: Lexington Books.

Bifulco, A., Harris, T., and Brown, G.W. (1993). Mourning or early inadequate care: Reexamining the relationship of maternal loss in childhood with adult depression and anxiety. *Development and Psychopathology, 4*(3), 433-449.

Black, D. (1998). Bereavement in childhood: Coping with loss, Part 2. *British Medical Journal, 316*(7135), 931.

Bowlby, J. (1980). Disordered variants and some conditions contributing. In *Attachment and loss: Loss, sadness, and depression,* Volume 3 (pp. 350-380). New York: Basic Books.

Boyer, B.A., Bubel, D., Jacobs, S.R., Knolls, M.L., Harwell, J.D., Goscicha, M., and Keegan, A. (2002). Posttraumatic stress in women with breast cancer and their daughters. *American Journal of Family Therapy, 30*(4), 323-338.

Brody, E. (1985). Parent care as a normative stress. *The Gerontologist, 25,* 19-29.

Brown, G.W., Harris, L., and Copeland, J. (1977). Depression and loss. *British Journal of Psychiatry, 130,* 1-18.

Brown, L.M. and Gilligan, C. (1992). *Meeting at the crossroads: Women's psychology and girls' development.* Cambridge, MA: Harvard University Press.

Cancer causes relationship changes (1994). *USA Today,* 123(2592), p. 9.

Caplan, P.J. (1989). *Don't blame mother: Mending the mother-daughter relationship.* New York: HarperCollins.

Carter, B. and McGoldrick, M. (1988). Women and the family life cycle. In Carter, B. and McGoldrick, M. (Eds.), *The changing family life cycle* (pp. 29-68). Boston: Allyn and Bacon.

Chodorow, N. (1999). *The reproduction of mothering: Psychoanalysis and the sociology of gender.* Berkeley, CA: University of California Press.

Christ, G.H. (2000). *Healing children's grief: Surviving a parent's death from cancer.* New York: Oxford University Press.

Christ, G.H., Siegel, K., Freund, B., Langosch, D., Hendersen, S., Sperber, D., and Weinstein, L. (1993). Impact of parental terminal cancer on latency-age children. *American Journal of Orthopsychiatry, 63*(3), 417-425.

Christ, G.H., Siegel, K., Mesagno, F.P., and Langosch, D. (1991). A preventive intervention program for bereaved children: Problems of implementation. *American Journal of Orthopsychiatry, 61*(2), 168-178.

Christ, G.H., Siegel, K., and Sperber, D. (1994). Impact of parental terminal cancer on adolescents. *American Journal of Orthopsychiatry, 64,* 604-613.

Claus, E.V., Risch, N., and Thompson, W.D. (1994). Autosomal dominant inheritance of early-onset breast cancer. *Cancer, 7,* 643-651.

Clingempeel, W., Brand, E., and Ievoli, R. (1984). Stepparent/stepchild relationships in stepmother and stepfather families: A multimethod study. *Journal of Applied Family and Child Studies, 33*(3), 465-473.

Cohen, P., Dizenhuz, I.M., and Winget, C. (1977). Family adaptation to terminal illness and death. *Social Casework, 58,* 223-228.

Coleman, M. and Ganong, L.H. (1987). The cultural stereotyping of stepfamilies. In Pasley, K. and Ihinger-tallman, M. (Eds.), *Remarriage and stepparenting: Current research and theory* (pp. 19-41). New York: Guilford Press.

Compas, B.E., Worsham, N.L., Epping-Jordan, J.E., Grant, K.E., Mireault, G., Howell, D.C., and Malcarne, V.L. (1999). When mom or dad has cancer: Markers of psychological distress in cancer patients, spouses, and children. In Suinn, R.M. and VandenBos, G.R. (Eds.), *Cancer patients and their families: Readings on disease course, coping, and psychological interventions* (pp. 291-308). Washington, DC: American Psychological Association.

Coontz, S. (1992). *The way we never were: American families and the nostalgia trap*. New York: Basic Books.

Croyle, R.T., Smith, K.R., Botkin, J.R., Baty, B., and Nash, J. (1997). Psychological responses to BRCA1 mutation testing: Preliminary findings. *Health Psychology, 16,* 63-72.

Dautzenberg, M.G.H. (2000). The competing demands of paid work and parent care. *Research on Aging, 22*(2), 165.

Debold, E. (1991). The body at play. *Women in Therapy, 11*(3/4), 169-183.

DeMaris, A. and Greif, G.L. (1992). The relationship between family structure and parent-child relationship problems in single father households. *Journal of Divorce and Remarriage, 18*(1/2), 55-77.

Diefenbavch, M.A., Miller, S.M., and Daly, M.B. (1999). Specific worry about breast cancer predicts mammography use in women at risk for breast and ovarian cancer. *Health Psychology, 18*(5), 532-536.

Dilworth, J.L. and Hildreth, G.J. (1998). Long-term unresolved grief: Applying Bowlby's variants to adult survivors of early parental death. *Omega—The Journal of Death and Dying, 36*(2), 147.

Dorval, M., Patenaude, A.F., Schneider, K.A., Kieffer, S.A., DiGianni, L., Kalbrenner, K.J., Bromberg, J.I., Basili, L.A., Calzone, K., Stopfer, J., et al. (2000). Anticipated versus actual emotional reactions to disclosure of results of genetic tests for cancer susceptibility. *Journal of Clinical Oncology, 18*(10), 2135-2142.

Easton, D.F., Bishop, T., Ford, D., and Crockford, D.C. (1995). The breast cancer linkage consortium, 1993: Genetic linkage in familial breast and ovarian cancer. *American Journal of Human Genetics, 52,* 678-701.

Edelman, H. (1994). *Motherless daughters*. New York: Addison-Wesley.

Ell, K., Nishimoto, R., Mantell, J., and Hamovitch, M. (1988). Longitudinal analysis of psychological adaptation among family members of patients with cancer. *Journal of Psychosomatic Research, 32*(4-5), 429-438.

Ell, K. and Northern, H. (1990). *Families and health care: Psychosocial practice*. New York: Aldine de Gruyter.

Epstein, S.A., Lin, T.H., Audrain, J., Stefanek, M., River, B., and Lerman, C. (1997). Excessive breast self-examination among first-degree relatives of newly diagnosed breast cancer patients. High Risk Cancer Consortium. *Psychosomatics, 38*(3), 253-261.

Erblich, J., Bovbjerg, D.H., and Valdimarsdottir, H.B. (2000). Looking forward and back: Distress among women at familial risk for breast cancer. *Annals of Behavioral Medicine 22*(1), 53-59.

Erikson, E.H. (1963). Childhood and society (Second edition). New York: Norton.

Erikson, E.H. (1968). *Identity: Youth and crisis*. New York: Norton.

Facione, N.C. (2002). Perceived risk of breast cancer: Influence of heuristic thinking. *Cancer Practice, 10*(5), 256-262.

Fanos, J.H. (1996). *Sibling loss.* Mahwah, NJ: Lawrence Erlbaum Associates.

Fanos, J.H. and Wiener, L. (1994). Tomorrow's survivors: siblings of human immunodeficiency virus-infected children. *Journal of Developmental and Behavioral Pediatrics, 15*(3), S43-S48.

Fischer, L.R. (1986). *Linked lives: Adult daughters and their mothers.* New York: Harper & Row.

Fitch, J. (1999). *White oleander.* New York: Little Brown and Co.

Freud, S. (1917). *Mourning and melancholia,* Volume 14. London: Hogarth Press.

Furman, E. (1974). *A child's parent dies: Studies in childhood bereavement.* New Haven, CT: Yale University Press.

Gersten, J.C., Beals, J., and Kallgren, C.A. (1991). Epidemiology and preventive interventions: Parental death in childhood as a case example. *American Journal of Community Psychology, 19*(4), 481.

Gilbar, O. (1998). Coping with threat: Implications for women with a family history of breast cancer. *Psychosomatics: Journal of Consultation Liaison Psychiatry, 39*(4), 239-339.

Gilligan, C. (1982a). Adult development and women's development: Arrangements for a marriage. In Giele, J. (Ed.), *Women in the middle years* (pp. 89-114). New York: Wiley.

Gilligan, C. (1982b). *In a different voice: Psychological theory and women's development.* Cambridge, MA: Harvard University Press.

Gilligan, C., Lyons, N.P., and Hammer, T.J. (Eds.) (1990). *Making connections: The relational world of adolescent girls at Emma Willard School.* Cambridge, MA: Harvard University Press.

Glaser, B.G. and Strauss, A.L. (1967). *The discovery of grounded theory: Strategies for qualitative research.* Chicago: Aldine.

Goldberg, J.E. (1994). Mutuality in mother-daughter relationships. *Families in Society: Journal of Contemporary Human Services, 75*(4), 242-248.

Gray, R.E. (1989). Adolescents' perceptions of social support after the death of a parent. *Journal of Psychosocial Oncology, 7*(3), 127-144.

Harris, M. (1995). *The loss that is forever: The lifelong impact of the early death of a mother or father.* New York: Dutton/Dutton Signet.

Hatter, B.S. (1996). Children and the death of a parent or grandparent. In Corr, C.A. and Corr, D.M. (Eds.), *Handbook of childhood death and bereavement* (pp. 131-148). New York: Springer.

Hetherington, E.M. and Stanley-Hagan, M.M. (1999). Stepfamilies. In Lamb, M.E. (Ed.), *Parenting and child development in 'nontraditional' families* (pp. 137-159). Mahwah, NJ: Lawrence Erlbaum Associates.

Hewitt, H., Herdman, R., and Holland, J. (Eds.) (2004). *Metting psychological of women with breast cancer.* Washington, DC: Institute of Medicine and National Research Council, National Academies Press.

Hilton, B.A., Crawford, J.A., and Tarko, M.A. (2000). Men's perspectives on individual and family coping with their wives breast cancer and chemotherapy. *Western Journal of Nursing Research, 22*(4), 438-459.

Hoke, L.A. (2001). Psychosocial adjustment in children of mothers with breast cancer. *Psycho-Oncology, 10*(5), 361-369.

Hopwood, P., Long, A., Pool, C., Evans, G., and Howell, A. (1998). Psychological support needs for women at high genetic risk of breast cancer: Some preliminary considerations. *Psycho-Oncology, 7*(5), 402-412.

Horowitz, A. (1985). Family caregiving to the frail elderly. In Eisendorfer, C. (Ed.), *Annual Review of Gerontology and Geriatrics, 5,* 194-246.

Hudson, K.L., Rothenberg, K.H., Andrews, L.B., Kahn, M.W., and Collins, F.S. (1995). Genetic discrimination and health insurance: An urgent need for reform. *Science, 270,* 391-393.

Ihinger-Tallman, M. and Pasley, K. (1987). Divorce and remarriage in the American family: A historical review. In Pasley, K. and Ihinger-Tallman, M. (Eds.), *Remarriage and stepparenting: Current research and theory* (pp. 3-18). New York: Guilford Press.

Jemal, A., Murray, T., Samuels, A., Kaplan, A.G., Miller, J.B., Stiver, I.P., and Sorrey, J.L. (2003). Cancer statistics, 2003. *CA: A Cancer Journal for Clinicians, 53,* 5-26.

Jordan, J.V., Kaplan, A.G., Miller, J.B., Stiver, I.P., and Surrey, J.L. (1991). *Women's growth in connection: Writings from the Stone Center.* New York: Guilford.

Kaplan, G., Gleason, N., and Klein, R. (1991). Women's self development in late adolescence. In Jordan, J. et al. (Eds.), *Women's growth in connection: Writings from the Stone Center* (pp. 123-140). New York: Guilford Press.

Karp, J., Bown, K.L., Sullivan, M.D., and Massie, M.J. (1999). The prophylactic mastectomy dilemma: A support group for women at high genetic risk for breast cancer. *Journal of Genetic Counseling, 8*(3), 163-173.

Keitel, M.A., Cramer, S.H., and Zevon, M.A. (1990). Spouses of cancer patients: A review of the literature. *Journal of Counseling and Development, 69,* 163-166.

Kerr, R.B. (1994). Meanings adult daughters attach to a parent's death. *Western Journal of Nursing Research 16*(4), 347-365.

Kissane, D.W., Bloch, W., Burns, I., McKenzie, D.P., and Posterino, M. (1994). Psychological morbidity in the families of patients with cancer. *Psycho-Oncology, 3,* 47-56.

Kissane, D.W., Bloch, S., Dowe, D.L., Snyder, R.D., Onghena, P., McKenzie, D.P., and Wallace, C.S. (1996). The Melbourne Family Grief Study I: Perceptions of family functioning in bereavement. *American Journal of Psychiatry, 153,* 650-658.

Kissane, D.W., Bloch, S., Onghena, P., McKenzie, D.P., Snyder, R.D., and Dowe, D.L. (1996). The Melbourne Family Grief Study II: Psychosocial morbidity and grief in bereaved families. *American Journal of Psychiatry, 153,* 659-666.

Klass, D., Silverman, P.R., and Nickman, S.L. (Eds.) (1996). *Continuing bonds: New understandings of grief.* Bristol, PA: Taylor and Francis.

Kleinman, A. (1980). *Patients and healers in the context of culture.* Berkeley: University of California.

Kliman, G. (1968). *Psychological emergencies of childhood.* New York: Grune and Stratton.

Kroll, L., Barnes, J., Jones, A.S., and Stein, A. (1998). Cancer in parents: Telling children. *British Medical Journal, 316*(7135), 880.

Krupnick, J.L. and Solomon, F. (1987). Death of a parent or sibling during childhood. In Bloom-Feshbach, J. and Bloom-Feshbach, S. (Eds.), *The psychology of separation and loss: Perspective on development, life transitions, and clinical practice* (pp. 345-374). San Francisco: Jossey-Bass.

Lederberg, M.S. (1998). The family of the cancer patient. In Holland, J.C. (Ed.), *Psycho-Oncology* (pp. 981-993). New York: Oxford University Press.

Lerman, C., Croyle, R.T., Tercyak, K.P., and Hamann, H. (2002). Genetic testing: Psychological aspects and implications. *Journal of Consulting and Clinical Psychology, 70*(3), 784-797.

Lerman, C., Kash, K., and Stephanek, M. (1994). Younger women at increased risk for breast cancer: Perceived risk, psychological well-being, and surveillance behavior. *Monographs of the National Cancer Institute, 1,* 171-176.

Lerman, C., Narod, S., Schulman, K., Hughes, C., Gomez-Caminero, A., Bonney, G., and Gold, K., Trock, B., Main, D., Lynch, J. (1996). BRCA1 testing in families with hereditary breast-ovarian cancer: A prospective study of patient decision making and outcomes. *JAMA, 275*(24), 1885-1892.

Lerner, H.D. and Lerner, P.M. (1987). Separation, depression and object loss: Implications for narcissism and object relations. In Bloom-Feshbach, J., Bloom-Feshbach, S., and Associates (Eds.), *The psychology of separation and loss.* San Francisco: Jossey-Bass.

Lerner, H.G. (1993). *The dance of deception: Pretending and truth-telling in women's lives.* New York: HarperCollins.

Lewis, F.M. (1996). The impact of breast cancer on the family: Lessons learned from the children and adolescents. In Baider, L., Cooper, C.L., and Kaplan De-Nour, A. (Eds.), *Cancer and the family* (pp. 271-287). New York: John Wiley and Sons.

Lewis, F.M., Behar, L.C., Anderson, K.H., Shands, M.E., Zahlis, E.H., Darby, E., and Sinshimer, J.A. (2000). Blowing away the myths about the child's experience with the mother's breast cancer. In Baider, L., Cooper, C.L., and Kaplan De-Nour, A., (Eds.), *Cancer and the family,* Second edition (pp. 201-221). New York: John Wiley and Sons.

Lewis, F.M. and Hammond, M.A. (1992). Psychosocial adjustment of the family to breast cancer: A longitudinal analysis. *Journal of the American Medical Women's Association, 47*(5), 194-200.

Lewis, F.M. and Hammond, M.A. (1996). The father's, mother's and adolescent's functioning with breast cancer. *Family Relations, 45,* 456-465.

Lichtman, R.R., Taylor, S.E., Wood, J.V., Bluming, A.Z., Dosik, G.M., and Liebowitz, R.L. (1984). Relationships with children after breast cancer: The mother-daughter relationship at risk. *Journal of Psychosocial Oncology, 2,* 1-19.

Lindberg, N.M. and Wellisch, D. (2001). Anxiety and compliance among women at risk for breast cancer. *Annals of Behavioral Medicine, 23*(4), 298-303.

Lindemann, E. (1944). Symptomalogy and management of acute grief. *American Journal of Psychiatry, 101,* 141-148.

Lynch, H.T., Lemon, S.J., Durham, C., Tinley, S.T., Connolly, C., Lynch, J.F., Surdam, J., Orinion, E., Slominski-Caster, M.S., and Watson, P. (1997). A descriptive study of BRCA1 testing and reactions to disclosure of test results. *Cancer, 79*(11), 2219-2228.

Mailick, M. (1979). The impact of severe illness on the individual and the family: An overview. *Social Work in Health Care, 5*(2), 117-128.

Marwit, S.J. and Klass, D. (1996). Grief and the role of the inner representation of the deceased. In Klass, D. and Silverman, P.R., and Nickman, S.L. (Eds.), *Continuing bonds: New understandings of grief. Series in death education, aging, and health care* (pp. 311-328). London: Taylor and Francis.

Maxwell, Joseph A. (1996). *Qualitative research design: An interactive approach.* Thousand Oaks, CA: Sage.

McCloskey, L.A. and Walker, M. (2000). Posttraumatic stress in children exposed to family violence and single-event trauma. *Journal of American Academy of Child Adolescent Psychiatry, 39*(1), 108-115.

Meiser, B., Butow, P., Schneiden, V., Gattas, M., Gaff, C., Harrop, K., Bankier, A., Young, M.A., and Tucker, K. (2000). Psychological adjustment of women at increased risk of developing hereditary breast cancer. *Psychology, Health and Medicine, 5*(4), 377-388.

Meiser, B. and Halliday, J.L. (2002). What is the impact of genetic counseling in women at increased risk of developing hereditary breast cancer? A meta-analytic review. *Social Science and Medicine, 54*(10), 1463-1470.

Miki, Y., Swensen, B., Shattuck-Eidens, D., Futeral, A., Harshman, K., and Tautigian, S., Liu, Q., Cochran, C., Bennett, L.M., and Ding, W. (1994). A strong candidate for the breast and ovarian cancer susceptibility gene BRCA1. *Science, 266,* 66-71.

Miller, J.B. (1986). *Toward a new psychology of women* (Revised edition). Boston: Beacon.

Miller, M.A. (1995). Re-grief as narrative: The impact of parental death on child and adolescent development. In Adams, D.W. and Deveau, E.J. (Eds.), *Beyond the innocence of childhood: Helping children and adolescents cope with death and bereavement* (pp. 99-113). Amityville, NY: Baywood Publishing Co.

Mills, D.M. (1988). Stepfamilies in context. In Beer, W.R. (Ed.), *Relative strangers: Studies of stepfamily processes* (pp. 1-28). Totawa, NJ: Rowman and Littlefield.

Mirkin, M.P. (1994). Female adolescence revisited: Understanding girls in their sociocultural contexts. In Mirkin, M.P. (Ed.), *Women in context: Toward a feminist reconstruction of psychotherapy* (pp. 77-95). New York: Guilford.

Moss, M.S., Resch, N., and Moss, S.Z. (1997). The role of gender in middle-age children's responses to parent death. *Omega, 35*(1), 43-65.

Muus, R.E. (1996). *Theories of adolescence.* New York: McGraw-Hill.

Narod, S.A., Brunet, J.S., Ghadirian, P., Robson, M., Heimdal, K., Neuhausen, S.L., Stoppa-Lyonnet, D., Lerman, C., Pasini, B., and de los Rios, P. (2000). Tamoxifen and risk of contralateral breast cancer in BRCA1 and BRCA2 mutation carriers: A case-control study. *The Lancet, 356,* 1876-1881.

National Breast Cancer Coalition (2003). <http://www.natlbcc.org/>.

National Cancer Institute (2002). Cancer survivorship: Improving treatment outcomes and quality of life. <http://plan.cancer.gov/public/survivor.htm>.

Newman, B.M. and Newman, P.R. (1995). *Development through life: A psychosocial approach.* Pacific Grove, CA: Brooks/Cole.

Nolen-Hoeksema, S. and Larson, J. (1999). *Coping with loss.* Mahwah, NJ: Lawrence Erlbaum Associates.

Normand, C.L., Silverman, P.R., and Nickman, S.L. (1996). Bereaved children's changing relationships with the deceased. In Klass, D., Silverman, P.R., and Nickman, S.L. (Eds.), *Continuing bonds: New understandings of grief. Series in death education, aging, and health care* (pp. 311-328). London: Taylor and Francis.

Northouse, L. (1984). The impact of cancer on the family: An overview. *International Journal of Psychiatry in Medicine, 14*(3), 215-242.

Oktay, J. (1998). Genetics cultural lag: What can social workers do to help? *Health and Social Work, 23*(4), 310-315.

Oktay, J.S. and Walter, C.A. (1991). *Breast cancer in the life course: Women's experiences.* New York: Springer.

Osterweis, M., Solomon, F., and Green, M. (Eds.) (1984). *Bereavement reactions, consequences and care.* Washington, DC: National Academy Press.

Padgett, D. (1998). *Qualitative methods in social work research: Challenges and rewards.* Thousand Oaks, CA: Sage.

Padgett, D.K., Yedidia, M.J., Kerner, J., and Mandelbatt, J. (2001). Emotional consequences of false positive mammography: African-American women's reactions in their own words. *Women and Health, 33*(3-4), 1-14.

Parkes, C.M. (1987). *Bereavement: Studies of grief in adult life.* New York: Penguin Books.

Pasley, K., Ihinger-Tallman, M., and Lofquist, A. (1994). Remarriage and stepfamilies: Making progress in understanding. In Pasley, K. and Ihinger-Tallman, M. (Eds.), *Stepparenting: Issues in theory, research and practice* (pp. 1-14). Westport, CT: Greenwood Press.

Patenaude, A.F. (2000). A different normal: Reactions of children and adolescents to the diagnosis of cancer in a parent. In Baider, L., Cooper, C.L., and Kaplan

De-Nour, A. (Eds.), *Cancer in the family,* Second edition (pp. 239-254). New York: John Wiley and Sons.

Patenaude, A.F. (2004). *Genetic testing for cancer: Psychological approaches for helping patients and families.* Washington, DC: American Psychological Association.

Patten, Scott B. (1991). Are the Brown and Harris "vulnerability factors" risk factors for depression? *Journal of Psychiatry and Neuroscience, 16*(5), 267-271.

Pill, C.J. and Zabin, J.L. (1997). Lifelong legacy of early maternal loss: A women's support group. *Clinical Social Work Journal, 25*(2), 179-195.

Pipher, M. (1994). *Reviving Ophelia: Saving the selves of adolescent girls.* New York: Putnam.

Preto, N.G. (1988). Transformations of the family system in adolescence. In Carter, B. and McGoldrick, M. (Eds.), *The changing family life cycle* (pp. 255-283). New York: Gardner Press.

Pruett, C.L., Calsyn, R.J., and Jensen, F.M. (1993). Social support received by children in stepmother, stepfather and intact families. *Journal of Divorce and Remarriage, 19*(3-4), 165.

Quick, D.S., McKenry, P.C., and Newman, B.M. (1994). Stepmothers and their adolescent children: Adjustment to new family roles. In Pasley, K. and Ihinger-Tallman, M. (Eds.), *Stepparenting: Issues in theory, research and practice* (pp. 105-125). Westport, CT: Greenwood Press.

Quindlen, A. (1995). *One true thing.* New York: Dell.

Rando, T.A. (1984). *Grief, dying, and death: Clinical interventions for caregivers.* Champaign, IL: Research Press Corp.

Reinharz, S. (1992). *Feminist methods in social research.* New York: Oxford University Press.

Rolland, J.S. (1994). *Families, illness and disability: An integrative treatment model.* New York: Basic Books.

Rosenblatt, P.C. (1996). Grief that does not end. In Klass, D., Silverman, P.R. and Nickman, S.L. (Eds.), *Continuing bonds: New understandings of grief. Series in death education, aging, and health care* (pp. 311-328). London: Taylor and Francis.

Rosenheim, E. and Reicher, R. (1985). Informing children about a parent's terminal illness. *Journal of Child Psychology and Psychiatry and Allied Disciplines, 26,* 995-998.

Rosenstock, I. (1966). Why people use health services. *Milbank Memorial Fund Quarterly, 44,* 94-127.

Ross, G. E. (1987). The role of the surviving parent in the adaptation of bereaved adolescents. *Journal of Palliative Care, 3*(1), 30-34.

Rossi, A.S. and Rossi, P. (1990). *Of human bonding: Parent-child relations across the life course.* New York: Aldine de Gryter.

Rothemund, Y., Paepke, S., and Flor, H. (2001). Perception of risk, anxiety and health behaviors in women at high risk for breast cancer. *International Journal of Behavioral Medicine, 8*(3), 230-239.

Rubin, L.B. (2000). *Tangled lives: Daughters, mothers, and the crucible of aging.* Boston: Beacon Press.

Saler, L. and Skolnick, N. (1992). Childhood parental death and depression in adulthood: Roles of surviving parent and family environment. *American Journal of Orthopsychiatry, 62*(4), 504.

Sanders, C.M. (1998). *Grief: The mourning after: Dealing with adult bereavement.* New York: Wiley.

Santrock, J.W. and Sitterle, K.A. (1995). Parent-child relationships in stepmother families. In Pasley, K. and Ihinger-Tallman, M. (Eds.), *Stepparenting: Issues in theory, research and practice* (pp. 273-299). Westport, CT: Greenwood Press.

Schwartz, M.D., Peshkin, B.N., Hughes, C., Main, D., Isaacs, C., and Lerman, C. (2002). Impact of BRCA1/BRCA2 mutation testing on psychologic distress in a clinic-based sample. *Journal of Clinical Oncology, 20*(2), 514-520.

Secunda, V. (1991). *When you and your mother can't be friends: Resolving the most complicated relationship of your life.* New York: Dell.

Sharpe, S. (1994). *Fathers and daughters.* Routledge: London.

Sheehan, N.W. and Donorfio, L.M. (1999). Efforts to create meaning in the relationship between aging mothers and their caregiving daughters: A qualitative study of caregiving. *Journal of Aging Studies, 13*(2), 161-176.

Shulman, S. and Seiffge-Krenke, I. (1997). *Fathers and adolescents: Developmental and clinical perspectives.* Routledge: London.

Siegel, K., Karus, D., and Raveis, V.H. (1996). Adjustment of children facing the death of a parent due to cancer. *Journal of the American Academy of Child and Adolescent Psychiatry, 35*(4), 442-450.

Siegel, K., Raveis, V.H., and Karus, D. (1996). Pattern of communication with children when a parent has cancer. In Baider, L., Cooper, C.L., and Kaplan De-Nour, A. (Eds.), *Cancer in the family* (pp. 109-128). New York: John Wiley and Sons.

Sigman, M. and Wilson, J.P. (1998). Traumatic bereavement: Post-traumatic stress disorder and prolonged grief in motherless daughters. *Journal of Psychological Practice, 4*(1), 34-50.

Silverman, P.R. (1987). The impact of parental death on college-age women. *Psychiatric Clinics of North America, 10*(3), 387-404.

Silverman, P.R. and Klass, D. (1996). Introduction: What's the problem? In Klass, D., Silverman, P.R., and Nickman, S.L. (Eds.), *Continuing bonds: New understandings of grief. Series in death education, aging, and health care* (pp. 311-328). London: Taylor and Francis.

Silverman, P.R. and Worden, J.W. (1992). Children's reactions in the early months after the death of a parent. *American Journal of Orthopsychiatry, 62*(1), 93-104.

Smith, M.Y., Redd, W.H., Peyser, C., and Vogl, D. (1999). Post-traumatic stress disorder in cancer: A review. *Psycho-Oncology, 8*(6), 521-537.

Spira, M. and Kenemore, W. (2000). Adolescent daughters of mothers with breast cancer: Impact and implications. *Clinical Social Work Journal, 28*(2), 183-195.

Stantrock, J.W. and Sitterle, K.A. (1987). Parent-child realtionships in stepmother families. In Pasley, K. and Ihinger-Tallman, M. (Eds.), *Remarriage and stepparenting: Current research and theory* (pp. 273-299). New York: Guildford Press.

Steiner-Adair, C. (1991). When the body speaks: Girls, eating disorders and psychotherapy. *Women and therapy, 11*(3/4), 253-266.

Stinson, K.M. (1991). Adolescents and their fathers. In Stinson, K.M. (Ed.), *Adolescents, family and friends: Social support after parent's divorce or remarriage* (pp. 71-96). New York: Praeger.

Stoppelbein, L. and Greening, L. (2000). Posttraumatic stress symptoms in parentally bereaved children and adolescents. *Journal of the American Academy of Child and Adolescent Psychiatry, 39*(9), 1112-1119.

Strauss, A. and Corbin, J. (1998). *Basics of qualitative research: Techniques and procedures for developing grounded theory.* Thousand Oaks: Sage.

Strewing, J., Hartge, P., Wacholder, S., Baker, S.M., Berlin, M., McAdams, M., Timmerman, M.M., Brody, L.C., and Tucker, M.A. (1997). The risk of cancer associated with specific mutations of BRCA1 and BRCA2 among Ashkenazi Jews. *The New England Journal of Medicine, 336,* 1401-1408.

Stroebe, M., Gergen, M., Gergen, K.J., and Stroehe, W. (1992). Broken hearts or broken bonds: Love and eath in historical perspective. *American Psychologist, 47,* 1205.

Suleiman, S.R. (Ed.) (1986). *The female body in Western culture.* Cambridge, MA: Harvard University Press.

Surrey, J.L. (1991). The self in relation: A theory of women's development. In Jordan, J.V., Kaplan, A.G., Miller, J.B., Stiver, I.P., and Surrey, J.L. (Eds.), *Women's growth in connection: Writings from the Stone Center* (pp. 51-66). New York: Guilford Press.

Swensen, C.H. and Fuller, S.R. (1992). Expression of love, marriage problems, commitment and anticipatory grief in the marriages of cancer patients. *Journal of Marriage and the Family, 54*(1), 191-196.

Tarkan, L. (1999). *My mother's breast: Daughters face their mothers' cancer.* Dallas, TX: Taylor.

Tennant, C. (1988). Parental loss in childhood: Its effect in adult life. *Archives of General Psychiatry, 45,* 1045-1049.

Thompson, M.P., Kaslow, N.J., Price, A.W., Williams, K., and Kingree, J.B. (1998). Role of secondary stressors in the parental death-child distress relation. *Journal of Abnormal Child Psychology, 26*(5), 357.

Tracy, G.E. (2004). Breast cancer—The disease many women fear the most. *South Dakota Journal of Medicine, 57*(4), 148.

Trask, P.C., Paterson, A.G., Wang, C., Hayasaka, S., Milliron, K., Blumberg, L.R., Gonzalez, R., Murray, S., and Merajver, S.D. (2001). Cancer-specific worry interference in women attending a breast and ovarian cancer risk evaluation program: Impact on emotional distress. *PsychoOncology, 10*(5), 349-360.

Troll, L. (1987). Mother-daughter relationships through the life span. In Oskamp, S. (Ed.), *Applied social psychology annual 7* (pp. 284-305). Newbury Park, CA: Sage.

Tudiver, F. (1991). Psychosocial characteristics of recently widowed men. *Family Medicine, 23,* 501.

Tyson-Rawson, K. (1996). Relationship and heritage: Manifestations of ongoing attachment following father death. In Klass, D., Silverman, P.R., and Nickman, S.L. (Eds.), *Continuing bonds: New understandings of grief. Series in death education, aging, and health care* (pp. 311-328). London: Taylor and Francis.

Umberson, D. and Chen, M.D. (1994). Effects of a parent's death on adult children: Relationship salience and reaction to loss. *American Sociological Review, 59*(1), 152-168.

U.S. Cancer Statistics Working Group (2003). *United States cancer statistics: 2000 Incidence.* Atlanta, GA: Department of Health and Human Services, Centers for Disease Control and Prevention, and National Cancer Institute.

VanEerdewegh, M., Bieri, M., Parilla, R., and Clayton, P. (1982). The bereaved child. *British Journal of Psychiatry, 140,* 23-29.

Veach, T.A. and Nicholas, D.R. (1998). Understanding families of adults with cancer: Combining the clinical course of cancer and stages of family development. *Journal of Counseling and Development, 76*(13), 144.

Vollman, R.R., Ganzert, A., Picher, L., and Williams, W.V. (1971). The reactions of family systems to sudden and unexpected death. *Omega, 2,* 101-106.

Walsh, F. and McGoldrick, M. (1991). *Living beyond loss: Death in the family.* New York: Norton.

Weil, J. (2000). *Psychosocial genetic counseling.* New York: Oxford University Press.

Weingarten, K. (1994). *The mother's voice: Strengthening intimacy in families.* New York: Guilford.

Weiss, R.S. (1994). *Learning from strangers: The art and method of qualitative interview studies.* New York: The Free Press.

Welch, A.S., Wadsworth, M.E., and Compas, B.E. (1996). Adjustment of children and adolescents to parental cancer: Parents' and children's perspectives. *Cancer, 77,* 1409-1418.

Weller, R.A., Weller, E.B., Fristad, M.S., and Bowes, J.M. (1991). Depression in recently bereave prepubertal children. *American Journal of Psychiatry, 148*(11), 1536.

Wellisch, D.K. (1979). Adolescent acting out when a parent has cancer. *International Journal of Family Therapy, 1*(3), 230-241.

Wellisch, D.K., Gritz, E.R., Schain, W., Wang, H.J., and Siau, J. (1991). Psychological functioning of daughters of breast cancer patients. Part I. Daughters and comparison subjects. *Psychosomatics 32*(2), 324-336.

Wellisch, D.K., Gritz, E.R., Schain, W., Wang, H.J., and Siau, J. (1992). Psychological functioning of daughters of breast cancer patients. Part II. Characterizing the distressed daughter of the breast cancer patient. *Psychosomatics, 33*(2), 171-179.

Wellisch, D.K., Hoffman, A., and Gritz, E. (1996). Psychological concerns and care of daughters of breast cancer patients. In Baider, L., Cooper, C.L., and Kaplan De-Nour, A. (Eds.), *Cancer and the family* (pp. 289-304). New York: John Wiley and Sons.

Wellisch, D.K. and Lindberg, N.M. (2001). A psychological profile of depressed and nondepressed women at high risk for breast cancer. *Psychosomatics: Journal of Consultation Liaison Psychiatry, 42*(4), 330-336.

Wellisch, D.K., Schains, W., Gritz, E.R., and Wang, H.J. (1996). Psychological functioning of daughters of breast cancer patients. Part III. Experiences and perceptions of daughters related to mother's breast cancer. *Psycho-Oncology, 5,* 271-281.

Wells, R. (1997). *Divine secrets of the ya-ya sisterhood.* New York: Harper Perennial.

Wilcox-Rittgers, C.A. (1997). Maternal death in late adolescence/early adulthood and psychological development in women. *Dissertation Abstracts International, 58,* 5B, 2706.

Wooster, R., Bignell, G., Lancaster, J., Swift, S., Seal, S., Mangion, J., Collings, N., Gregory, S., Gumbs, C., and Micklem, G. (1995). Identification of the breast cancer susceptibility gene BRCA2. *Nature, 378,* 789-791.

Worden, J.W. (1996). *Children and death: When a parent dies.* New York: Guilford.

Wortman, C.B. and Dunkel-Schetter, C. (1979). Interpersonal relationships and cancer. *Journal of Social Issues, 35*(1), 120-155.

Zakowski, S.G., Valdimarsdottir, H.B., Bovbjerg, D.H., Borgen, P., Holland, J., Kash, K., Miller, D., Mitnick, J., Osborne, M., and Van Zee, K. (1997). Predictors of intrusive thoughts and avoidance in women with family histories of breast cancer. *Annals of Behavioral Medicine, 19,* 362-369.

Zax, B. and Poulter, S. (1998). *Mending the broken bough: Restoring the promise of the mother-daughter relationship.* Pittston, PA: Berkley Publishing Group.

Index

Page numbers followed by the letter "b" indicate boxed material; those followed by the letter "f" indicate figures; and those followed by the letter "t" indicate tables.